# FAT FUNERAL

## The Scientific Approach to Long-Term Weight Loss

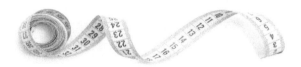

Daniel E. Dell'uomo, MS, CPT
Daniel S. Dell'uomo, DDS, PhD

Cover Design: Alex Udarbe and Christopher Andrews
Interior Design: Christopher Andrews and Daniel E. Dell'uomo

FatFuneralBook.com
ISBN: 978-0-578-45237-1 (paperback)
ASIN: B07MKSXW22 (Kindle ebook)
Copyright Registration Number: TX 8-719-341

Title Page Image Credit: Sergey Mironov/Shutterstock.com

First Edition

*To Judy*

# CONTENTS

# Part 2 · Exercise

# Part 3 · Sleep

# Part 4 · Checks & Balances

# Part 5 · Stairway to Heaven

Blind belief in authority is the greatest enemy of truth.
—Albert Einstein

# 1

# YOU AND I

It's not your fault. The weight thing, I mean. Gaining weight usually isn't a choice. If it were, there wouldn't be 1.9 billion overweight people.[1]

It's not your fault. Losing weight isn't as easy as tic-tac-toe—"eat less, move more." If it were, there wouldn't be 600 million obese people.[2] This isn't a simple problem with an obvious solution.

It's not your fault. The forces that lead to weight gain aren't well-understood. If they were, there wouldn't be 42 million obese children under the age of five.[3]

No, confusion abounds. There's confusion about why people get fat, nutrition in general, the role of exercise, and which weight-loss strategies really work. There's so much confusion that many people throw up their hands, giving up on making sense of it.

But sense is out there.

A bit of background. I've been there. One sunny day in the summer of 2009, my two best friends told me that I'd gotten fat. To my horror, I realized they were right. I was 230 pounds.

The next day, I devoted all my willpower to losing weight. I dropped 50 pounds in two months, and kept most of them off ever since.

That was almost ten years ago.

If you've never been in a relationship, you shouldn't give relationship advice. If you've never worked on plumbing, you shouldn't give plumbing advice. And if you've never been fat, gotten thin, and stayed thin for years, you shouldn't give weight-loss advice. It's a required credential.

Another required credential for giving weight-loss advice is science. There's a lot of science in this book. There has to be.

When I set out to lose weight, I was close to finishing a degree in biology. Aside from briefly consulting a trusted cousin, I didn't seek any outside advice. I just thought about my weight problem from a cold biological perspective, drew conclusions from solid premises, and zealously acted on them.

It worked wonders. In no time flat, I went from 230 pounds to 180 pounds, and felt a spiritual change in my health and self-confidence. After that, I didn't think about weight loss for a while.

It wasn't until I was studying physiology and genetics in grad school that I stumbled on an article on the front page of Yahoo! offering weight-loss tips.

I read the article, mostly out of boredom.

I was shocked. The tips were a lazy mix of vague platitudes, misconceptions from the '90s, and a plug for some supplement. The list seemed to have been thrown together in no particular order, with no particular thought. I pictured thousands of struggling people being misled by this drivel.

But after reading forty weight-loss books and countless weight-loss articles and blog posts, I realized that this lousy Yahoo! article was the *norm*, not the exception. Something serious was missing from the weight-loss industry.

More effort went into marketing and recipes than careful

analysis. More focus was placed on arbitrary short-term programs than on building effective habits.

And everything dripped with bias.

It's not your fault. If you've failed to lose weight in the past, it's probably because the weight-loss industry failed you. You didn't have the right knowledge, or the right approach.

I thought you deserved a better weight-loss book. Around six years ago, I set my homepage to Google Scholar, pushed off from shore, and pored over the primary literature of nutrition, metabolism, physiology, exercise physiology, biochemistry, pathology, psychology, epidemiology, obesity research, anthropology, and philosophy of science, stitching diverse insights into a coherent quilt.

I ate textbooks, scientifically oriented books, and scientifically oriented blogs.

I interviewed trainers (and got certified myself), weight-loss coaches (and coached people myself), bodybuilders, and ordinary folks who'd lost a good deal of weight, seeking diverse perspectives and common themes and matching them against my own experience.

To cut costs and focus on the book, I moved back in with my parents at an advanced age. It was there that my dad, an eternally fit and clever dentist with a PhD in physiology, decided to come on as a coauthor.

This book was my life.

This is *your* life, and it's ending one second at a time.

It's time to learn about the most effective ways to lose weight.

# 2

# LITTLE NUMBERS

Get ready for a lot of little numbers. They'll look like this[4,5,6] perched like birds on the upper-right corner of words. Each little number is a citation. If you look it up in the back of the book, you'll find the source of the information in the sentence.

Don't worry. You don't have to look any of these up. But if you *did* look one up, you'd find that it probably points to a peer-reviewed scientific study—a *human* study—published in a peer-reviewed scientific journal. (Sometimes it might lead to a credible book, institutional website, or nutrition database.)

These little numbers caused me untold suffering, but they were necessary. Because above all else, weight-loss arguments should be based on science. Science isn't perfect, but it's the best we have.

Instead of science, you've probably seen other forms of evidence used in weight-loss arguments.

Like success stories. Success stories and other anecdotes are just *stories*.

Stories get embellished, changed, and made up. Stories may be entertaining and even inspiring, but you can't trust them. As a form of evidence, stories are almost completely worthless. Even if a success story is true, what worked for someone else might not work for you. For you, it might be *counter*productive.

Even arguments like "this worked for a lot of my clients" aren't meaningful. Maybe the coach or trainer is lying. Maybe they're subconsciously ignoring clients it didn't work for. Maybe what *really* worked was their personality, which inspired their clients over and above their program.

We can't know.

Before-and-after pictures could have been photo-shopped, or even different people. Or maybe the transformation was due to something other than what's being claimed—maybe those same pictures have already been used to sell another diet or program. Or maybe they paid the person $2000 not to eat for a week before the after-picture. Or maybe the person just decided to do that on their own, without telling anyone. How would you know?

Whatever its flaws, at least science *attempts* to control for things like that. At least science *attempts* to be deliberate and objective. At least science *attempts* to describe specific protocols that can be reproduced.

But science and titles are not the same thing. "I'm a doctor" or "I'm an expert" are not scientific arguments. Instead, they are logical fallacies known as "appeals to authority."[7]

And they can lead to trouble.

Dr. Mehmet Oz, for instance, went to Harvard before getting his MD at the University of Pennsylvania in 1986 and becoming a cardiothoracic surgeon, professor of medicine at Columbia, and TV personality. You can't get better credentials.

But a 2014 study in the *British Medical Journal* found that 54% of Dr. Oz's health recommendations—many of which concern weight loss—were either based on no scientific evidence at all, or were *directly contradicted* by the best available evidence.[8]

In short, any valid weight-loss argument should be based on science, no matter who makes it. Science is the only authority figure. Not a degree, not a title, and not a story. No one is above citing science. Beware those who don't. (And saying "studies suggest..." is *not* citing science. *Which* studies suggest?)

Still, citing studies is no guarantee. You may look up the reference for an enticing claim in a diet or health book and find a mouse study, or a small observational study from the '90s. This sort of thing, especially in nutrition, has undermined people's faith in science. There's a popular attitude that you can find a study to support almost any argument.

And it's true.

That's why you'll be seeing the term *meta-analysis* a lot.

A *meta-analysis* is a study of studies. It's a statistical study performed by a group of scientists who evaluate all the relevant studies on a certain topic, and form a summary conclusion.

This grouping of studies irons out a lot of the bias and chance inherent in individual studies, and affords the clearest window to truth. Even a meta-analysis can't escape bias, but you can't find a meta-analysis of randomized controlled trials to support any odd argument you want to make in nutrition.

If you look up one of the little numbers, there's a good chance it will point to a meta-analysis. Whenever possible, I gave precedence to meta-analyses—even if it meant renouncing cherished beliefs.

So science. Science and meta-analyses. But if you're still here, don't worry. I tried very hard not to be boring. The little numbers *stand* for relevant scientific studies so I don't have to bore you with the details. Do you really care what all the scientists' names were, or what they look like? This style allows us to cover a lot of ground without getting bogged down in minutiae.

But rest assured: every point, every concept, and every argument was meticulously, painstakingly researched.

Because weight loss is that important.

# 3

# WHY HABITS ARE SUPREME

There is no program in this book. There are no recipes.

There are only science, facts, and a few simple habits.

Habits are what life generally amounts to. Your day-in, day-out, run-of-the-mill habits play a crucial role in your success at just about anything. People think weight loss is an exception to this rule.

You see it all the time. Everyone is "trying to lose weight." Everyone is on a diet. Everyone is starting a 21-day cleanse.

These little affairs might work for a bit, but they're ultimately destined to fail by their very nature: they're *short-term* strategies.

After the program or diet ends, all that's left is your *habits*. William James, the father of American psychology, once wrote,

> *All our life, so far as it has definite form, is but a mass of habits.* [9]

As we'll see, your mass is literally determined by your eating habits.

Research indicates that we make over 200 eating decisions per day.[10] If this seems high, it's because most of these "decisions" are actually unconscious, automatic reactions.

In other words, they're habits.

People gain weight because of their habits. Then they try to lose weight with a short-term strategy—a diet, cleanse, workout program, etc.—without addressing the very habits that made them fat. That's what yo-yo dieting is: ignoring habits in favor of Band-Aids.

## The Five Golden Weight-Loss Habits

You probably don't want to lose weight temporarily. I'm guessing you want it gone for good. Well, the only way to do that is changing your habits.

We have a limited amount of willpower to make any big changes in life. And the same limited pool of willpower gets drained by many different activities.[11,12]

Since you have limited willpower to devote to weight loss, this brings up *willpower allocation theory*: the study of the optimal way to use your limited willpower to achieve a certain goal.

What is the optimal way to use your limited willpower to lose weight?

Most people blow all their weight-loss willpower on arbitrary diets and programs. Instead, it's best to spend your willpower on changing your habits.

But which habits?

That was the point of this book: a short, focused, practical list of the most effective habits the average person can reasonably develop in order to lose a lot of weight and keep it off—with the habits carefully ranked in order of importance.

Let's learn the science behind The Five Golden Weight-Loss Habits.

# PART 1

# Lucid Nutrition

# 4

# THE STATE OF NUTRITION

Despite the overwhelming consensus that a good diet is pivotal to good health, MDs are barely trained in nutrition. 75% of American medical schools, including Harvard,[13] don't require a nutrition class for graduation.[14]

In four years of medical school, the average US doctor spends 19.6 hours on the entire field of nutrition.[15] This number varies widely; some medical schools don't even offer nutrition.[16]

The students are innocent. A 2017 study found that medical students were "dissatisfied with their current education in nutrition" and "felt inadequately prepared to provide nutrition care."[17]

Apparently medical schools don't consider nutrition to be something a doctor should know about.

If your doctor *did* learn some nutrition, it was mostly in the first two years of medical school.[18] This means they had two more years of school to forget most of what they learned, three to seven years of residency to forget all of it, and however long they've been practicing medicine to forget that they forgot.

When the average doctor talks about food, they're drawing on a knowledge base equivalent to a two-day seminar they attended over a decade ago. As the US Public Health Office put it, "physicians are woefully undertrained in nutrition."[19]

In short, *MD* doesn't entail any knowledge of food.

If MDs don't know nutrition, who does? Dietitians? People with PhDs in nutrition? Perhaps. At least these people *studied* nutrition.

But look at the news. Nutrition experts can't seem to agree on very basic things, like whether carbs or meat are "bad" for people or not. Carbs and meat comprise the majority of the food eaten by humans. That would be like physicists disagreeing on Newton's Laws of Motion.

In fields like chemistry or mechanics, there's a foundation of systematic knowledge that was laid down over hundreds of years and thousands of experiments. This foundation is made of laws and equations that were rigorously proven, and are now accepted beyond a shadow of a doubt. (*Insert famous equation.*)

From this foundation, new laws are proposed, tested, and verified—and knowledge grows. Progress is usually slow and plodding. But in a few hundred years, our growing grasp of nature took us from celebrating crossing an ocean in a sailboat to landing on the moon—and then making self-driving cars.

But it's not that simple. The time it takes a field to get a firm foundation in place is highly variable, and depends on the field. For example, advanced knowledge of astronomy has existed for thousands of years.[20] To test predictions, all you had to do was look at the stars.

But in fields with less accessible data, foundations took far longer to form. Molecular biology only came into its own in the last century.

Nutrition still hasn't.

In the early days of a field, before it has a foundation, there are competing theories about very basic things. In 18th-century chemistry, for example, there were opposing ideas about what electricity was. Some early chemists thought it was a force of attraction and friction, while others thought it was a kind of fluid that ran through objects.[21]

Similarly, today's nutrition experts disagree on whether meat or carbs are bad, and whether it's better or worse to eat at certain times of the day.

These are fundamental questions. And when experts clash on fundamentals, it's a sign of a field without a foundation.

## Staggering Complexity

The main problem with nutrition science is that it's more or less impossible to fully isolate the long-term health effects of eating different foods. We don't have the technology to peer inside the body and see what different foods are doing to us in the long term. (Not yet.)

All we *can* do is look at associations between eating certain foods and getting different health outcomes.

But foods aren't eaten alone. People eat many foods, with changing, seasonal menus. And diseases can take decades to develop. How do you isolate the health effects of any one food?

And how do you isolate those health effects from genetics, environmental factors, lifestyle factors, social factors, stress, the patterns associated with specific foods (for instance, did you know people who eat red meat are more likely to smoke, drink excessively, not exercise, and eat fewer fruits and vegetables?[22,23]), as well as from other, *unknown* factors?

It's a hopeless task. This is why foods go from "good" to "bad" depending on the study, the news article, and the day of the week.

## Limitations of Nutrition Studies

The best we can do is split people into random groups, put them on different diets, and measure their health outcomes— the *randomized controlled trial* (RCT). This is the high-flying gold standard of health research. The bald eagle. Nothing else really compares. The only thing better would be a *meta-analysis* (a study of studies) of randomized controlled trials. A meta-analysis of RCTs from 2001 is much stronger evidence than an observational study published tomorrow.

But nutrition RCTs are far from perfect.

Unlike drug trials, there's no placebo control in a nutrition trial. If someone is eating a banana, they know it. And while diseases can take decades to develop, nutrition trials are necessarily rather short-term. And they have serious ethical limitations that limit their value—you can't lock people in cages and micromanage their diets. You basically just have to trust them to follow the rules.

But we *can* lock animals in cages and micromanage their diets, so we do. Then we trumpet the results of these animal studies as if they applied to humans. Like when *Time Magazine* referenced research showing that cholesterol was bad for rabbits in their famous cholesterol-condemning cover story of 1984.[24]

This was faulty reasoning. Cholesterol only exists in animal food, and rabbits are obligate herbivores. Saying that cholesterol is bad for rabbits and implying that cholesterol might therefore be bad for humans is the same as saying that a vegan diet is bad for tigers, and that vegetables might therefore be bad for humans.

But instead of rabbits, most animal nutrition studies are done on mice. Mice are great for clarifying physiological mechanisms, but as someone who used to work in a mouse lab, I can tell you that basing a human diet claim on mice is a mistake.

A mouse can fit in your hand. The last time we shared a common ancestor with mice was *80 million* years ago.[25]

What can mice tell us about what to eat?

Take chimps. Compared to mice, chimpanzees are about *sixty* times closer to us, genetically.[26] Chimp nutrition studies would be a big upgrade over mouse studies, right?

But even chimp nutrition studies—which are rare, due to ethical issues and the long lifespan of chimps—would prove absolutely nothing about *human* nutrition.

Despite being so close to us genetically, chimps have much bigger large intestines than us.[27] That's typical of a species that eats lots of plants that we can't digest. Chimps eat lots of leaves, for example.[28]

Chimps can digest cellulose. We can't. That's a profound difference—not the sort of thing you can brush off with "eh, close enough."

And yet chimps share 99% of our DNA.[29] This is a species that *looks* like us, and can partially *communicate* with us. And yet this a species adapted to eating different foods, in different amounts, with a fundamentally different digestive tract. What holds true for chimp nutrition does *not* necessarily hold true for human nutrition.

What does this say about mouse studies?

## The Perils of Observation

In *observational studies*, people are passively tracked and their health outcomes are recorded, with no intervention. Scientists try to figure out what foods people eat, then they let them live their lives. After enough time has passed, the scientists use statistical tests to show that eating different foods was associated with different health outcomes. Then news outlets trumpet these associations with sexy headlines.

But when two variables—A and B—are associated, that's

it. That's as far as it goes. A may cause B, B may cause A, or C may cause both. The association doesn't say which, and isn't evidence of cause, effect, or anything, really. To beat a dead horse, correlation isn't causation.

Making matters worse, these studies often rely on *food frequency questionnaires* (FFQs) to determine what foods people eat. These FFQs are just a series of multiple-choice questions about the foods you eat and how often you eat them. Much of what we know about nutrition is directly based on food frequency questionnaires—FFQs are one of the most common tools used in big nutritional population studies.[30]

There's just one problem: What did you eat six days ago?

No one else can remember, either.

Memory is notoriously unreliable. Eyewitness testimony in court cases often leads to misidentification of criminals,[31] which means people can't even be trusted to remember the face of someone they saw commit a crime. But scientists trust people to accurately remember their diets over long stretches of time. And they assume that people are capable of giving reliable, unbiased, objective assessments of their diets in the first place.

Food-frequency questionnaires have drawn serious criticism from scientists.[32] A 2015 paper in *Mayo Clinic Proceedings* called food-frequency questionnaires "error-prone…pseudo-scientific and highly edited anecdotes," concluding that they should be "inadmissible in scientific research."[33]

But even if food-frequency questionnaires were perfectly valid and reliable—and we had an accurate picture of what people were really eating—there would still be major problems with drawing conclusions from such studies.

Diet is not the only thing that affects health. Instead, diet occurs in a fiendishly intricate web of outside, health-influencing factors known as *confounding variables*.

Here are a few confounding variables: whether someone

exercises (and the type and amount of exercise), stress levels, spirituality, age, ethnicity, alcohol consumption (and *past* consumption), whether someone smokes (and *past* smoking), drug use (and *past* drug use), gender, known medical conditions (and *past* medical conditions, and *unknown* medical conditions), height, weight, air quality, water quality, family disease history, family relationships, social relationships, social standing, mental health, blood type, job satisfaction, and exposure to toxins (and *past* exposure).

And then there are the *unknown* confounding variables.

And then there are the mind-boggling idiosyncrasies of a person's genome, whose full complexity we are nowhere close to grasping.

But don't worry. Researchers "control" for all these things.

And they can apparently control for all these things with questions like this:

*Are you basically satisfied with your life?* ☐Yes ☐No[34]

This was on a questionnaire in the Nurses' Health Study, one of the most cited and influential nutrition studies of all time.

## Take-Home

Due to the ridiculous complexity of nutrition science, nutrition still doesn't have a solid foundation, and being a "nutrition expert" doesn't mean all that much.

# 5

# INDUSTRIAL NUTRITION ADVICE

What's the biggest industry in the world? Take a guess.

Healthcare? Banking? Oil?

Nope. It's food.[35] The food industry services over seven billion customers a day. It's been estimated that half of all the world's assets, labor, and consumer expenditures belong to the food industry.[36]

Just think of all the world's supermarkets, restaurants, fast-food chains, food stands, food trucks, vending machines, food corporations, farmers, agricultural conglomerates, and meat-packing companies. Taken together, these entities bring in *trillions* of dollars each year.

Does this ocean of money affect official diet advice?

In 2016, it made headlines that a review on heart-disease risk factors published by Harvard researchers in 1967 in the prestigious *New England Journal of Medicine* had been the result of blatant industry corruption.[37]

Evidence that sugar was associated with heart disease had

been mounting since the 1950s, but this 1967 review blamed heart disease almost entirely on saturated fat, minimized the role of sugar, downplayed and ignored conflicting evidence, and helped frame the heart-disease discussion for decades to come.

It turns out that the sugar industry, through their Sugar Research Foundation, had paid three of these Harvard researchers—including Mark Hegsted, who would later help shape US dietary guidelines—the modern equivalent of $50,000 to write an explicitly pro-sugar review.[38]

No industry funding was disclosed in the study.

Speaking of hearts, the American Heart Association recommends that we avoid saturated fat,[39] and cook with vegetable oil instead of butter.[40] Vegetable oils are by far the biggest dietary source of *n-6 fatty acids*,[41] a type of polyunsaturated fat. And in 2009, the AHA released an advisory to the public on n-6 fatty acids.

In other words, they released an advisory on vegetable oil.

The lead author of this AHA advisory was William Harris. At the time, Harris was a consultant for Monsanto,[42] the world's biggest producer of the seeds used to make vegetable oil.[43] Harris was also a consultant for Unilever, maker of I Can't Believe It's Not Butter!—the first ingredient of which is vegetable oil.[44]

Unilever also employed another author on the advisory, as well as one of its three official reviewers.[45]

This advisory concluded that at least five to ten percent of all our calories should come from n-6 fatty acids (vegetable oil) if we want to lower our risk of heart disease—and that "higher intakes appear to be safe and may be even more beneficial."[46]

So paid consultants for vegetable-oil companies concluded that vegetable oils are safe, and that we should eat more of them.

It turns out that over 90% of industry-sponsored nutrition

studies produce results favorable to that industry.[47] Compared to studies with no industry funding, industry-funded studies are almost eight times more likely to produce favorable results.[48]

A 2007 study found that if a nutrition study pertained to a certain food industry—but had no industry funding—there was a 37% chance it would produce a bad result for that industry. With industry funding, however, that number dropped to 0%.[49]

Back to the AHA advisory. Unsurprisingly, there were other scientists—who *weren't* paid vegetable-oil consultants—who strongly disagreed with the AHA's conclusion. One commentary published in the *British Journal of Nutrition* questioned whether the advisory was "evidence based or biased evidence?"[50]

The next year, the *British Journal of Nutrition* published a meta-analysis of randomized controlled trials (the Holy Grail of evidence) on fatty acids and heart disease. It specifically addressed the AHA advisory, concluding:

> *Advice to specifically increase n-6 PUFA intake…is unlikely to provide the intended benefits, and may actually increase the risks of coronary heart disease and death.*[51]

The researchers accused the AHA advisory of ignoring relevant studies and including studies with serious limitations to support its conclusions.

Who to believe? Scientists with no obvious agenda, or scientists employed by vegetable-oil companies?

## The USDA

The United States Department of Agriculture (USDA) decides the official nutrition advice of the United States government.

The USDA was the builder of the Food Pyramid, and the spinner of MyPlate. It is www.nutrition.gov.

If you think about it, it's a bit strange that the United States Department of *Agriculture* would have this power. Listed under "What We Do" on the USDA website, you'll find "provide economic opportunity through innovation," and "promote agriculture production."

The only time you see the word "health" is "healthy private working lands."[52]

Based on their own words, then, the USDA is an organization concerned with the *business* of food, not with health. And it is *business* that has continually shaped the USDA dietary guidelines—and thus, the official dietary guidelines of America.

It all started with *Dietary Goals for the United States*, a 1977 document released by the Senate's Select Committee on Nutrition.[53] The basic message of this document was to eat more grains, eat less total fat, and eat more polyunsaturated fat—a message the USDA still endorses today.

But right from the start, this advice came under fire. A 1979 review in the *American Journal of Clinical Nutrition* said:

> *Regarding humans, no evidence exists, either observational or experimental, that demonstrates a causative relationship between dietary fat per se and human atherosclerotic disease… The benefits of a low-fat, low-saturated fat, low-cholesterol diet have never been adequately tested… There are few precedents for use of diets high in polyunsaturated fats* [vegetable oil], *and scientists question the advisability of such diets.*[54]

The American Medical Association was also staunchly opposed to this advice.[55]

But the biggest uproar came from food corporations. The

cattle and salt industries were particularly livid—*Dietary Goals* specifically told people to eat fewer of their products.

So they unleashed their lobbying power on the Senate.[56]

It worked. The very same year, the Committee released an emergency "Second Edition" of *Dietary Goals*. To placate the salt industry, the maximum advisable salt intake was increased from three grams a day to five grams a day. To appease the cattle industry, the original advice to "decrease consumption of meat" was changed to "choose meats, poultry, and fish which will reduce saturated fat intake."[57]

Disgusted by such corruption, the original author of *Dietary Goals*, Nick Mottern, resigned.[58]

The following year, the USDA wrested official-nutrition-advice power from the Senate Committee, and appointed a new Administrator of Human Nutrition: Mark Hegsted.[59]

That's the same Mark Hegsted who accepted a bribe from the sugar industry. And since then, every five years, the USDA has released *Dietary Guidelines for Americans*, a publication that mirrors the original *Dietary Goals* in form, content, and the tendency to cave to industry pressure.

In the early 1980s, the USDA assembled a team of nutrition experts to create the Food Pyramid. At the head of the team was a nutritionist named Luise Light, a professor at NYU.

Light and her team consulted with experts and scoured the literature for months to produce the best food guide they could. Their original advice was to ruthlessly cut down on junk food, eat a base of vegetables and fruits, eat reasonable amounts of "protein foods" like meat, eggs, and nuts, and eat two to three servings of both dairy and whole grains each day.[60]

Satisfied, they submitted their guidelines to the Secretary of Agriculture.

But the Secretary sent the Pyramid back, with several...*edits*.

Dr. Light and her team were horrified. Their original advice to eat three to four servings of *whole grains* each day had been changed to *six to eleven* servings of *grains*, which now made up the base of the Pyramid. Refined grains had previously occupied the top-most, "Use Sparingly" section; the Secretary had completely reversed their advice.

According to Dr. Light, this edit was "a concession to the processed wheat and corn industries."[61]

Fruits and vegetables were slashed from five to nine servings a day to two to three servings a day. The general message went from cutting out junk food to eating junk food in moderation.

According to Dr. Light, all these changes were "calculated to win the acceptance of the food industry."[62]

Light goes on:

> *I vehemently protested that the changes, if followed, could lead to an epidemic of obesity and diabetes—and couldn't be justified on either health or nutritional grounds…Over my objections, the Food Guide Pyramid was finalized…ultimately, the food industry dictates the government's food advice, shaping the nutrition agenda delivered to the public.…nutrition for the government is primarily a marketing tool to fuel growth in consumer food expenditures.*[63]

Dr. Light is not alone in her view. According to Walter Willett, MD, PhD, chair of Harvard's nutrition department, and the second-most cited author in all of clinical medicine, the Food Pyramid was "out of date from the day it was printed" and "not compatible with good scientific evidence."[64]

According to the Harvard School of Public Health, the Food Pyramid as well as more current guidelines are "based on out-of-date science and influenced by people with business interests."[65]

Take the official advice on sugar. The American sugar lobby

gained ever more power in the '80s and '90s as US sugar consumption skyrocketed.[66] Here's how the sugar advice in *Dietary Guidelines* changed over that time:

1985: "Avoid too much sugar"

1990: "Use sugars only in moderation"

1995: "Choose a diet moderate in sugars"

2000: "Choose beverages and foods to moderate your intake of sugars"[67]

Look at those verbs. We go from being told to "avoid" sugars in '85 to being told to "use" them in '90, and finally, to actually "choose" sugars in 1995—a stretch of time when the negative health evidence on sugary drinks was mounting almost as quickly as sugar revenues.

## Nutrition Professionals

What about dietitians? They seem knowledgable about food and diets, and many dietitians have helped countless people eat healthier and lose weight.

But are dietitians immune from industry influence?

Sadly, one look at the corporate sponsors page of the Academy of Nutrition and Dietetics—the official licensing body of American dietitians—tells us otherwise.

In 2014 and 2015, some of the Academy's esteemed sponsors included General Mills, Kellogg's, Pepsi, Coke, Unilever (I Can't Believe It's Not Butter! and Ben and Jerry's) and Conagra (Slim Jims, Reddi-wip, and Orville Redenbacher's).[68]

Not coincidentally, the Academy's advice—and thus, that of many dietitians—is aligned with these corporate interests.

In fact, the Academy merely echoes the nutrition advice of the USDA, which it readily admits.[69]

For example, dietitians urge us to "eat at least half of all grains as whole grains each day"[70]—just like the USDA does.[71]

On the surface, this advice sounds reasonable.

*Eat at least half of all grains as whole grains each day.*

They're encouraging us to eat whole grains, right?

But if you read between the lines, what this advice is *really* saying, in a diabolically subtle way, is that it's okay to eat lots of refined grains. Because if we follow the above advice—and "at least half" of all the grains we eat are *whole* grains—then the rules of logic tell us it's okay if the other 50% are *refined*.

Refined grains are universally reviled among credible nutrition authorities. So why would the Academy—and thus, many dietitians—be so lenient on them?

Could it be because the Academy is sponsored by General Mills and Kellogg's?

Similarly, instead of supporting the proposed ban on large sodas in New York City in 2012, the Academy encouraged "moderation."[72] Indeed, according to the Academy of Nutrition and Dietetics, when it comes to sugary drinks, "the key is to moderate, not eliminate."[73]

The key is to *moderate*—despite overwhelming evidence that sugary drinks are unhealthy and fattening.[74,75]

Why would the Academy be so lenient on soda?

Could it be because it's sponsored by Coke and Pepsi?


Industry corruption of nutrition advice is not a uniquely American problem. In 2010, the food industry spent over a billion dollars to crush a European initiative that would have required unhealthy foods to be labeled with a red-light symbol.[76]

## Take-Home

We can't count on physicians to know nutrition, or on nutrition science to give us definitive answers, or on governments and dietitians to give us nutrition advice that isn't tainted by industry.

So where can we turn?

A foundation.

# 6

# THE FOUNDATION OF NUTRITION

Humans are biological organisms. We're a species made of cells. We have DNA that's transcribed into RNA which is translated into proteins that do the plethora of life's functions. We are living things that grow, reproduce, and die. We are part of biology.

And as lauded genetics researcher Thedosius Dobzhansky said, "nothing in biology makes sense except in the light of evolution."[77]

Nothing, indeed. Evolution sculpted every species on Earth. Different environments selected for different genes, and the best-adapted organisms were more likely to survive the endless meat-grinder of natural selection that wiped out 99% of all the species that ever lived.[78]

Nature has been in continual flux for billions of years, and species continually adapted to changing surroundings, often becoming entirely new species in the process. That's how a single ancient cell exploded into all the life-forms that ever existed on Earth.

Evolution is a "theory" to the same extent that gravity is a "theory." You can't technically call evolution and gravity "facts" because scientific theories can never be proven absolutely—they can only be falsified. As Stephen Hawking said:

> *You can never prove it* [a theory]...*on the other hand, you can disprove a theory by finding even a single observation that disagrees with the predictions of the theory.*[79]

And no theory has withstood more attacks than evolution. For over a hundred years, armies of creationists have desperately searched for a shred of evidence to falsify evolution.

They've failed miserably.

Like gravity, evolution has been rigorously established beyond a shadow of a doubt by enormous bodies of evidence converging from many different fields.[80]

At this point, evolution is simply bulletproof. If anything, there's more controversy among physicists about the nature of gravity than there is among biologists about evolution.[81]

Evolution is the fundamental force of biology.

## Nutrition = Biology

Nutrition is the study of how food affects health. We usually think of *human* nutrition, but nutrition applies to any species that eats food. "Health" is the proper physiological function of an organism, and "food" is typically a plant or an animal—genes eating genes.

Since nutrition is only a function of *living* things, and since biology is the study of living things, nutrition is just a part of biology. There is no part of nutrition that isn't also a part of biology.

Thus, nutrition is a sub-discipline, or *subset* of biology—a *part* of biology completely contained in the *whole* of biology. It looks like this:

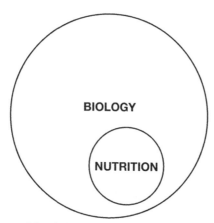

*Nutrition is a subset of biology.*

All of human culture and technology—like modern food processing—haven't changed this. While we humans may be the most advanced species, we haven't transcended biology. We're still made of cells that grow, reproduce, and die. We're still DNA that is transcribed into RNA that is translated into proteins. We're still phenotypes arising from genotypes.

Most of our cells aren't even technically *ours*. There are a hundred trillion microbes in your gut.[82] This means there are more cells from *other* species in your body than human cells.

We aren't separate, special, extra-biological snowflakes. Instead, we are pulsing plethoras of interconnected life, and everything about us—including our nutrition—is governed by the same gene-environment interactions that determine the fate of every other species on Earth.

And our genes are *caused* by evolution.

Which brings us to the foundation.

# The Foundation of Human Nutrition

Evolution explains biology.

↓

Human nutrition is a subset of biology.

↓

**Evolution explains human nutrition.**


That's it. Three lines. If you accept the first two premises, the conclusion is irrefutable. That's the power of logic.

(You could substitute "human" with any other species.)

To challenge the first or second premise would be to say that evolution does not explain biology, or that humans or human nutrition are somehow outside of biology.

Either one is an obvious mistake.

So this is proof that evolution explains human nutrition.

What does this mean? It means that, like any other species, what makes up a "healthy diet" for humans is explained by evolution.

Foods aren't innately "healthy" or "unhealthy." The health status of a food depends on the species, and ultimately on the individual organism. If a particular organism is sufficiently adapted to eating a particular type of food, then that food is *much* less likely to cause health problems for that organism than a food it's *not* sufficiently adapted to eating.

Evolutionary adaptation explains how the same food can be nutritious for one species and poisonous for another. For example, there are species of bacteria that thrive on a diet of cyanide (which is poisonous to humans).[83]

Carnivores like cheetahs and tigers would suffer terrible health effects on a vegan diet, and herbivores like cows and deer would suffer terrible health effects on a meat diet—because these species are not sufficiently adapted to eating these types of food in large quantities.

Humans are no different: whether a food is healthy for you or not depends on whether you are sufficiently adapted to eating that type of food.

## The Foundation of Human Nutrition

Evolution explains biology.

↓

Human nutrition is a subset of biology.

↓

**Evolution explains human nutrition.**

# 7

# PALEO FANTASIES

Whatever its flaws, the "Paleo Diet" was the first popular dietary framework to recognize the importance of evolution in human nutrition. It was the first diet to try to guide food decisions with evolutionary reasoning. For this, it deserves a lot of credit.

Most nutrition authorities rarely if ever use evolutionary reasoning. They almost proceed as if people were created 6,000 years ago by God.

To be sure, experimental evidence is the strongest kind, and takes precedence over evolutionary logic. But given the lack of quality controlled trials addressing so many important questions in nutrition (and the limitations of nutrition trials in general) practicing blind nutritional empiricism—forming nutrition positions *solely* based on experimental evidence—is a pale and sickly approach.

Blind empiricists ignore the fact that evolution is the fundamental force of biology, and the root of all biologic variation (including human nutrition). And they ignore the fact that evolution was established with far more rigorous and exacting standards than most nutrition theories ever were.

At least Paleo *attempts* to use evolutionary logic.

But based on several faulty premises, there are serious flaws in the basic Paleo Diet—*Don't eat grains, legumes, or dairy!* —which have made others wary of Paleo, and have given Paleo a bit of a bad name.

Nevertheless, Paleo has a very strong track record in diet trials. Versions of the Paleo Diet have generally been found to cause significant weight loss and big improvements in major health markers like cholesterol, blood pressure, triglycerides, and insulin sensitivity.[84,85,86]

Head-to-head, the Paleo Diet has been shown to improve glycemic control and reduce waist circumference more than the Mediterranean diet.[87] It's been found to cause more weight loss, lower blood pressure, more satiety (the "full" feeling), higher HDL (good) cholesterol, and lower triglycerides than a standard diabetes diet.[88,89] And it's been shown to cause more weight loss and bigger improvements in various health markers than several other traditional diets.[90,91,92]

So Paleo is clearly an effective way to eat.

*That's* not the problem.

The problem with Paleo is that, based on flawed evolutionary logic, it's too restrictive of a diet, which makes it impractical for many people.

Which is a *big* problem.

Let's see where Paleo goes wrong.


## The Paleo Argument

There are many variations of "Paleo," but they're usually based on the following premises: that people started practicing agriculture about 10,000 years ago, that 10,000 years is an "eye-blink" in evolutionary terms, and that since agriculture began, we've hardly evolved at all.

Instead (*the Paleo argument goes*), the relevant period of our evolution was the "Paleolithic Era," which spanned from 2.6 million years ago to 10,000 years ago. People today basically have the same genes that people had in the Paleolithic Era. Thus, we're not adapted to eating foods that only became widely available *after* the dawn of agriculture—like grains, dairy products, legumes, and potatoes—because our genes haven't had sufficient time to adapt to them. And since genetic differences between people are trivial, we'd *all* be better off avoiding those foods and eating a "Paleolithic diet" of meat, fruits, vegetables, etc.

Every single one of these premises is wrong.

## Debunking Paleo

First, to say that 10,000 years is an "eye-blink" is to misunderstand evolution. Evolutionary timescales are not absolute—they're relative. If the environment of a species doesn't change, that species may stay almost exactly the same for an extremely long time. For example, horseshoe crabs have hardly changed in hundreds of millions of years.[93]

On the other hand, when selective pressures change, a species can evolve extremely quickly.

For example, it only took around 15,000 years for this:

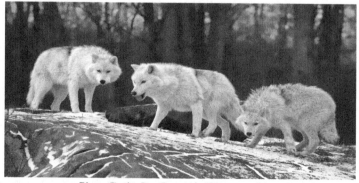

Photo Credit: Jim Cumming/Shutterstock.com

To evolve into this:

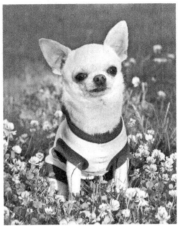

*All dogs are direct descendants of wolves.*[94]
Photo Credit: Little Moon/Shutterstock.com

Some people will argue that this wolf-to-dog transition was caused by "artificial" selective pressure, since it was imposed by humans (implying that it was artificially strong).

But if we're going that route, we'll have to say that the transition from hunter-gatherers to farmers was also caused by "artificial" selective pressure (since it was imposed by humans).

In any case, the agricultural transition was a time when we were forced to adapt to drastically different lifestyles, drastically different climates, and drastically different diets.

Selective pressures don't come much stronger than that.

And increasing selective pressures accelerate evolution.

Based on genetic evidence, some scientists have concluded that—contrary to the main premise of the Paleo diet—not only *have* humans evolved in the last 10,000 years, but our rate of evolution may have accelerated about *100-fold* during this time.[95]

How is that possible? Well, evolution largely proceeds

through *beneficial mutations*. The vast majority of mutations are neutral. Of the mutations that aren't neutral, the *vast* majority are harmful. Beneficial mutations are unicorn rare.[96]

But beneficial mutations are major drivers of evolutionary change. Most of evolution's all-time greatest hits—wings, vision, opposable thumbs, etc.—started out as beneficial mutations.

And the thing is, during the Paleolithic Era, the total human population was quite small. 60,000 years ago, there were only about a quarter million human-like creatures walking the Earth.[97] That's the population of Buffalo, NY.

With a population that small, beneficial mutations might happen once in a blue moon. But by 3,000 years ago, the human population had exploded to 60 million people.[98] This 240-fold increase in population size meant a 240-fold increase in the frequency of beneficial mutations in our gene pool. So there were *240 times* more beneficial mutations. And they could now spread far and wide in a world increasingly connected by trade and war.

These rare and helpful mutations were the raw material for our recent spate of evolution.

*What* recent spate of evolution?

How are we different than cavemen?

Let me count the ways.

- **Skin color.** Paleolithic people generally had dark skin. The mutation in the gene that causes the "white" skin of Europeans—SLC24A5—is only 5,800 years old.[99]
- **Eye color.** It's likely that cavemen didn't have blue eyes. The genes that cause baby blues—HERC2 and OCA2, of course—likely originated between seven and ten thousand years ago near present-day Lithuania.[100,101]
- **Bones.** We have thinner bones than Paleolithic people.[102]
- **Cranial structure.** Paleolithic people had pronounced

brow ridges (the infamous "Neanderthal brow"), which
have mostly disappeared. Our jaw ridges and skull volumes
are smaller than those of Paleolithic people.[103] There's
actually evidence of enlarging craniums in Europeans
over just the last 1,000 years.[104] (Evolution is ongoing.)

- **Resistance to disease.** Malaria is only 4,000 years
old, and we've adapted several genetic defenses to it
since then. 400 million people have a red-blood-cell
disorder called *G6DP deficiency*, which—like sickle-cell
anemia—doubles as a defense to malaria. G6DP deficiency is only around 2,500 years old.[105]

   Malaria is likely just one of *many* diseases we've recently
adapted to. When Europeans first came to the Americas,
they brought infectious diseases that killed over 90% of
the native population in the following centuries.[106]

- **Ability to eat dairy.** Before 8,000 years ago, all adults
were probably lactose intolerant. (The enzyme needed
to digest lactose—*lactase*—was only produced by infants
and small children, who need it to digest breast milk.)
The mutation that led to *adult* lactase production was
beneficial for populations that herded cattle; using cattle
for dairy instead of just meat provides five times more
calories per acre.[107]

- **Blood-sugar regulation.** A variant of a gene that
protects against diabetes (TCF7L2) has seen positive
selective pressure in several populations which began
right around the time they started agriculture.[108]

- **Saliva proteins.** A 2015 study found that the gene
that codes for a protein called salivary agglutinin (which
affects cavity formation) is different in populations with
a longer history of agriculture.[109]

In other words, we look different than cavemen, we're
adapted to different diseases than cavemen, and we process

food differently than cavemen. And these are just the *known* differences. There are likely other important differences—including dietary ones—that we're not yet aware of.

## Is a Person a Person?

Aside from the mistaken idea that modern humans are identical to cavemen, another Paleo fantasy is that modern humans are identical to each other.

The phrase "10,000 years" is bandied about the Paleo-sphere as the time span that "we humans" have been farming for—the bright red line dividing hunting and gathering from farming.

But this is a cartoon simplification.

While agriculture *did* start around 10,000 years ago in the Middle East, it took another 5,000 years for agriculture to spread through Europe. Amerindians (Indians from America) only started farming around 1,000 years ago.

Australian Aborigines never started farming at all.[110]

So "we humans" didn't start farming at any one time.

These variable farming start dates almost certainly mean that some populations are less adapted to agricultural foods than others. Diabetes seems to be a diet-related disease,[111] and Amerindians—who, again, have only been farming around 1000 years—are 2.5 times more likely to get diabetes than people of European descent. Aborigines—who, again, never started farming—are four times more likely to get diabetes than other Australians.[112]

Population differences are even more striking with dairy, a major food group that's only about 8,000 years old. There has been a tremendous range of adaptation to dairy. For example, 95% of the population of Denmark and Sweden are able to digest the lactose in dairy,[113] while 98% of Southeast Asians are *unable* to digest lactose—they're lactose intolerant.[114]

So the vast majority of people in certain countries have no problem with a major food group, while this same major food group gives the vast majority of people in *other* countries diarrhea, nausea, and cramps.

These striking modern differences in response to dairy products almost certainly reflect big differences in the amount of dairy in ancestral diets.

Humans also vary widely in their number of copies of a gene called AMY1, which codes for *salivary amylase*—an enzyme that starts digesting starch in the mouth. People have anywhere from one to *fifteen* copies of this gene.

That's a tremendous range.

Populations with traditionally high-starch diets tend to have much higher copy numbers of AMY1 than populations with traditionally *low*-starch diets. And the higher your copy number of AMY1, the more amylase your mouth releases when there's starch in it.[115]

A 2012 study showed that, seventy-five minutes after eating starch, people with high copy numbers of AMY1 had significantly lower blood sugar than people with low copy numbers. The scientists concluded that people with low copy numbers "may be at greater risk for insulin resistance and diabetes if chronically ingesting starch-rich diets."[116]

(Starch makes up over half the carbs eaten in the US.[117])

In short, people clearly aren't the same, nutritionally.

The "Ideal Human Diet" doesn't exist.

But along with many other diet ideologies, Paleo falsely assumes that one diet can be optimal for everyone, and makes cookie-cutter recommendations that don't begin to encompass the vagaries of the human genome.

And forget population differences. What about *you*? It's highly likely that even within a genetic population, different diets are better for different people based on *individual* factors like gender, body-fat level, age, food preferences, medical history, insulin sensitivity, and exercise patterns.

Not to mention *genetics*.

In any case, by banning all agricultural foods, Paleo contradicts facts of recent nutritional selection and advocates a strict diet that's impractical for many people (*no grains, no dairy, no legumes*).

And *practical* is the word of the day.

## Take-Home

Paleo is a healthy diet, but it's too restrictive, and is based on several fallacies.

# 8

# THE MYTH OF "HEALTHY" FOODS

Forget *super*—no food is even universally "good." As in, *good for everyone, in large amounts.* Not one.

Show me any food on Earth. I'll show you a surprising number of people who probably shouldn't make it a staple.

You already know about lactose and gluten. There are five billion people (two-thirds of everyone[118,119]) who may get gastro-irritated from milk.

Milk is high in protein, calcium, potassium, selenium, riboflavin, and vitamin B-12.[120] But if milk gives you a stomach ache whenever you drink it, it's not healthy for you.

Likewise, whole wheat is high in fiber, several B-vitamins, and lots of minerals.[121] But it has gluten, and for the 1% of people with Celiac disease, according to a 2010 review in *Nature*:

> *A strict life-long gluten-free diet is the only safe and efficient available treatment.*[122]

They didn't mince words.

*One percent* may sound tiny, but that's **75 million humans** who shouldn't eat wheat, barley, rye, or brewer's yeast—basically all bread, pasta, pastries, baked goods, crackers, cereal, pancakes, waffles, french toast, breadcrumbs, couscous, and beer[123]—*ever again.*

Poor souls. For them, there's no such thing as "healthy whole wheat." But in a very real sense, *any* food is a foreign substance entering your body.

## An Ocean of Allergies

Roughly eight percent of all kids and five percent of all adults (that's hundreds of millions of people) have food allergies.[124] Many of these allergies are to "healthy" foods. Some of the most common food allergies are to fish, crustaceans (shrimp, crab, lobster), peanuts, tree nuts, wheat, soy, eggs, and milk.[125]

And there are two more basic food groups that commonly cause allergies. Maybe you've heard of them: fruits and vegetables.[126]

That's right. A 2010 study of Canadian adults found that, after milk and shellfish, fruits and vegetables were respectively the third- and fourth-most-common food allergies.[127]

Apparently some people are allergic to health.

Seeds, in particular, can provoke especially severe reactions.[128]

The point is, *any* food can be an allergen.[129] And if you're allergic to a food, no matter how *healthy* and *organic* and *antioxidant-packed* it may otherwise be, then that food is not healthy for you.

Sorry to burst your superfood.

## Can the Healthiest Food Be Unhealthy?

What's considered the healthiest food on Earth? Probably a green vegetable, right? Kale? Maybe broccoli? Brussels sprouts? Let's take all three—kale, broccoli, and Brussels sprouts. It's hard to go wrong there.

These three foods are *cruciferous vegetables*—plants of the *Brassica* genus, which also includes collard greens, turnips, and bok choy. Cruciferous vegetables were "superfoods" before that word existed. They've often been associated with a reduced risk of cancer,[130] heart disease,[131] and death.[132]

You'd be hard-pressed to name a more immaculate food group than cruciferous veggies.

But for many people, eating large and regular amounts of cruciferous vegetables is probably *not* healthy. I speak of *hypothyroidism*, a disease where the thyroid gland (located at the base of the neck) spits out too little thyroid hormone (many important functions). Hypothyroidism can cause heart disease, obesity, joint pain, and infertility.[133] And cruciferous vegetables contain *goitrogens*,[134] which are substances that mess with the thyroid gland.

People with healthy thyroids probably have nothing to lose—and everything to gain—by eating gobs of cruciferous veggies every day. (As long as they're not iodine deficient,[135] at least.)

But if you have hypothyroidism, some medical professionals will actually tell you to avoid overeating kale, broccoli, and Brussels sprouts.[136] There is hard evidence that eating large and regular amounts of several types of raw cruciferous veggies—like Brussels sprouts, certain collards, and a type of kale—could cause problems for people with hypothyroidism.[137]

Nor is hypothyroidism some fringe disease. Based on the results of a well-known 2000 study,[138] there are roughly 1.3 million Americans with overt hypothyroidism, most of whom are undiagnosed.[139] There are another 27 million Americans with *subclinical hypothyroidism*, which puts you at risk for the overt kind.[140]

The numbers may be even higher overseas. Hypothyroidism is far more common in India,[141] for example.

Skeptics will say that even people with hypothyroidism would have to eat very large amounts of raw cruciferous veggies every day to cause problems—implying that no sane person would do this. For instance, no one would ever stuff large amounts of raw kale in a blender every morning and make a smoothie.

*Right.* And isn't the definition of a "healthy food" something we *could* eat as a daily staple—*without* potential health problems?

Listen to your body.

Not people who prefix foods with "super."

## Take-Home

People can have health issues with almost any food, including large amounts of kale and Brussels sprouts. No food is universally healthy for everyone in large amounts.

# 9

# SATIETY:
# WHY PEOPLE GET FAT

In the land of weight loss, satiety is king.

"Satiety" is science-talk for feeling full. Satiety is caused by eating food. Information about the amount of food in your GI tract—like how much it's stretching your stomach ("gastric distension")—is communicated to your brainstem and hypothalamus by peptide signals with arbitrary names like cholecystokinin, glucagon-like peptide 1, and peptide YY.[142,143]

If these signals are strong enough, *voila!* Your appetite is curbed.

Satiety is critical to weight loss because we're always getting hungry, we're always eating, and we're always getting full—one of the great circles of life.

And when it comes to satiety, wait for it...*foods are not equal.* **Per calorie, some foods are *far* more filling than others.**[144,145,146,147]

It's hard to overstate the importance of this.

Just for the sake of argument, let's say you're not an ascetic monk who chooses to live with continual hunger pangs. In that case, you will generally, more or less, most of the time, often enough to count...*eat until you feel somewhat full.*

And if you consistently eat foods on the *less*-filling end of the spectrum, you'll have to eat more total calories to feel full.

So you *will* eat more total calories.

(Because you're not an ascetic monk who chooses to live with continual hunger pangs.)

And we all know what happens when you consistently eat more calories. You gain fat. And if you give it enough time, unless you're a genetic luck-pot, you *get* fat.

While some people are genetically disposed to be fat, **most people get fat because their regular diets contain less-filling foods**.

People can get skinny by removing these less-filling foods from their regular diets, and replacing them with more-filling foods (that still taste good; no ascetic monking required).

**The key is to base your diet on filling foods.**

But what foods are more filling, and which are less filling? Where *is* this spectrum of filling-ness?

It's very simple. You don't have to worry about any details. Just think of one, all-important, neon-bright dividing line:

# processed foods
# vs.
# whole foods

Processed foods (definition to come) are generally *much* less filling than whole foods.[148,149] *Because* processed foods are less filling, when people have unlimited access to processed foods (like most of us do) they tend to eat more total calories.[150,151,152]

Food processing is a science, an art, and an evolutionary novelty. It creates uber delicious foods that are aliens to our body's satiety system, which evolved regulating whole-food diets.

For all its alleged complexity, the obesity epidemic is very simple. People eat too much processed food. A 2015 study found that 77% of the food Americans buy is processed, and that 61% of it is "highly processed."[153]

This is why 71% of us are overweight.[154]

And in the cause lies the cure. **Get in the habit of eliminating processed food from your regular diet.**

(Your *regular diet* is the diet you eat *most* days of the week.)

But what exactly *is* "processed food," aside from the obvious junk foods? Great question. The term *processed food* isn't in the dictionary, so here's a useful, practical definition to bring to the supermarket:

> **processed food** *n* : *a food with an ingredients list longer than one item*

Let's see what makes processed food so bad.

# 10

# THE FAT FOUR

The Paleo Diet has given many people a bad impression of using evolutionary reasoning in nutrition. But when something isn't used correctly, you don't get a good idea of its value. It's like trying to cut a steak with a scalpel, and then concluding that a scalpel isn't a useful tool.

Skeptics of using evolutionary reasoning in nutrition will usually admit that evolution is integral to nutrition—*theoretically*. But they argue that it's impossible to determine exactly what our distant ancestors ate—and thus, what *we* should eat.

And they are completely correct.

But determining what we *should* eat isn't the strength of evolutionary reasoning. No, its strength lies in determining, with absolute certainty, something even more important: what we *shouldn't* eat.

What if I told you there are only four bad foods? (Just four.)

What if I told you these four foods are the root of the obesity epidemic, causing people to overeat and get fat on a massive scale?

What if I told you that no human population is adapted to these foods, so they probably aren't healthy for *anyone* to eat in large amounts—but that they make up a *staggering* proportion of our total food intake?

I'm going to tell you. After a systematic analysis of nutrition, anthropology, physiology, obesity research, metabolism, and the US food supply, without further adieu, I give you *The Fat Four*:

## 1. added sugar
## 2. added oil
## 3. white flour
## 4. processed meat

These are the only four foods that are unequivocally "bad," "unhealthy," and "fattening."

Just these four.

*Added sugar, added oil, white flour,* and *processed meat.*

The Fat Four.

If a food isn't made with one of these four, it's probably fine.

On the other hand, a food is "junk food" precisely *because* it has one or more of these four. A food is "fattening" precisely *because* it has one or more of these four.

Every. Single. Time.

Pizza? *White flour* and *added sugar* (the dough and the sauce).

Candy bars? *Added sugar* (and usually *white flour* and *vegetable oil,* too).

Chicken nuggets? *Processed meat* and *white flour.*

Cake? *White flour* and *added sugar* (and usually *vegetable oil*).

French fries? *Vegetable oil.* (Added oil.)
Potato chips? *Vegetable oil.* (Added oil.)
Any chip in a crinkly bag? *Vegetable oil.*
Bacon? *Processed meat.*
Pie? *White flour* and *added sugar* (and usually *oil*).
Muffins? *White flour* and *added sugar* (and usually *oil*).
Donuts? *White flour* and *added sugar* (and usually *oil*).
Slim Jims? *Processed meat.*
Chicken wings? *Vegetable oil* and *white flour* (and thus: *processed meat*).
Ice cream? *Added sugar* (and usually *vegetable oil*).

All of these foods are fattening *because* of the Fat Four. There is nothing else holding them together.

But it's hardly just obvious junk foods like these. Every day, due to misconceptions and deceptive marketing, untold millions of people around the world eat foods that they believe are basically "not fattening," "healthy," or even "slimming"—but that are actually infested with The Fat Four.

Let's see some examples.

Virtually every single breakfast cereal? *Added sugar.*

(This includes cereals marketed as healthy, like Kashi GOLEAN Crunch!, which is high in added sugar.[155])

Any non-whole-grain bread? *White flour.*

Most "100% Whole-Wheat" breads? *Added sugar* and often *added oil.*[156]

Almost any "bar"? *Added sugar.*

(Protein bars are candy bars with added protein.)

Granola? *Added sugar* (and *oil*, in Nature Valley's case[157]).

Most yogurt? *Added sugar.*

Any non-whole-grain pasta? *White flour.*

Most pasta sauce? *Added sugar.*

Most nuts? *Vegetable oil.*

Any salad dressing? *Vegetable oil.*

In other words, if you think you're *not* eating the Fat Four on a regular basis, you probably need to think again. Unless you make a specific effort not to eat the Fat Four, you almost inevitably will—because they're *everywhere*.

The Fat Four have slithered onto most of the shelves in your health-food store, almost every shelf of your supermarket, and every single shelf of your convenience mart.

*Ubiquitous* almost doesn't do them justice. Any food with a long ingredients list will almost always have one of the Fat Four. In fact, the Fat Four are such a fixture on ingredients lists that the easiest way to avoid them is simply to avoid foods that *have* ingredients lists.

Let's see what makes the Fat Four so bad.

## Barren Wastelands

The Fat Four are highly processed, and devoid of nutrients. Added sugar and refined vegetable oil are barren nutritional wastelands with nutrient tables so full of zeros that it makes you wonder if you're reading the vitamin and mineral content of a food or a piece of cardboard.[158,159]

White flour is marginally better, but it's still nutritionally bankrupt compared to whole-wheat flour.[160]

Every time you eat one of these ingredients, you're depriving your body of nutrients that it was evolved to have.

We're not evolved to eat nutritionally crippled foods.

## No One Is Adapted

While 10,000-odd years *was* enough time for many populations to adapt to grains and dairy, the Fat Four have only been widely eaten for about 200 years.

This wasn't *nearly* enough time for people to adapt.

There is no evolutionary precedent for these foods.

Added sugar has only been available to most people since the early 1800s.[161] White flour wasn't widely available until about 1880, when roller mills were introduced.[162] Refined vegetable oil wasn't eaten on a large scale until the early 20th century.[163]

(Canola oil was invented—yes, *invented*—in the 1970s.[164]) We are completely unadapted to these foods.

But these foods are the *majority* of what we currently eat.[165] See the problem?

## The Art of Processed Food

Not only are we not adapted to the Fat Four *themselves*, but we're also completely unadapted to the way they're processed into food. Added sugar, added oil, and white flour are the primary colors of the processed-food palette from which food corporations paint their tantalizing products.

These three ingredients are added to foods scientifically, in precise amounts derived from trial and error, food-testing panels, and countless prototypes to produce optimal "bliss points" that keeps us coming back again and again.[166]

And again.

For example, before Dr. Pepper unleashed their "Cherry Vanilla" flavor in 2004, they had tested 61 prototypes and conducted 3,904 taste tests. They carefully documented these taste tests and fed the data through advanced statistical software that helped them calibrate the *exact* amounts of sugar and flavorings to add.[167]

After all that, the new flavor wasn't even terribly successful. (That's how stiff the competition is.)

We're not adapted to this sort of food engineering. Like addictive drugs, processed foods are designed to hit our pleasure centers in unnatural ways.

And they are less filling per calorie.[168]

This makes them *fattening*.

## Easy to Break Down

It takes energy—*calories*—to digest food. The amount of calories it takes ranges from 0% to 30% of the total calories in the food itself, depending on the food's allotment of fat, carbs, and protein (protein takes the most calories to digest).[169]

Added sugar, white flour, and vegetable oil are so heavily refined that they're relatively easy for our bodies to digest.

This isn't good. It means we burn significantly fewer calories digesting them. A 2010 study found that people burned 47% fewer calories (73 calories vs. 137 calories) digesting a meal of processed food versus a meal of whole food.[170] (The meals were matched for calories, and close in macros.)

Those differences add up.

## Processed Meat

Unlike the other members of the Fat Four, processed meat isn't usually an *ingredient*, but a *type* of food—like chicken nuggets, bologna, salami, bacon, General Tso's chicken, etc.

Processed meat is bad because it has astronomical amounts of salt. And it's bad because it's often significantly lower in protein than unprocessed meat, which makes it less filling[171] (and more fattening). And it's bad because it's often doused in white flour and sugar and fried in oil to make something like General Tso's chicken or chicken tenders with barbecue sauce.

Processed meat is bad because it has nitrite, which can produce nitrosamines in the stomach, which might cause cancer.[172,173,174]

Processed meat is bad because it's consistently associated with terrible health outcomes.[175,176,177,178,179]

## *Most* of the Time

Cutting the Fat Four from your regular diet is probably the best nutritional decision you can ever make—for your weight, health, and life. It's *far* more powerful than simply eating more of some "superfood" plant.

Focus on cutting the Fat Four from your *regular* diet. This means the diet you eat *most* of the time—most days of the week. You don't have to be some kind of puritan to do this.

You can still eat anything you want, sometimes.

In practice, "sometimes" means once or even twice a week.

Our metabolisms seem to be regulated by what we eat *most* of the time. You just have to make sure your *regular, most-days* diet is good. (That it doesn't contain the Fat Four.)

Eating whole foods on work days and letting loose a bit on the weekend can be a helpful guide.

If your regular diet doesn't contain the Fat Four, you might be surprised with what you can get away with.

## Take-Home

A good diet is more defined by what you *don't* eat than what you *do* eat. Eliminating the Fat Four from your regular diet is the foundation of a healthy diet and a healthier body weight.

The Fat Four have transformed our diets, created a new constellation of diseases, and made hundreds of millions of people fat.

No one is adapted to eating the Fat Four in large amounts.

Get them in your head, and out of your regular diet.

## 1. added sugar
## 2. added oil
## 3. white flour
## 4. processed meat

The Fat Four don't usually go by these names, or show up in red on ingredients lists. Instead, they're deceitful, full of serpent wiles, often hiding in places we don't expect—like healthy-looking food.

Let's get into the gory details of the Fat Four.

# 11

# SWEET NOTHING

## The History of Sugar

Sugarcane looks like bamboo. It was domesticated around the dawn of agriculture in New Guinea.[180] For the first few thousand years, people just squeezed the juice from the stem.

Modern granulated sugar wasn't invented until 400 AD.[181] It was an instant classic.

But until the 19th century, granulated sugar was strictly a luxury item. For most people, table sugar might as well have been a Lamborghini. It was so expensive that they used to call it "white gold." In the 16th century, relative to today's prices, sugar cost as much as caviar. As late as the early 19th century, people who could afford sugar stored it in boxes with locks.[182]

The huge demand for sugar led to the hellish Triangular Slave Trade, in which slaves bought in West Africa were shipped to sugar plantations in the Caribbean where they were literally worked to death producing sugar that was shipped back to Europe, with the handsome profits used to buy more slaves to ship across the Atlantic.

It wasn't until the early 19th century that industrial processing made granulated sugar widely available to the masses.[183] But even then, sugar was only a shadow of what it would become. Here's how US sugar consumption changed since the early 19th century:

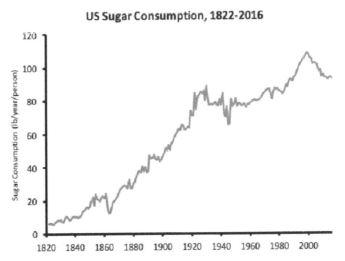

**US Sugar Consumption, 1822-2016**

*This looks like Apple's stock price after Steve Jobs returned.*
Source: Stephan Guyenet, Whole Health Source.[184]

In 1822, the average American ate six pounds of sugar per year. That number doubled by 1850, and doubled again by 1900. Save for a brief hiccup during the Great Depression and World War 2, the American sweet tooth grew ever sweeter. By 2005, the average American was eating 100 pounds of sugar per year.

Instead of storing it in lock-boxes, sugar is so cheap today that fast-food chains offer free refills on giant sugary drinks (and turn a blind eye to thieves).

Unfortunately, we're completely unadapted to this

sort of sugar. It's sugar isolated from all natural context, concentrated into an alien form that wasn't part of our evolutionary environment (in either the Paleolithic or Agricultural Eras).

## Sugar, Obesity, and Heart Disease

How has all this sugar affected our health? According to a 2007 paper in *The American Journal of Clinical Nutrition*:

> *The first documentation of hypertension, diabetes, and obesity occurred in the very countries (England, France, and Germany) where sugar first became available to the public.*[185]

In the US, obesity rates rose in lockstep with our intake of added sugar.[186] It took longer for added sugar to invade developing countries, but once it did, their rates of obesity and heart disease quickly caught up with ours.[187]

A 2013 meta-analysis concluded that intake of added sugar and sugary drinks was a "determinant of body weight."[188] In other words, consuming more added sugar generally makes people weigh more, and consuming less added sugar generally makes people weigh less.

It's pretty cut and dried.

A 2014 study looked at added sugar intake and rates of heart disease in 11,733 Americans. It found a dose-response relationship—the more added sugar someone ate, the greater their risk of heart disease. Compared with someone who ate little added sugar, a person with a diet of at least 25% added sugar had a **275% increased risk of heart disease**.[189]

Added sugar has also been tied to Crohn's disease,[190] colon cancer,[191] and breast cancer.[192]

## Natural Sugar

With all the extravagant problems caused by added sugar, many people have begun to condemn *all* sugar—even natural sugar in whole foods like fruit.

But sweet foods are not inherently bad. Anthropological data, nutrition studies, and evolutionary reasoning assure us that it's not necessarily the *quantity* of sugar that makes people fat and sick. Instead, it's the *quality*.

Fruit, for instance, has lots of sugar. Our early primate ancestors were probably eating fruit as long as sixty million years ago.[193] Our lineage has likely been eating fruit ever since. In fact, we don't have a longer working relationship with any other food. (Fruit, by the way, is the only food that *wants* to be eaten; its evolutionary strategy is for animals to eat it and spread its seeds.)

So we're definitely adapted to eating sugar. And despite some of the outrageous claims you may see online, eating more fruit is generally associated with weight loss.[194]

The sugar in fruit isn't added sugar. Instead, it comes ensconced in *fiber*. Throughout our evolution, sugar and fiber usually went hand in hand. Fiber is filling (*satiating*).[195,196]

Fiber has lots of bulk, but few calories.

It's very good to eat foods with lots of bulk but few calories. (Like fruit.)

It's very bad to eat foods with little bulk but lots of calories. (Like added sugar.)

Honey is an exception to this rule—a natural food that's high in sugar, low in fiber, and dense in calories. And honey probably wasn't an evolutionary trifle; extant hunter-gatherer tribes in warm climates eat honey whenever they can.

(So do chimps, bonobos, orangutans, and gorillas.[197])

The Hadza, for example, are a tribe of hunter-gatherers in Tanzania (Africa) whose diet is fifteen percent honey.[198]

That's a lot, fifteen percent. It's the same percentage that added sugar takes up in the typical American diet.[199] Honey may seem like an important exception to our added-sugar rule. (In fact, it kept me up at night.)

But at the end of the day, the Hadza's honey is not "added sugar," either. Humans have a long evolutionary relationship with honey. Honey comes from nectar and bees, not metal factories. Honey is composed of at least 181 natural substances, and may have some positive effects on triglycerides, cholesterol, and weight control.[200]

The Hadza don't use software to analyze data from taste tests to figure out the precise amount of honey to add to their foods to maximize "bliss points" and "crave-ability."

In fact, the Hadza don't add honey to their food at all. They mostly eat it plain.[201] This is a *far* cry from the way added sugar has been systematically and surgically injected into our food supply.

It's funny, though. Despite all the honey the Hadza eat, honey isn't even their main source of sugar. The rest of their calories come from berries (20%), a tropical fruit called baobab (14%), tubers (19%), and meat (32%).[202]

This makes the Hadza diet **almost 50% sugar**.

The Hadza eat *triple* the amount of sugar we do.

Are they fat, like us?

The average Hadza BMI is just over 20.[203] (Very low.)

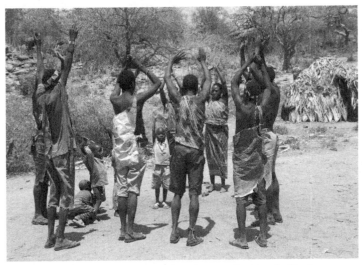

*The fattening effects of a high-sugar diet in the Hadza.*
Photo Credit: franco lucato/Shutterstock.com

But wait. Do the Hadza burn off all these sugar calories with their hyperactive hunter-gatherer lifestyles? Is *that* their secret?

Scientists recently compared the Hadza's daily calorie expenditures with those of typical Westerners. They found that:

> *Contrary to expectations, measures of TEE* [total energy expenditure] *among Hadza adults were similar to those in Western (U.S. and Europe) populations.*[204]

In other words, adjusted for weight, a Hadza person doesn't burn more calories than the average Western couch potato.

How is that possible? Well, while the Hadza are much more active than we are, it turns out that we Western couch potatoes burn so many more calories *at rest*—again, adjusted for weight—that it all evens out. The Hadza burn more calories through physical activity, but we burn more calories at rest.

(Your body is always burning calories, even when you're not moving. Depending on body size, almost anyone would burn between 1000 and 3000 calories lying still in bed all day.[205])

According to the scientists, the similarity in total calorie burning between Westerners and the Hadza:

> *challenge the view that Western lifestyles result in abnormally low energy expenditure, and that decreased energy expenditure is a primary cause of obesity.*[206]

The Hadza undermine the notion that the obesity epidemic is a result of people not burning enough calories. This casts doubt on the idea that people get fat because they don't exercise enough.

Further undermining that idea is the inconvenient fact that, while obesity levels have skyrocketed in recent decades, we've actually been exercising *more*.[207]

(So there's that.)

Long-term weight loss is mostly about changing your regular diet.

## In Defense of High-Fructose Corn Syrup

It's time that someone took a stand for high-fructose corn syrup. It has an abysmal reputation, which isn't fair—to the average person. Vilifying high-fructose corn syrup as a uniquely evil slime is a huge distraction from added sugar in general.

First, the name. "High-fructose" is a misnomer. Most high-fructose corn syrup is 55% fructose and 41% glucose (and 4% other sugars).

Sucrose—also known as *sugar, cane sugar, table sugar, beet sugar, evaporated cane juice, organic evaporated cane juice,* etc.—is 50% fructose and 50% glucose.[208]

So the difference in fructose between normal sugar and "high"-fructose corn syrup is only 5%. A more accurate name would be "marginally-higher-fructose corn syrup." The "high" makes it sound like some appalling fructose bomb. But it really isn't. Especially when you consider that the sugar in apple juice is 66% fructose.[209]

Or that the sugar in agave is around *90%* fructose.[210] *That's* high-fructose. (For reference, the sugar in orange juice is 51% fructose.[211])

There's nothing especially "high" about high-fructose corn syrup. But enough semantics. More importantly, study after study has found no significant difference between high-fructose corn syrup and sucrose ("sugar") in terms of short-term metabolic effects,[212] satiety,[213] or association with obesity.[214]

They're equally bad.

But even if you accept all this, you may note a lingering stink around high-fructose corn syrup, perhaps wafting from a subconscious belief that what we call "sugar" is somehow "more natural" than high-fructose corn syrup.

Let's see how "sugar" is made.

## How "Sugar" Is Made

In the beginning, there is sugarcane. The cane is harvested, diced up, and trucked to a mill.

At the mill, the cane is dumped into a belt-conveyor that leads to a "crusher," a whirlwind of mechanical hammers that pulverize the cane into tiny pieces.

Then another belt conveyor sends the pulverized cane to a "milling tandem" to extract the juice. (A *milling tandem* is a series of giant rotating cylinders that compress the pulverized cane, squeezing out the juice.)

This cane juice is dumped down a 33-foot tower pumped full of sulphur-dioxide vapors, which bleach the juice as it falls down. (Just your standard sulphur-dioxide tower.)

Next, the bleached cane juice is mixed with a bunch of calcium hydroxide in an "agitator tank" for six hours, which is just what it sounds like. This mixing process is known as "alkalization," and the juice's color changes from brown to yellow.

Then the bleached, alkalized cane juice is dumped into a "clarifier tank" for two hours, which separates the juice from a sediment that collects at the bottom of the tank.

This bleached, alkalized, clarified cane juice is sent through a series of giant cylindrical "evaporators" for boiling, which raise the juice's sugar concentration from fifteen percent to sixty percent.

Then the juice is poured into 15-ton tanks for further "clarification." At this stage, there's another sediment that floats to the *top* of the tank, where it's skimmed off by rotating paddles.

The bleached, alkalized, double-clarified, evaporated cane juice is then mixed with a solution of microscopic sucrose crystals suspended in alcohol, which binds to the sugar and "helps draw it out," according to the video.

Then the bleached, alkalized, double-clarified, evaporated, alcohol-drawn cane juice is placed in large vacuum pans to boil, *further* concentrating the sugar.

Then it's fed to a high-speed centrifuge machine that spins at 1200 revolutions per minute, which draws the "molasses" to the outer rim, leaving the cane-juice crystals in the inner basket.

Finally, these crystals are washed (in washing machines) and blow-dried, drying them to the industry-standard humidity of 0.02%.

And there you have it.

Bleached, alkalized, double-clarified, evaporated, alcohol-drawn, boiled, centrifuged, washed, blow-dried cane juice crystals.

Also known as *table sugar*.

Just like grandma used to make.

(Source: [215])

For the record, "brown sugar" is made by taking these white sugar crystals and coating them with brown syrup.[216]

## Added Sugar by Any Other Name

On ingredients lists, food companies like to use creative synonyms for added sugar. One of their favorites is "evaporated cane juice." According to Judy Sanchez, a spokesperson for US Sugar Corp., "All sugar is evaporated cane juice. They just use that for a natural-sounding name."[217]

The FDA discourages food companies from using the phrase "evaporated cane juice."[218] Mostly because it's grossly misleading. It's not even juice.

Food companies also like to replace plain old added sugar with healthy-sounding alternatives—like honey, agave nectar, or "organic brown rice syrup." While these added sugars may seem like healthier options, *any* added sugar is a problem.

Sugar is never added to a food to make it healthier. The only reason that sugar is added to a food (whatever the sugar, whatever the food) is to make it *taste* better—so it will *sell* more.

That's the only motivation.

The science-word for "tastiness" is *palatability*.

Palatability is inversely related to satiety—the more tasty a food is, on average, the *less* filling it is.[219] This is why added sugar is fattening: foods with added sugar drip with palatability (tastiness), so they're less filling. Which means we eat more of them.

Which means we get fat.

Controlled feeding trials have shown that when people have access to palatable processed food, they eat far more calories than they need to maintain their weight—and they gain weight.[220,221,222]

*Any* added sugar will hit your sweet receptors and make a food more palatable and more fattening, even if it's a "healthy" added sugar. Try to think of "organic brown rice syrup" as a synonym for "fattening added sugar."

And eating a spoonful of honey is not the same thing as eating a processed food with honey as a listed ingredient.

Don't let "health-food" companies fool you.

With that in mind, here are some synonyms for *added sugar* you'll see on ingredients lists:

> *sugar, raw sugar, cane sugar, coconut sugar, brown sugar, palm sugar, invert sugar, confectioner's sugar, dextrose, maltose, high-fructose corn syrup* (and almost anything that ends in "ose"), *corn syrup, maple syrup, rice syrup, brown rice syrup, cane syrup, dried cane syrup, malt syrup, cane crystals* (and almost anything with "syrup" or "cane"), *evaporated cane juice, fruit juice concentrate* (anything with "juice"), *barley malt extract, honey, molasses, blackstrap molasses, molasses powder, agave nectar, date paste, dates*

(And, of course, any of the above terms preceded by "*organic.*")

What's in a name? Added sugar by any other name will taste as sweet, and make you just as fat. But rather than memorizing a big list of synonyms to help you navigate ingredients lists, it's easier just to avoid foods that *have* ingredients lists (processed foods).

## The Scope of Sugar

Adding sugar is the easiest way to make food taste better. To be sure, adding fat or salt (or both) is also highly effective. But there's something different about adding sugar. Ordinary people don't snack on salt cubes or butter balls or glasses of vegetable oil. They will, however, consume *pure* sugar: sugary drinks, certain candies, certain desserts, etc.

So sugar, *by itself*, can independently drive calorie intake. That's a profound difference.

And when you consider that sugar doesn't spoil, is very cheap, and goes with almost any food, and when you consider that the main goal of food corporations is to sell food, and that tasty food sells better, and that adding sugar is an insanely effective way to make food taste better, you start to realize that adding sugar to almost every processed food is an economic inevitability.

Every candy? *Added sugar.*

Every dessert? *Added sugar.*

Every "bar"? *Added sugar.* (Okay, 99.9% of bars.)

Every cereal? *Added sugar.* (Okay, 99.9% of cereals.)

Every baked good? *Added sugar.*

Added sugar is in countless snack foods, most yogurts, and many places you might not expect—like "whole wheat" bread, most dressings, and most sauces.

Added sugar is so ubiquitous in the US food supply that when the American Heart Association urged Americans to drastically cut their intake of added sugar in 2009, representatives from every sector of the processed-food industry went to an AHA summit in Washington the following spring to protest.

They argued that added sugar was so integral to their manufacturing processes that, if they were to significantly reduce it, it would jeopardize the US food supply.[223]

But it didn't matter. Consumers paid little attention to the AHA, and the food industry did little to cut back.

## Sugar Nutrition

White rice is infamous for being low in nutrients—a cardboard carbohydrate. Let's use white rice as a benchmark.

Here are the stats for 28 grams (102 calories) of uncooked, un-enriched white rice:

### WHITE RICE, 28G

| vitamin | RDA% | mineral | RDA% |
|---------|------|---------|------|
| vitamin A | 0% | calcium | 1% |
| vitamin C | 0% | iron | 1% |
| vitamin D | 0% | magnesium | 2% |
| vitamin E | 0% | phosphorus | 3% |
| vitamin K | 0% | potassium | 1% |
| thiamin | 1% | sodium | 0% |
| riboflavin | 1% | zinc | 2% |
| niacin | 2% | copper | 3% |
| vitamin B6 | 2% | manganese | 15% |
| folate | 1% | selenium | 6% |
| vitamin B12 | 0% | | |
| vitamin B5 | 3% | | |
| choline | 1.6mg | | |

Source: [224]

White rice won't win any health awards. But imagine you're lost at sea and forced to live on white rice. Let's say you're eating twenty servings—about 2000 calories—of white rice per day. In this scenario, you'd actually end up getting a decent amount of most minerals and B vitamins.

Now imagine you're forced to live on sugar.

Here are the numbers for 28 grams of sucrose (104 calories):

## SUCROSE, 28G

| vitamin | RDA% | mineral | RDA% |
|---|---|---|---|
| vitamin A | 0% | calcium | 0% |
| vitamin C | 0% | iron | 0% |
| vitamin D | 0% | magnesium | 0% |
| vitamin E | 0% | phosphorus | 0% |
| vitamin K | 0% | potassium | 0% |
| thiamin | 0% | sodium | 0% |
| riboflavin | 0% | zinc | 0% |
| niacin | 0% | copper | 0% |
| vitamin B6 | 0% | manganese | 0% |
| folate | 0% | selenium | 0% |
| vitamin B12 | 0% | | |
| vitamin B5 | 0% | | |
| choline | 0mg | | |

*It's a ghost town.*

Source: [225]

This "food" makes up 15% of the American diet. No calorie is emptier. Compared to sucrose, white rice might as well be kale. You could eat 2000 calories of sucrose per day for a month without catching a glimpse of a nutrient.

Now, let's see how we likely experienced sugar during most of our evolutionary past.

Here are the stats for one small banana (90 calories):

## BANANA, SMALL

| vitamin | RDA% | mineral | RDA% |
|---|---|---|---|
| vitamin A | 1% | calcium | 1% |
| vitamin C | 15% | iron | 1% |
| vitamin D | 0% | magnesium | 7% |
| vitamin E | 1% | phosphorus | 2% |
| vitamin K | 1% | potassium | 10% |
| thiamin | 2% | sodium | 0% |
| riboflavin | 4% | zinc | 1% |
| niacin | 3% | copper | 4% |
| vitamin B6 | 19% | manganese | 14% |
| folate | 5% | selenium | 1% |
| vitamin B12 | 0% | | |
| vitamin B5 | 3% | | |
| choline | 9.9mg | | |

Source: [226]

A banana crushes white rice, nutrient-wise.
But compared to sucrose:

> "*Here grows the cure of all, this fruit divine.*"
> -John Milton, *Paradise Lost*

Sugar in whole food isn't the same as sugar in processed food.

## Processed Fructose Problems

I'm sure you've heard about the evils of fructose. While fructose in a natural context—fruit, honey, etc.—is nothing to worry about due to the colossally ancient evolutionary relationships involved, there's reason to think the large amounts of fructose in processed foods and sugary drinks (evolutionary novelties) could be a problem.

As we've seen, added sugar is usually around half fructose and half glucose. (The "starchy carbs"—bread, pasta, potatoes, rice, etc.—are mostly glucose, with negligible fructose.)

You may have heard that any cell can metabolize glucose, but only your liver can metabolize fructose. This is mostly true.[227] But contrary to popular belief, this *doesn't* mean all fructose is converted into fat. Human isotope tracer studies tell us that over 92% of the fructose we eat is converted into glucose, lactate, or glycogen, or is oxidized directly.[228]

Only a small fraction is converted into fat.

The *real* issue with fructose is that, unlike glucose, fructose doesn't cause much insulin secretion.[229,230] *Insulin* is secreted by the pancreas when blood sugar (glucose) is elevated. Insulin helps move blood sugar into cells, where it's used for fuel.

(Contrary to popular belief, carbs aren't unique in causing insulin secretion. Protein does, too. Calorie for calorie, fish and beef both cause greater insulin spikes than white or brown pasta.[231])

In any case, you *want* insulin secretion when you eat carbs, because contrary to another popular belief, insulin promotes satiety,[232,233,234,235,236,237] making you feel full. The reason insulin is filling is because it causes *leptin* to be secreted.[238,239,240,241]

Leptin is the hormone that makes you feel full.

$$\text{glucose} \;\rightarrow\; \text{insulin} \;\rightarrow\; \text{leptin} \;\rightarrow\; \textbf{\textit{full}}$$
$$\text{fructose} \;\neq\; \text{insulin}$$

## Leptin

Leptin is secreted by fat cells, and acts on receptors in the hypothalamus.[242] Leptin is the master satiety hormone—it's the hormone that makes you feel full. Feeling "full" is feeling leptin.

Leptin reduces fat mass by encouraging energy expenditure, limiting food intake, and ramping up fat burning ("fatty-acid oxidation"). Less leptin causes overeating and weight gain. All known types of monogenic (*one-gene*) obesity syndromes are caused by mutations in leptin genes.[243]

To recap, insulin causes leptin secretion. And since fructose doesn't cause insulin secretion, fructose ultimately causes less leptin secretion than glucose. This is why a 2013 study found that people felt fuller after drinking a glucose drink than a fructose drink, even though both drinks had equal calories.[244]

You want your food to release leptin. Eating food that releases too little leptin—*processed food*—makes people fat. Fructose doesn't release leptin.

In fructose-containing whole foods, this isn't really a problem: these whole foods have fiber and other healthy compounds that balance things out, satiety-wise.

But in processed foods, all bets are off. In controlled human trials, unnatural forms of fructose—like the kind in sugary drinks and processed foods—have been shown to raise triglycerides,[245] raise blood sugar,[246] raise blood pressure,[247] cause weight gain,[248] increase abdominal fat,[249] and increase both LDL ("bad") cholesterol and total cholesterol.[250] Unnatural forms of fructose have also been associated with non-alcoholic fatty liver disease[251] (literally a fattening of the liver, the body's central metabolic organ).

But again, these studies were based on *unnatural* fructose, stripped of fiber and natural context. Higher intakes of fruit—which is also high in fructose—have been associated with a *lower* risk of metabolic disorders like obesity, high blood sugar, high blood pressure, high triglycerides, and high LDL cholesterol.[252]

And even though honey is 51% fructose and very low in fiber,[253] honey seems to release more satiety hormones than sucrose,[254] and has various health benefits.[255] Our guts have a long history with the 181 substances in honey.

We don't know exactly *why* honey might be better than sucrose, but it probably has to do with a food being more than the sum of its parts.

Sugar in whole food isn't the same as sugar in processed food.

## Dessert: The Sugar on Top

What is dessert, really? When you strip it down to bare essentials, *dessert* is basically just using added sugar to stuff more calories into a full stomach.

(A great feeling, admittedly.)

Before we eat dessert, leptin is telling our brain that we're full—that we have enough food, that we don't need any more.

Then we purposely allow the unnatural allure of added sugar (ice cream, cake, pie, etc.) to overwhelm our innate satiety system and trick us into eating more calories than we need.

It's hard to imagine a more fattening habit.

And the essence of dessert is added sugar. Can you think of a single popular dessert that doesn't have sugar?

I can't.

True, most desserts also have fat. But not all. For example, jello, angel food cake, and many candies are fat-free. On the other hand, added sugar is part of *every single* traditional American dessert, with no exceptions.

Sugar, not fat, is king of dessert.

## Addicted to Sugar

There's a robust literature showing that sugar is addictive to rats. Sugar-fed rats have shown all the classic signs of drug dependency: bingeing, withdrawal, craving, and cross-sensitization to other drugs. When rats are intermittently fed lots of sugar, it can cause the same type of brain changes as drugs like cocaine.[256]

Both food and drugs have powerful reinforcing effects which are partly caused by dopamine spikes in the brain. And just like drug addicts, alcoholics, and problem gamblers, obese people tend to have fewer dopamine receptors than normal-weight people. Specifically, all these groups have fewer D2 dopamine receptors in a brain region called the striatum.[257]

With fewer dopamine receptors, to get the same pleasure as a normal person, these people need *more*—more drugs, more alcohol, more gambling, more sugar, etc.

And dopamine receptors *themselves* seem to be affected by hyper-rewarding stimuli. For example, in one experiment, rats were given intermittent access to sugar for a month. The rats gradually *doubled* their sugar intake. At the same time, the binding capacity of their D2 receptors significantly decreased[258]—they needed more sugar to get the same high.

When humans regularly eat lots of sugary junk food, it probably causes a similar reduction in D2 receptor binding. We gradually need more and more sugary junk food to get the same high.

There's also evidence that internal opioids mediate both the amount of food we consume and our food preferences, particularly for foods high in sugar.[259] One look at the news tells us the dangers of anything related to opioids.

In short, sugar is ensconced in the same addictive reward pathways as cocaine and opiates.

Isn't "sweet tooth" just a euphemism for "sugar addiction"?

## Take-Home

For both health and long-term weight loss, eliminating added sugar from your regular diet is supremely important.

# 12

# THE MOST EFFECTIVE WEIGHT-LOSS HABIT

"Awake, arise, or be forever fallen."
-John Milton, *Paradise Lost*

Get ready.

Real weight loss—the kind that *lasts*—means making changes. Making changes takes willpower.

And willpower is limited. So it's critical to spend it wisely.

Most people blow their willpower on diets and exercise programs. Don't blame yourself if diets and exercise programs haven't worked out. Diets and exercise programs *never* work out. Not long-term, anyway.

No matter how great the diet or program, it's *always* destined to fail in the long term—because it's *short*-term. Short of surgery, nothing you do in the short term will achieve *long*-term weight loss. (And even surgery can fail.)

Your habits led you here. And unless you change them,

your habits will keep pulling you back. They're all-powerful like that.

Instead of going on a diet, it's far more effective to spend your willpower changing your habits.

But *which* habits?

Since life is short, it makes the most sense to start with the most effective weight-loss habit you can possibly develop.

So which habit—if you're not already doing it, of course—will melt fat the quickest, keep it off the longest, and do the most to change your life?

For the average person, what's the most effective weight-loss habit in the world?

## Habit 1: Cut out all sugary drinks.

This is the lowest-hanging fruit. The 800-pound gorilla. If you regularly drink any form of sugary drink, then quitting that habit is the most effective thing you can possibly do to lose a lot of weight and keep it off.

Bar none.

As long as you regularly drink things that taste sweet and don't have zero calories, there's no need to talk about anything else. There's no need to talk food. There's no need to talk exercise or other strategies. No need to discuss attitudes.

Those would be a waste of time.

Why? As we've seen, it's fiendishly hard to isolate the health effects of a particular food. Despite these inherent difficulties, sugary drinks—including juice and sports drinks—have been consistently, convincingly, and independently implicated in human weight gain.[260,261,262,263,264,265,266,267,268,269,270,271,272,273,274,275,
276,277,278,279,280,281,282,283,284,285,286,287,288,289,290,291,292,293,294,295,296,297,298,299]

Men and women. Young and old. Black and white. They're all fatter, on average, when they drink sugar. They're all skinnier, on average, when they drink less sugar.

Nutrition experts agree on surprisingly little. But there's a wide consensus among credible nutrition authorities that sugary drinks are bad.

Very, *very* bad.

The mechanism, of course, involves satiety. As we've seen, at least in unnatural contexts, fructose is less filling than glucose. And basically every sugary drink (juice, soda, sweet tea, etc.) has lots of fructose—and no fiber.

But it gets worse. There's evidence that liquid calories simply aren't as filling as calories from solid food (even junk food).[300] Controlled trials indicate that people feel more full if they *eat* a given number of calories than if they *drink* them, and that drinking calories causes significantly less dietary compensation.[301]

In other words, sugary drinks have calories, but they're extremely *un*-filling.

## Uniquely Fattening

Sugary drinks are even more fattening than junk food. At least with junk food, you're ingesting calories when you feel like eating something. But not only are sugary drinks full of calories and less filling than junk food, but people often drink sugary drinks *when they don't even feel like eating.*

Hunger and thirst are two completely different things. You can be thirsty but not hungry. And you can be hungry but not thirsty. We're evolved to sate our hunger with calories, and quench our thirst with zero-calorie water.

But sugary drinks throw a wrench in this ancient metabolic formula. People drink sugar to quench their thirst with lots of calories that don't fill them up—when they're not even hungry.

Could there be a more obvious cause of obesity?

During the 1980s and '90s, the percentage of obese Americans roughly doubled.[302] What changed? Among other things, between 1977 and 2001, US calorie intake from sugar-sweetened beverages increased by 135%.[303]

## Sugary Drinks and Evolution

We've seen that evolution is the foundation of nutrition. And the fact is that humans are not adapted to sugary drinks. It's extremely likely that sugary drinks (including fresh-squeezed juice) formed *no* significant part of our evolutionary past.

True, *some* populations are adapted to drink milk. Milk has lactose, and lactose is a sugar.

But milk is not a "sugary drink." For one, milk doesn't have any fructose.[304] And unlike sugary drinks, milk has significant protein, the most filling macronutrient.[305] Milk also has natural minerals, and isn't *nearly* as high in sugar as juice, soda, or other sugary drinks. No, unless it's chocolate or strawberry milk, milk is not a sugary drink.

## Juice: Highly Unnatural

Juice is a wolf in sheep's clothing. It may seem "natural" because you can squeeze it from a fruit, but it's extremely unlikely that drinking juice formed any part of the evolutionary environment that shaped our genes. This is why juice helps shape our jeans to XXL+ today.

Chimpanzees, gorillas, and orangutans are our close Hominid relatives. These species eat lots of fruit—*far* more than the average human. If any species were adapted to drink juice, it would be them. But there's no evidence of any of these species drinking juice the way that modern humans do.

Similarly, the diets of hundreds of modern-era hunter-gatherer tribes have been studied in detail. While there are many qualifiers, it's thought that these modern tribes provide some approximation of our ancient diet.[306]

I've studied many of these diets in excruciating detail. Different tribes eat wildly different diets. Many eat large amounts of fruit. But I'm not aware of a *single case* of hunter-gatherers drinking juice as a significant portion of their natural diet. *Or of drinking juice at all.*

Seriously. Not one case. The closest thing I found was a tribe of Native Americans in northern Mexico who would occasionally roast and chew wild Agave, suck the molasses-like juice from the leaves, and then spit out the leaves.[307]

This is hardly a tall glass of orange juice with breakfast every morning.

If you think about it, throwing away most of a fruit to make juice only makes sense if you live in a post-industrial, food-saturated society like ours—*with refrigerators.*

Until very recently, humans who didn't live near the equator couldn't even eat *fruit* for much of the year, let alone drink juice. Fresh-squeezed juice spoils very quickly at room temperature (or turns into wine). Before refrigerators, it would have been exceedingly difficult for the average person to drink fruit juice on a regular basis.

The earliest evidence of what we'd call "juice" appeared in 16th-century Italy, with lemonade.[308] Large-scale production of commercial orange juice didn't start until the 1920s.[309]

While it's been theoretically *possible* to drink juice for some time, there's no reason to think juice was *ever* an important calorie source until this past century. And if juice wasn't an important calorie source, there were no selective pressures around it—and no adaptation to it.

So just because juice is a *natural* part of a *natural* food doesn't mean it was ever a *natural* part of our diet. Fruit juice isn't fruit. Nor does being *part* of fruit make juice healthy. (Cocaine is a natural part of an edible plant, too.[310])

Eating fruit has been associated with a reduced risk of obesity and diabetes.[311,312]

Drinking juice has been associated with weight gain,[313] obesity,[314] and diabetes.[315]

According to a 2006 study on juice consumption in children:

> *Increased fruit juice intake was associated with excess adiposity* [fat] *gain, whereas parental offerings of whole fruits were associated with reduced adiposity gain.*[316]

Fruit was slimming, juice was fattening.

We're adapted to fruit, not fruit juice.

In one important way, juice is even worse than soda. People know soda is bad. There's no confusion here. But there persists a stubborn, toxic belief that juice—or at least *some* juice—is "healthy."

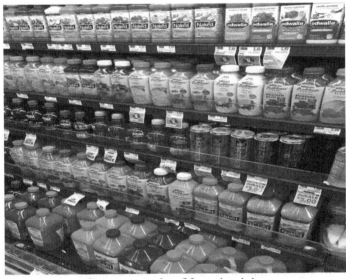

*Prime examples of fattening juice.*
Photo Credit: Jeramey Lende/Shutterstock.com

Don't be fooled by expertly crafted food packaging. If a food needs packaging to make it look healthy, it's probably not healthy. (Is broccoli *advertised* as being healthy?)

Take "not from concentrate" orange juice, which can sit in million-gallon aseptic storage tanks for an entire year before being pumped with flavor packs and shipped to your supermarket.[317] *Simply orange.*

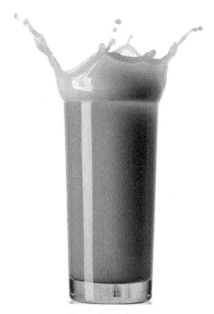

*Pure liquid sugar.*
Photo Credit: Alex Staroseltsev/Shutterstock.com

What about vitamin C? Juice usually has lots of it. Sometimes it even has the natural kind of vitamin C (not added ascorbic acid, like many drinks have). But given the omnipresence of vitamin C in fruits, vegetables, and vitamin pills, unless you're lost at sea and dying of scurvy with nothing but juice, vitamin C is a pathetic excuse to drink juice.

Juice is an alien to the human metabolism.

Habit 1 means no juice. Of any kind.

Period.

Note: what comes out of a blender is a *smoothie*, not juice—the fiber hasn't been lost. Smoothies made from whole foods are fine, if you're into that. On the other hand, what comes out of a juicer *is* juice—and Habit 1 applies.

What about juice fasts? Don't they work for a lot of people? Perhaps. But so would Coke or Pepsi fasts. Consuming only 500 calories per day of *any* food or drink will cause substantial weight loss. It has nothing to do with juice.

Lastly, the whole "detox" thing is more or less a myth created by people trying to sell things. There isn't a shred of hard scientific evidence (a randomized trial, etc.) supporting any commercial detox diet.[318] The body is great at eliminating toxins on its own. If it weren't, you'd be dead.

## Alcohol

Since we're on the topic of drinks, a word about alcohol. Alcohol is the only recreational drug that is universally accepted in secular society. Sadly, it's also the only drug with significant calories.

When it comes to body weight, alcohol is a mixed bag. It can definitely be fattening, especially if it's done immoderately, mixed with sugar, or leads to bad eating decisions.

A five-year prospective study of drinking habits in 7,608 British men found that heavy alcohol intake "contributes directly to weight gain and obesity, irrespective of the type of alcohol consumed."[319] A similar association between heavy drinking and weight gain was found in a study of 49,324 women a year later.[320]

Alcohol has lots of calories, lowers inhibitions, and lowers leptin levels[321]—a trio that often makes for a dangerous cocktail of drunk eating. "Drunk food" is junk food.

Habit 1 assumes you're not drinking heavily every day.

If you are, you'll probably want to change that first.

But what about *moderate* drinking?

That study of 49,324 women found that "light to moderate drinking (up to 30 g/d) is not associated with weight gain."[322] That's around two drinks a day.

Interesting. It's worth noting that the average American's alcohol intake was declining significantly at exactly the same time our obesity levels were surging the fastest (the '80s and '90s).[323,324] This strongly suggests that alcohol wasn't an important factor in the obesity epidemic.

(Unless it was caused by people drinking less.)

In fact, a 2010 study on the drinking habits of 19,220 American women concluded that:

> *Women who consumed a light to moderate amount of alcohol gained less weight and had a lower risk of becoming overweight and/or obese during 12.9 years of follow-up.*[325]

Another study of 7,230 US adults concluded that "both men and women drinkers tended to gain less weight than did nondrinkers."[326]

It seems that it's the *dose* of alcohol that makes the fattening poison—or the slimming potion.

But unless you regularly drink heavily, there are simply more important things to focus on than alcohol.

## In Defense of Diet Drinks

It's time that someone stood up for diet soda. Look, I haven't been living under a rock. I've read the science. I've read the news articles allegedly based on science. I'm fully aware that diet soda is not "ideal" or "healthy" or "good."

I understand that water would be better.

But people aren't perfect. Sometimes we want to drink something that tastes sweet. Diet drinks are controversial, and there is little scientific consensus about their efficacy for weight loss. It's difficult to disentangle confounding variables and industry funding from many of these studies. So we'll let the National Weight Control Registry decide. The National Weight Control Registry (NWCR) is made up of people who've lost at least 30 pounds and kept them off at least a year. I'm one of over 10,000 members.

We're the small minority of weight losers who managed to lose weight and keep it off. Scientists regularly survey us about what we do.

According to a 2014 survey, few people in the NWCR touch sugary drinks. But 53% of us regularly drink artificially sweetened beverages.[327] (I drink them once or twice a week.) This suggests that artificially sweetened beverages are compatible with losing weight and keeping it off.

And an objective look at the sprawling science on the topic tells us that diet drinks are better than sugary drinks. Several controlled trials—a *far* stronger form of evidence than association studies—have shown that diet drinks lead to less weight gain and more weight loss than sugary drinks.[328,329,330,331]

Some trials have even found artificially sweetened drinks to be better than water for weight loss.[332] According to a 2014 meta-analysis of randomized controlled trials on artificial sweeteners:

> *Data from RCTs* [randomized controlled trials], *which provide the highest quality of evidence... indicate that substituting LCSs* [low-calorie sweeteners] *for calorically dense alternatives results in a modest reduction of body weight, BMI, fat mass, and waist circumference.*[333]

Similarly, a 2015 meta-analysis in *The International Journal of Obesity* found that replacing sugar with artificial sweeteners leads to reduced calorie intake and weight loss.[334]

At the end of the day, sugary drinks have lots of calories, and most artificially sweetened drinks have none. This isn't a minor difference.

Nevertheless, some scientists propose that diet drinks mess with our hormones, trick our brains, and lead to sugar cravings that cause us to overeat later—negating the calorie difference.

This theory remains somewhat speculative. Some studies support it,[335] but many don't.[336] Even if it does happen to an extent, such an indirect mechanism seems preferable to the *directly* fattening mechanism of sugary drinks.

Ultimately, if you have a decent diet, diet drinks probably pose a greater risk to your teeth—with their citric acid—than your waistline.

## Health Concerns of Diet Drinks?

Do artificially sweetened drinks cause health problems? While some observational studies have tied them to metabolic problems like diabetes,[337] according to a 2013 review on the metabolic risks of artificially sweetened beverages (ASB):

> *Higher-quality studies suggest either no effect of ASB or perhaps a protective effect through replacement of calorically dense alternatives.*[338]

A 2016 study found that sugary drinks—but *not* diet soda—were associated with insulin resistance and prediabetes.[339]

Diet wins. What about cancer? Let's talk about aspartame, since people think it's one of the worst sweeteners. Aspartame is the main sweetener in Diet Coke.

According to a review in *Annals of Oncology*:

> *Despite some rather unscientific assumptions, there is no evidence that aspartame is carcinogenic* [cancer-causing]*...according to the current literature, the possible risk of artificial sweeteners to induce cancer seems to be negligible.*[340]

Another review of aspartame in *Critical Reviews of Toxicology* in 2007 concluded that "studies provide no evidence to support an association between aspartame and cancer in any tissue."[341]

The "aspartame causes cancer" meme was based almost entirely on media sensationalism of early mouse studies. Not only is it a mistake to extrapolate from mice to humans, but a 2015 meta-analysis of mouse studies found that aspartame doesn't even cause cancer in mice.[342]

For decades, aspartame has been continually declared safe by regulatory agencies in accordance with strict international standards. Aspartame has repeatedly been approved by the leading toxicologists in the world, as well as the National Cancer Institute[343] and the American Cancer Society, whose website states that:

> *Aside from the effects in people with phenylketonuria, no health problems have been consistently linked to aspartame use.*[344]

There's no conspiracy here.

What about "chemicals"? It's worth noting that everything is a chemical—every part of your body and every part of the Earth. Matter is made of chemicals. Regarding the "chemicals" in diet soda, the only difference between Coke and Diet Coke is that the high-fructose corn syrup in Coke has been swapped with aspartame, acesulfame K (another artificial sweetener), and some citric acid.[345]

High-fructose corn syrup is a chemical, too.

And not a good one.

## Green Light

Given all the above evidence, and given that many people are going to drink sweet-tasting drinks no matter what they're told, it's a gross injustice to lump soda and diet soda together.

*Not great* is better than *very bad*.

While hardly ideal, diet drinks are better than sugary drinks. Period.

If you have to pick, choose diet soda over soda (or juice). Every single time.

Think of artificially sweetened drinks as the sugar version of the nicotine patch. Use them as a tool to help you transition from sugary drinks to water, and to help manage cravings for sugary drinks.

Just try not to make them a daily staple.

Stick to water most days.

## Habit 1: The Killer App

Aside from scientific evidence, there are other reasons Habit 1 is so effective. First, *there is never any social pressure against it.*

There is often social pressure to eat junk food. Think about it. Declining a piece of cake at a birthday or homemade cookies at dinner or pizza at a work party can sometimes be seen as rude. We humans often eat together. We like the taste of the Fat Four, and we like others to share in our dietary debauchery.

While it's always *possible* to say no, it isn't always easy.

It can get old being the self-righteous, finger-wagging prude

who constantly turns up their nose and says, "I don't eat that."
So we often get pressured into eating it.

To this day, I have aunts who try to feed me baked goods
with their hands, as if I were an infant.

They often succeed.

On the other hand, one's choice of beverage (except for
alcohol, sometimes) is utterly personal. Has anyone ever pressured you to drink juice or soda?

Choosing water instead of liquid sugar hardly ever meets
an ounce of resistance. No one cares what you drink.

And unlike healthy food—which isn't always available—you
can *always* drink water. It's always around.

You can be a healthy island in your beverage choices.

Another reason Habit 1 is king is that it's black and white.
There's little room for interpretation. Any beverage with calories—unless it's white milk or alcohol—is forbidden. All you
have to do is look at the drink label. If it has calories and it's
not white milk, don't drink it.

(Coffee and tea have so few calories that you can count
them as zero-calorie drinks. Just don't add sugar.)

It can be hard to tell how processed and fattening a certain
food may be, but drinks are crystal clear. And clear is good.

Clear leads to automatic decisions and automatic habits.

## Life Lessons

I used to drink blue Powerade with lunch and dinner every
day. I got fat. After I lost weight, I more or less returned to
my old eating habits—with one important exception: no more
sugary drinks.

I've maintained this weight loss since 2009.

I still drink blue Powerade sometimes, but only the kind
with zero calories.

Habit 1 isn't about cutting out sugary drinks for a month

or two. It's about cutting them out forever. While you can occasionally eat any junk food you want, unless you don't care about your weight, there's really no reason to ever quench your thirst with added sugar.

It comes down to deciding what's more important to you: significantly less fat on your body, or sugar in your drinks. You probably can't have both.

You can try other approaches to lose weight, but if you're regularly drinking sugar, you're spinning your wheels—like a smoker trying to heal their lungs with something *other* than quitting smoking.

If you're not willing to give up sugary drinks, you might want to stop reading. But if you *are* willing, and you're used to drinking a lot of sugar, Habit 1 will be like going on a permanent diet—without the hunger or effort.

It's the golden ticket to long-term weight loss.

## Take-Home

Habit 1 means nothing to drink except water, white milk, unsweetened tea, unsweetened coffee, any drink with zero calories on the label (diet drinks in moderation), and alcohol (in moderation).

It means no juice of *any* kind.

It means no soda, no caloric energy drinks, no sports drinks, no lemonade, no Snapple, no Capri Sun, no sweet tea, no Gatorade, no Powerade, no Odwalla, no Vitamin Water, no milkshakes, no chocolate milk, no strawberry milk, and no sugar in your coffee—which means no Pumpkin Spice Lattes, Frappuccinos, Caramel Macchiatos, Caffe Mochas, etc.

(These coffee-shop drinks are particularly gruesome. A Starbucks White Chocolate Mocha has more sugar than a Coke,[346,347] and plenty of added fat on top.)

Habit 1 can be hard at first, but nothing is more worth the effort. Before long, water will start to taste good. And whenever you drink eight fluid ounces of water (just two-thirds of a can) instead of juice or soda, you'll save yourself around 100 of the world's most fattening calories.[348,349]

Every.

Single.

Time.

Your drinks won't have sugar, but life will be sweeter.

## The Five Golden Weight-Loss Habits

### Habit 1: Cut out all sugary drinks.

# 13

# HOW FOOD TRANSFORMED

## Diet, Not Exercise

Many people like to implicate a lack of exercise in the obesity epidemic. But in 2008, scientists compiled data on the average energy expenditures of people in North America and Holland between 1982 and 2006.[350] This was a stretch of time when obesity levels were skyrocketing around the world.

They calculated energy expenditure with the *double-labeled water method*, where you feed people isotopes, calculate $CO_2$ production based on how fast the isotopes leave their bodies, and use that number to calculate how many calories they burned.

This technique is slightly more accurate than asking "How much do you exercise?"

The scientists found that, contrary to popular belief, while the world was getting fat, average physical activity levels had not decreased at all.

Instead, they had slightly *increased*.[351]

So much for the "lack of exercise" hypothesis.

While exercise is healthy and conducive to maintaining

weight loss, lack of exercise had little to do with the world getting fat in the first place. It simply wasn't the major factor.

If our physical activity levels didn't change in a fattening direction when the world was getting fat, then what did?

What caused the worldwide obesity epidemic?

Without a doubt, it was our diet. While other factors (increased stress, lack of sleep, inactivity, etc.) likely played a role, nothing changed as drastically as our diet did.

And I'm not talking about our diet since the dawn of agriculture, or since the Industrial Revolution.

I'm talking about our diet since the 1970s.

## The 1970s: When Food Transformed

The Fat Four existed before the 1970s, but it wasn't until this fateful decade that they finally came into their own. Among other things, the '70s gave birth to classics like the Denny's Grand Slam, Orville Redenbacher's, Hamburger Helper, Starbucks, Snapple, the Happy Meal, the Egg McMuffin, Yoplait, Cup Noodles, Mrs. Fields, Country Time Lemonade, Extra Crunchy Jif Peanut Butter, Ruby Tuesday, Famous Amos, Twix, Ben & Jerry's, Reese's Pieces, and the Arby's Beef 'N Cheddar sandwich.[352,353]

But it wasn't just sexy new combinations of the Fat Four. The Fat Four *themselves* evolved. High-fructose corn syrup (added sugar) and canola oil (added oil) were both invented in the 1970s.[354,355]

(You generally want to avoid foods that were invented in the 1970s.)

It goes further. The '70s saw the evolution of the entire eating *climate*. The plastic soda bottle, the Crock-Pot, the first standard nutrition label, the plastic grocery bag, Cuisinart home appliances, and the supermarket checkout scanner were all introduced in the '70s.[356,357,358]

Our food system has only continued evolving since then. In 1978, only 8% of American households had microwave ovens. By 1999, 83% had microwaves.[359] Food that used to take hours to prepare could now be nuked in minutes. An entire new *genre* of food evolved: microwave dinners.

The problem is, *we* haven't evolved since then.

All these changes took an obvious toll. Before the '70s, US obesity rates were only slightly increasing—the slope on the graph was gentle and meandering.

Then, suddenly, towards the end of the 1970s, the slope got steep.

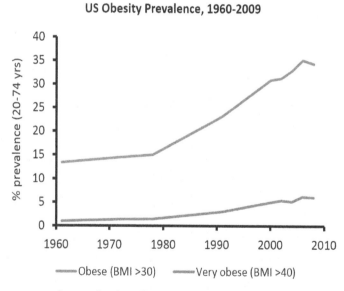

**US Obesity Prevalence, 1960-2009**

Source: Stephan Guyenet, Whole Health Source.[360]

The cause of this obesity uptick is not mysterious. Data indicate that the average American started eating significantly more calories somewhere around the late 1970s.

**Calories in the US food supply, per person per day, 1909-2000**

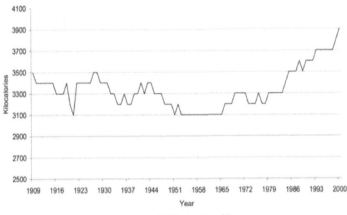

Source: USDA, 2004.[361]

We got fat because we ate more calories.
But *why* did we eat more calories?

## Of Mice and Overweight Men

It was during the 1970s that a graduate student in biopsychology named Anthony Sclafani accidentally figured out an easy way to make rats fat. One day at his lab at the University of Chicago, on a whim, Sclafani fed his rats some Froot Loops. They devoured the cereal (first ingredient: added sugar[362]) with such savagery that he was taken aback.

Obesity researchers had been struggling to find a quick, reliable way to fatten rats. But they hadn't tried feeding rats *human* food. Thinking he might be on to something, Sclafani fed rats an assortment of sugary supermarket foods like cookies, Froot Loops, and sweetened milk.[363]

According to Sclafani:

> *The rats virtually ignored the lab chow and overate the supermarket foods to extreme obesity. This finding*

*stimulated renewed interest in the role of diet in promoting overeating.*[364]

The "cafeteria diet," as it came to be known, is still fed to rats today,[365] and is more effective at inducing rodent obesity than traditional high-fat diets.[366] Rats will voluntarily endure extreme cold and electrocution to eat cafeteria food, "even when standard chow is freely available in unlimited amounts."[367] Something similar is happening to humans.

## Humans on a Cafeteria Diet

What happens when you give people unlimited access to processed food? We have that data.

In three separate trials, subjects were kept in metabolic wards and had their baseline calorie intake measured over four days. Then, for five to seven days, as their sole source of food, they were given unlimited access to special computerized vending machines that were stocked with processed junk food like pancakes, Doritos, white bread, potato chips, spaghetti, M&M's, jelly beans, cake, chocolate pudding, and sugary drinks.[368]

On these vending-machine diets, the subjects in all three trials ate far more calories than normal. And they gained weight. To be precise, they ate between 27% and 54% more calories than normal, and gained two to five pounds.[369,370,371]

According to one of the studies:

> *Volunteers overfed themselves from Day 1 of ad libitum* [unlimited] *intake and continued overfeeding themselves until the end of the protocol.*[372]

Many of us eat the types of food in those vending machines on a *daily* basis. Is it any wonder that we're overweight?

These results are consistent with a fundamental principle: **weight gain is caused by an excess of calories.** The people in these trials ate far more calories than they normally did, and *they gained weight.*

And these results are consistent with another fundamental principle: fattening foods are fattening because they *inherently* lead people to eat more calories—because they are weakly satiating (filling).[373]

When processed food is involved, even the best laid plans of mice and men go awry. To feel full, we need to eat more total calories of vending-machine food.

So we do.

## Sugar Teeth

Everyone knows that added sugar causes cavities. More technically, added sugar spurs the plaque bacteria that cause tooth decay.[374] Less technically, added sugar rots our teeth.

Think about that. Physiology isn't a collection of separate parts. It's a dynamic whole of living interconnection. It's unlikely that a food would rot our teeth, but leave the rest of our bodies completely unscathed. Sure enough, added sugar is linked to heart disease and other maladies.[375,376,377,378]

But it was a dentist living in the early 20th century who most vividly demonstrated what a diet full of added sugar, white flour, and vegetable oil could do to the human body.

## Weston Price: A Nutrition Giant

It was the early 1930s. America's dental health was deplorable. Tooth decay was rampant, our rate of cavities alarmingly high. Modern dental hygiene was still developing, and fluoride hadn't yet been added to public water.

But these dental problems weren't global. Surprisingly,

there were many accounts of primitive populations around the world who had superb teeth, despite no access to dental care whatsoever.

This seeming paradox wasn't lost on Weston Price, the director of the American Dental Association's Research Institute. Price had spent the last 25 years studying *pulp infection*, a disease at the center of teeth that was usually caused by tooth decay. He had 60 scientists at his disposal.[379]

Dr. Price realized that the solution to America's dental problems lay not in American research labs, but in the populations of the world with great teeth. There must have been something that made these populations immune to the tooth decay then ravaging the United States.

Price decided to find out what that was. In 1931, he embarked on a long odyssey to study isolated populations in every corner of the globe, hoping to shed new light on tooth decay.

He had a unique, unprecedented, and long-lost opportunity. At that time, the world was quickly modernizing, and "modern" food—specifically, added sugar, white flour, and vegetable oil—had only recently been introduced in many populations for the first time. But critically, there were still large segments of these populations who *didn't* have access to modern processed foods.

Dr. Price documented eleven of what he called "racial stocks" (it was a different time)—ethnic groups such as Swiss, North American Indians, Gaelics, Melanesians, and Australian Aborigines—who'd naturally been divided into two groups: one group who was eating a "modern" diet full of white flour, added sugar, and oil, and another group who was still eating the traditional, whole-food diet of their ancestors.[380]

Other than diet, these "stocks" of people were quite similar. They shared the same ethnicity, very similar cultures, and similar lifestyles. The main difference between them was diet.

This was big. Genetic, cultural, and lifestyle differences seriously confound most nutrition studies, making it hard to isolate the effects of diet. But other than diet, these people were more or less the same. This meant that if there were any major differences in dental or general health between the two groups, it was likely that diet had played a role.

Price had seized a golden opportunity to isolate the health effects of processed food (added sugar, white flour, and vegetable oil) on a massive scale. It was a sort of giant, naturally controlled trial.

While it lacked the rigor of a formal controlled trial, it was stronger in other ways. It takes time for the health effects of diet to emerge, but controlled trials are necessarily short-term. This natural trial, however, had lasted decades. And it hadn't interfered with daily life the way normal trials do.

It was a special moment for nutrition.

## The Results

After years of carefully documented research in various populations around the globe, Price found that, compared to people eating traditional, whole-food diets, people eating modern processed diets had a thirty-five-fold increase in cavities.[381]

For perspective, that's *one* cavity in all the teeth at a large social gathering, versus *thirty-five* cavities.

The traditional, whole-food diets were rich in minerals and fat-soluble vitamins, and the people eating them had excellent, straight teeth with good arches and very few cavities.

On the other hand, the people eating processed diets had lots of cavities and mangled teeth.

(Diet seemed to affect the *straightness* of teeth, not just cavities.) Price said this about his 6,000-mile journey through Africa:

> *We studied six tribes in which there appeared to be not a single tooth attacked by dental caries* [cavities] *nor a single malformed dental arch. Several other tribes were found with nearly complete immunity to dental caries. In thirteen tribes we did not meet a single individual with irregular teeth.*

On the other hand, Price noted:

> *Where the members of these same tribes had adopted modern civilization many cases of tooth decay were found.*[382]

The dental problems usually began in the first generation raised on processed food, with children developing crooked teeth and lots of cavities.

But teeth were hardly the only difference.

Price found that people eating modern processed diets had much higher rates of cancer, heart disease, arthritis, and tuberculosis (a disease then ravaging the world).[383]

Here are some highlights.

Price visited a community in an isolated Swiss valley who ate mainly whole-rye bread, cheese, and whole milk. (All whole foods.)

> *Notwithstanding the fact that tuberculosis is the most serious disease of Switzerland, according to a statement given me by a government official, a recent report of inspection of this valley did not reveal a single case.*[384]

Tuberculosis simply didn't affect these people.

Price spoke to a doctor who'd been living among traditional Eskimos. They ate mostly fish and seal oil, along with some caribou, berries, ground nuts, and kelp. (All whole foods.)

> *He* [the doctor] *stated that in his thirty-six years of contact with these people he had never seen a case of malignant disease among the truly primitive Eskimos and Indians, although it frequently occurs when they become modernized.*

"Malignant disease" means cancer. The Eskimos eating whole foods didn't get cancer—or at least, they didn't get the big obvious cancers doctors knew how to diagnose in the early 20th century. Price went on:

> *He found similarly that the acute surgical problems requiring operation on internal organs such as the gall bladder, kidney, stomach, and appendix do not tend to occur among the primitive, but are very common problems among the modernized Eskimos and Indians.*[385]

People eating processed food needed far more surgeries. Price visited several traditional Alaskan populations. He recounted:

> *Careful inquiry regarding the presence of arthritis was made in the more isolated groups. We neither saw nor heard of a case in the isolated groups. However, at the point of contact with foods of modern civilization, many cases were found including ten bed-ridden cripples in a series of about twenty Indian homes.*[386]

People who ate processed food were far more likely to have arthritis or be cripples.

Price visited traditional pastoralists (cattle herders) in Kenya whose diet was cattle milk, cattle meat, and cattle blood, with some fruits and vegetables sprinkled in. (All whole foods.)

He spoke with a local doctor:

> [The doctor] *assured me that in several years of service among the primitive people of that district he had observed that they did not suffer from appendicitis, gall bladder trouble, cystitis and duodenal ulcer. Malignancy was also very rare among the primitives.*[387]

People eating whole foods didn't suffer from these common ailments.

Finally, Price spoke with a government doctor in the Torres Strait, which lies between Australia and New Guinea. People in this region traditionally ate mostly seafood and plants. (All whole foods.)

> *In his thirteen years with them he had not seen a single case of malignancy, and had seen only one that he had suspected might be malignancy among the entire four thousand native population. He stated that during this same period he had operated on several dozen malignancies for the white population, which numbers about three hundred. He reported that among the primitive stock other affections requiring surgical interference were rare.*[388]

Despite being less than a tenth of the size of the native population, the white population eating modern processed food had *far* more cases of cancer.

Modern research confirms Price's findings: diet significantly affects your chances of dying from many cancers.

Leading nutrition experts at Harvard have estimated that around 20% to 40% of all cancer deaths are basically attributable to a poor diet.[389]

Other researchers have documented nasty health effects following the transition to processed food.[390,391] For instance, scientists studying Zulu people around 1960 found that urban Zulu women (who ate lots of processed food) weighed over 30 pounds more, on average, than rural Zulu women (who ate a more traditional diet).[392]

To sum up, when a species eats lots of food it's not adapted to, problems ensue.

## The Definition of "Processed Food"

You hear the terms "whole food" and "processed food" a lot. Almost all nutrition experts agree that we should eat whole foods and avoid processed foods. It's almost a cliche.

But these are fuzzy terms. What do they mean, exactly? There isn't a bright red line separating *whole food* from *processed food*. There are obvious whole foods (spinach), and there are obvious processed foods (Oreos). But there's a big grey area in between that's been left open to interpretation.

*Merriam-Webster's Collegiate Dictionary* defines a *whole food* as "a natural food and especially an unprocessed one."[393]

This definition sounds reasonable, but it's hopelessly vague. The word "natural" gets thrown around too much to mean anything useful, and the word "unprocessed" assumes a definition of "processed."

So I looked up *processed food* in the same dictionary.

There wasn't a definition.

This needs to change.

We're not adapted to the plethora of processed foods that line our shelves and make us fat and sick. Worst of all, many people don't even realize their regular diet is filled with processed foods that are making them fat and sick.

We need a useful definition of "processed food" to bring to the supermarket. Here it is.

**processed food** *n* : *a food with an ingredients list longer than one item*

If you're holding a food at the supermarket, flip it over and look for the ingredients list. It's usually in a box near the bottom. If there's more than one item on that list, you're holding a processed food.

If there's only one item—or if there's no ingredients list at all—it's probably a whole food.

Simple. Clear. Practical.

There are very few exceptions to this rule. Other than the rare whole-food muesli, any time you see an ingredients list longer than one item, it almost always means there are items on that list that aren't whole foods. And the overwhelming majority of the time, that list will contain added sugar, added oil, or white flour. (Or all three.) There will often be a hodgepodge of obscure preservatives and texturizing and/or flavor-enhancing chemicals on there, too.

Added sugar, added oil, and white flour are processed ingredients that make us fat. They've been systematically added to most foods at the supermarket (and almost everywhere else) for the sole purpose of making food taste better—so we'll eat more, and the food companies will sell more.

Food manufacturers try to hide this fact with deceptive packaging slogans like *Whole Grain is the first ingredient*. But a food isn't "whole" just because its first ingredient is "whole." That slogan appeared on a box of Lucky Charms.

**A food is only as good as its *worst* ingredient.**

For example, *whole wheat flour* may be a solid first ingredient, but if it's followed by added sugar or oil, you're looking at a processed food.

In general, multiple ingredients mean that a food was altered from its natural state. Something was infused into it, mixed with it, or added to it—to make it taste better, so we'll eat more, and the company will sell more.

Here it is again:

> **processed food** *n* : *a food with an ingredients list longer than one item*

This definition accounts for every typical processed food at the supermarket. The only exception would be something like a bag of sugar—which is obviously processed, but technically has one ingredient. This is largely irrelevant, though. Most people don't snack on bags of sugar or white flour, or sip from cartons of vegetable oil.

Instead, they eat foods with these ingredients.

The only important exceptions to our definition of *processed food* are certain dairy products and canned goods. White milk, many cheeses, and some yogurts have more than one ingredient, but the other ingredients tend to be things like vitamin D, yogurt cultures, or a mild preservative—not added sugar or vegetable oil. These dairy products can be treated as whole foods. So can many canned goods that might only have an added preservative and a little salt.

As long as there isn't added sugar, oil, or flour, you're fine.

But remember: this definition only applies to the supermarket. Restaurants and bakeries don't list the ingredients on their processed food.

## The Definition of "Whole Food"

Used as an adjective, "whole" has seven senses in *Merriam Webster's Dictionary*,[394] but only four of them really apply to food:

*having all its proper parts or components:* **complete, unmodified**
*constituting the total sum or* **undiminished entirety: entire**
*constituting* **an undivided unit:** *unbroken,* **uncut**
*seemingly* **complete** *or* **total**

None of these definitions would seem to allow a "whole food" to have more than one ingredient, let alone a processed ingredient. With that in mind, here's a supermarket definition of *whole food*:

**whole food** *n : a food composed of a single unprocessed ingredient*

Whole foods have one ingredient that isn't processed. Oftentimes, they won't even bother to list that ingredient. Imagine how silly fresh fruit or wild-caught salmon would look with an ingredients list on the back.

Whole food: one, unprocessed ingredient.

*Healthy.*

These definitions will help you keep processed food out of your regular diet.

For our entire evolutionary past, we were eating simple, relatively unadorned whole foods—fruits, vegetables, tubers, meat, (and in recent millennia) dairy, whole grains, and legumes.

There was no one, "evolutionary diet." Our distant ancestors ate a wide range of foods. But there *was* a critical constant in all their various diets: *whole foods.*

Processed food didn't exist on any real scale until the 19th century.[395] This means our bodies are fundamentally adapted to whole foods, and fundamentally unadapted to processed foods. The satiety centers in our hypothalamus (which regulate total calorie intake via leptin binding[396]) evolved over the eons controlling the intake of *whole* foods.

Throw in the wrench of weakly satiating processed foods, and all bets are off.

## Ingredients, Not Calories

When most people want to judge a food's nutritional value, they look at the nutrition label, scanning for calories and grams and maybe a couple of vitamins to guide their choices.

But what they *should* be looking at is the ingredients list. The ingredients list is the most important piece of information on a food's packaging. It's what the food is actually *made* of, after all.

Calories and grams are secondary.

It may seem counterintuitive, but the reason processed food is fattening has little to do with calories. *All* food has calories. Everyone is constantly eating thousands upon thousands of calories each week. (If they didn't, they'd starve to death.) These thousands upon thousands of weekly calories have to come from somewhere.

A food isn't fattening or slimming because of the *quantity* of calories it contains, but because of the *quality* of those calories—and whether they fill us up. Processed food isn't fattening because it has "a lot of calories" or "a lot of fat" or "a lot of carbs." It's fattening because the calories and fat and carbs in processed foods don't fill us up as much as the calories and fat and carbs in whole foods.

When we eat processed foods, we eat *more* total calories and fat and carbs—and get fat. Processed food is fattening because it throws off our body's ancient, exquisite, finely-tuned system of weight control.

Weight loss *does* come down to calories, but when you're eating whole foods, your body counts calories for you. When you're eating whole foods, you'll naturally feel full on fewer calories.

And you won't have to deal with hunger.

And you'll naturally lose weight. (Maybe a lot of it.)

And other than sticking to whole foods most days, you won't have to do anything special to keep the weight off. Because losing weight wasn't a conscious choice—your body simply readjusted its food intake to a more appropriate level, on a more appropriate diet.

We're not meant to obsess over how much we're eating. And if you stick with whole foods most days, you won't have to.

**whole food** *n* : *a food composed of a single unprocessed ingredient*

**processed food** *n* : *a food with an ingredients list longer than one item*

Some people get caught up in the *length* of the ingredients list—*the more ingredients a food has, the more processed it is.* To their credit, a long list of obscure chemicals can't be good. All food started out alive, and a food is *processed* to the extent that this isn't obvious. For instance, fruit is clearly a plant. And meat is clearly an animal. But what's a Twinkie? Looking at its ingredients list, a Twinkie is about 30 different things.

Then again, there are only three ingredients in your standard potato chip: potatoes, vegetable oil, and salt. A long and tongue-twisting ingredients list, then, isn't necessary for a food to be processed and highly fattening.

**Any food with more than one ingredient is a processed food.**

## Marketing Sleaze

It's important to realize that a food's front packaging is an advertisement. It is nothing else. It is an ad to sell a product.

If you want to figure out if a certain food is healthy or not, it's best to **ignore the ad on the front, and look at the ingredients list on the back.**

Here's why this is necessary.

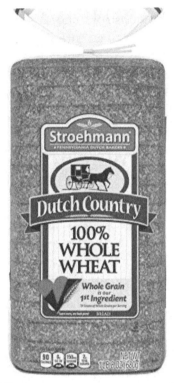

**INGREDIENTS:** Whole Wheat Flour, Water, **Sugar**, Wheat Gluten, Yeast, Wheat Bran, **Soybean Oil**, **Salt**, Enrichment (Calcium Sulfate, Vitamin E Acetate, Vitamin A Palmitate, Vitamin D3), Calcium Propionate (Preservative), Monoglycerides, Datem, Soy Lecithin, Citric Acid, Grain Vinegar, Potassium Iodate.[397]

Looking at the advertisement on the front of this bread, we see a quaint horse and buggy perched atop the phrases *Dutch Country* and *100% Whole Wheat*. These evoke an aggressively wholesome image, which is only enhanced by the ad's soothing beige color tones.

But it's *this* icon in the lower-left corner that seals the deal:

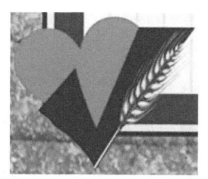

*Wholesome heart health.*

That's a wheat-chaff checkmark overlaying a big, vibrant cartoon heart. You feel healthier just looking at it.

*Well played,* Stroehmann.

But take a peek at that ingredients list.

As advertised, a whole grain—*whole wheat flour*—is the first ingredient. Stroehmann isn't outright lying to us.

But what *else* is lurking inside this fresh-baked loaf of wholesome, whole-wheat goodness?

**Added sugar, added oil, and seven obscure chemicals.**

How come these weren't on the front?

As this makes clear, the words *whole-wheat* and *whole-grain* don't necessarily mean *whole food.* A food's whole-ness is determined by its *ingredients list,* not the ad in front. (Whole grains aren't *whole* after they're injected with sugar and oil and additives.)

And as this makes clear, the point of food packaging is to sell food. It is an ad.

Depending on the target market, the ad will generally portray the food as healthy, traditional, or fun.

For instance, kids are even more attracted to sweet taste than adults.[398] From an early age, kids are bombarded with ads for added sugar. With predatory marketing full of friendly cartoon characters like Count Chocula and Tony the Tiger, cereal companies help teach our youngsters that the staple of a healthy breakfast is a bowl of candy mixed with milk.

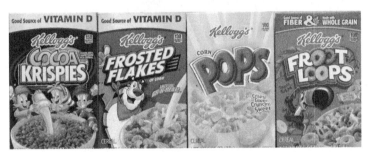

Photo Credit: LunaseeStudios/ Shutterstock.com

To woo parents and regulators, this candy is coated with vitamin dust and labeled "fortified." But the first or second ingredient is almost always added sugar.

Which makes it candy.

Many children carry their breakfast-candy habit to adulthood. To cater to grown-ups with a more health-conscious sweet tooth, food companies change the presentation of their candy.

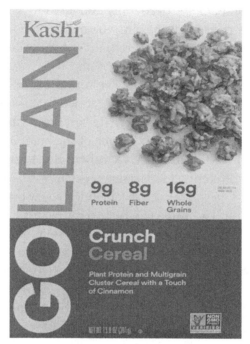

Photo Credit: Sheila Fitzgerald/ Shutterstock.com

**INGREDIENTS:** Kashi Seven Whole Grains And Sesame Blend (Whole: Hard Red Wheat, Brown Rice, Barley, Triticale, Oats, Rye, Buckwheat, Sesame Seeds), Soy Flakes, **Brown Rice Syrup**, **Dried Cane Syrup**, Chicory Root Fiber, Whole Grain Oats, **Expeller Pressed Canola Oil**, **Honey**, **Salt**, Cinnamon, Mixed Tocopherols For Freshness.[399]

This cereal looks healthy, right? The front ad boasts a hearty granola packed with a potent punch of protein, fiber, and whole grains (and possibly *LEAN*, too).

For reference, this cereal has 30% more sugar than Lucky Charms.[400,401]

More like "NO LEAN."

Food companies are federally obligated to list ingredients in order of prevalence, placing the main ingredient first, the second-most prevalent ingredient second, the third-most prevalent ingredient *third*, and so on.

But with added sugar, they've found a loophole. If they split up added sugar into *separate* added sugars and list them individually, they can hide them toward the bottom of the list.

For instance, added sugar is one of the main ingredients in that box of Kashi GOLEAN Crunch! But Kashi splits it up into *three* different added sugars (*brown rice syrup*, *dried cane syrup*, and *honey*). This way, each added sugar takes up less of the whole, and all three can be listed towards the bottom of the ingredients list—below the healthy-sounding *Kashi Seven Whole Grains and Sesame Blend* and *Soy Flakes*.

But who am I kidding? This assumes people even *read* ingredients lists on products like Kashi's. Instead, most of us get suckered in by the front of the box, duped by healthy buzzwords, "LEAN," and this non-GMO stamp.

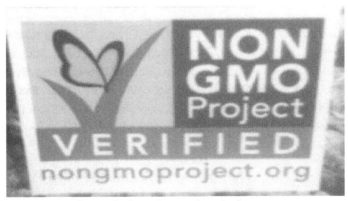

*Green checkmarks put the mind at ease.*

Kashi may sound like a quaint little mom-and-pop company, perhaps owned by a Mama and Papa Kashi.

Instead, Kashi is owned by Kellogg.

That's the same Kellogg that makes Cocoa Krispies, Apple Jacks, Froot Loops, and Pop-Tarts. These blockbuster junk foods are the reason you won't find the name *Kellogg* anywhere on Kashi's box.

That would be bad for business.

(Kellogg also owns Bear Naked, another brand of "healthy" granola.)

**Be extremely skeptical of food packaging.** It's safe to assume that any food that's *advertised* as healthy or slimming is probably precisely the opposite. Health claims and wholesome buzzwords on food packaging are no more genuine or sincere than the sleaziest late-night infomercial.

But food companies *are* obligated to list ingredients on the back, and can't outright lie here. That makes the ingredients list the most important part of a food's packaging.

## Organic Processed Food

The word *organic* may have meant something, once. But in the modern era of Big Organic, where the largest organic-food companies are owned by major junk-food corporations, all *organic* really means is that the food producer adhered to some rather arbitrary rules that must be followed to legally call a food "organic."

Ironically, these rules include a list of permissible **non-organic** synthetic food additives.[402] A food can have these synthetic, non-organic additives and still be "organic."

In 1995, there were 81 independent organic food companies in the United States. Between 1997 and 2010, the US organic food industry grew like a magic (organic) beanstalk, with sales increasing by 740%.[403]

When a market explodes like this, the number of companies in that market tends to increase. But due to consolidation by large junk-food corporations, there are only 15 independent organic-food companies in the US today.[404]

One is Cascadian Farm.

It's owned by General Mills (who also owns LaraBar).

Dagoba is a company that makes organic chocolate.

It's owned by Hershey.

Stonyfield is a company that makes organic yogurt.

It's owned by Dannon.

Post (maker of Cocoa Pebbles) bought three organic food companies in the last three years: Erewhon, Golden Boy, and New Morning.[405]

Odwalla, Honest Tea, Bolthouse Farms, and Naked Juice—those wholesome-looking beverages—are respectively owned by Coca-Cola, Coca-Cola, Campbell's Soup, and Pepsi.[406]

As much as we'd like to picture organic food growing on small family farms with battered old pickup trucks, organic food production is now controlled by the titans of processed junk food.

In *The Omnivore's Dilemma* (2006), Michael Pollan recounts his visit to a large organic grower in California:

> *My first stop was Greenways Organic, a successful two-thousand-acre organic produce operation tucked into a twenty-four-thousand-acre conventional farm in the Central Valley outside Fresno; the crops, the machines, the crews, the rotations, and the fields were virtually indistinguishable...*[407]

Organic food isn't special.

A meta-analysis in 2012 concluded that:

> *Our comprehensive review of the published literature on the comparative health outcomes, nutrition, and safety of organic and conventional foods identified*

*limited evidence for the superiority of organic foods.*
*The evidence does not suggest marked health benefits*
*from consuming organic versus conventional foods,*
*although organic produce may reduce exposure to*
*pesticide residues and organic chicken and pork may*
*reduce exposure to antibiotic-resistant bacteria.*[408]

Could this potential exposure to pesticide residues and antibiotic-resistant bacteria lead to cancer? A 2014 study tracked the organic-food habits and cancer rates of 623,080 women for 9.3 years.

It concluded:

*There was little or no decrease in the incidence of*
*cancer associated with consumption of organic food,*
*except possibly for non-Hodgkin lymphoma.*[409]

The health benefits of organic food are largely speculative. Regarding any positive health claims you may hear, it pays to remember that organic food is a 35-billion-dollar industry.[410]

And that's just in the United States.

If you want natural food grown with care, your best bet is a local farmers market, not Whole Foods.

The important distinction is between *processed* and *whole* food, not *organic* and *non-organic* food.

There's a great deal of "organic" processed food out there.

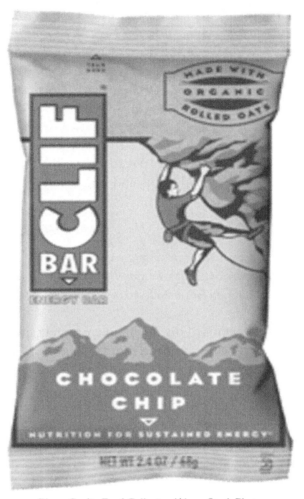

Photo Credit: Food Collection/Alamy Stock Photo

**INGREDIENTS: Organic Brown Rice Syrup**, Organic Rolled Oats, Soy Protein Isolate, **Organic Cane Syrup**, Organic Roasted Soybeans, **Rice Flour, Cane Sugar, Unsweetened Chocolate, Organic Soy Flour**, Organic Oat Fiber, **Organic High Oleic Sunflower Oil, Cocoa Butter**, Barley Malt Extract, **Sea Salt**, Natural Flavors, Soy Lecithin, Organic Cinnamon.[411]

In this healthy-looking Clif Bar (note the *organic* label) the first ingredient is added sugar (*organic brown rice syrup*). By definition, that makes this a candy bar.

Incidentally, the fourth, seventh, and thirteenth ingredients are also added sugars, the sixth and ninth ingredients are flours, and there's a vegetable oil (*organic high oleic sunflower oil*).

The motto of this candy bar is "nutrition for sustained energy," which is reinforced by the skinny extreme rock climber on the front wrapper.

Apparently this "nutrition" is coming from 25 grams of added sugar.[412]

For reference, a Kit Kat has 21 grams of added sugar.[413]

**Be extremely skeptical of food packaging.**

> **processed food** *n* : *a food with an ingredients list longer than one item*

This definition absolutely and unequivocally applies to "organic" foods.

## Engineering Food

Food companies have turned adding sugar into a science. Too much added sugar makes food cloyingly sweet, while too little makes it bland. So companies optimize their foods around "bliss points"—the exact amounts of added sugar that maximize eating pleasure for the average person.[414]

They do the same thing with vegetable oil and salt.

We are not adapted to this sort of food engineering.

If this weren't bad enough, there are companies with thousands of employees whose sole purpose is creating artificial flavorings. Through the marvels of modern chemistry, these companies are capable of producing any flavor under the sun, from strawberry, caramel, and vanilla, to chicken, citrus, and cheese.

These are the "artificial flavors" you see on ingredients lists.

To give you an idea of how big this industry is, there were six different artificial-flavor companies that each had over a billion dollars in revenue in 2013.[415]

*Six.*

These artificial flavors are added to enhance the already unnaturally seductive taste of processed food, for the sole purpose of selling more food.

And food products aren't just optimized for taste. Using computer analysis of extensive taste tests, foods are also optimized for color, smell, texture, and packaging. In *Sugar Salt Fat* (2014), Michael Moss recounts what he learned from a high-profile food engineer:

> *It's not simply a matter of comparing color 23 to color 24. In the most complicated projects, color 23 must be compared with syrup 11 and packaging 6, and on and on. Even in jobs where the only concern is taste and the variables are limited to the ingredients, endless charts and graphs will come spewing out of his computer. "I mix and match ingredients by this experimental design," he told me. "The mathematical model maps out the ingredients to the sensory perceptions these ingredients create, so I can just dial a new product. This is the engineering approach."[416]*

Technology has allowed us to artificially magnify the pleasures of eating, creating processed foods that overwhelm our body's innate system of weight control.

## Utter Convenience

Aside from simply making food taste better, it's hard to overstate the effect of technology on eating *convenience*. In today's world, all the major barriers between *wanting to eat* and *eating* have been completely removed.

It used to take a lot of time to prepare food. Even junk food. For example, Jell-O existed in the 1940s, but back then, it was a mix that came in a box. And it took *hours* to prepare.[417]

Today, preparing Jell-O usually entails reaching into the fridge and peeling the cover off—a cover that's been fitted with a convenient lip to make this step as painless as possible.

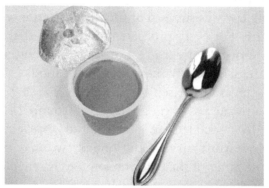

Photo Credit: mikeledray/Shutterstock.com

We're not adapted to added sugar to begin with—it's only been widely available since the early 1800s.[418]

But there's a world of difference between availability and *instant* availability. Modern technology has made a universe of taste-optimized processed food available at a moment's notice, nearly everywhere we go, 24 hours per day.

This is what's known as an *obesogenic environment*.[419]

## The Rumble Pit

The famous processed foods that line the center aisles of supermarkets and convenience stores—Pringles, Doritos, Chips Ahoy!, etc.—may seem like a random, merry hodgepodge of culinary delights.

But they aren't random.

These foods emerged from countless prototypes and careful testing. Their development was methodical and painstaking, involving huge amounts of corporate resources.

With millions of dollars in advertising at their backs, these products were released into the wild, catapulted onto shelves across the country to join the round-robin rumble pit of unbridled food capitalism. At stake was a piece of the world's biggest industry.[420]

The only law was survival of the fittest. And it was a fight to the death. For every processed food lining shelves today, countless more went extinct, beaten out by better-tasting, better-crafted, better-marketed processed foods.

And the cream has risen to the top.

But future success is no guarantee. Around 14,000 new processed-food products are launched into grocery stores each year.[421] Most won't survive. But one or two may claw their way into the ranks of the elite, forcing the current champions to adapt or die.

That's what you're up against with processed food.

Remember: Dr. Pepper released Cherry Vanilla after testing 61 prototypes and conducting 3904 taste tests.

And it was still a flop.

## Take-Home

Processed food was always fattening. But somewhere around the 1970s, it reached a tipping point. With better technology, the full potential of added sugar, added oil, and white flour began to blossom into a new breed of innovative, wildly seductive processed food. More than anything else, it's this modern processed food that caused the obesity epidemic.

And in the cause lies the cure.

## Habit 2: Only eat whole foods most days.

**processed food** *n* : *a food with an ingredients list longer than one item*

# The Five Golden Weight-Loss Habits

1. Cut out all sugary drinks.
2. Only eat whole foods most days.

   **processed food** *n: a food with an
   ingredients list longer than one item*

# 14

# DRIPPING WITH OIL

I'm not going to sugarcoat it: vegetable oil is just as bad as added sugar. In fact, it's probably even worse. Because unlike added sugar, people don't really know about vegetable oil.

They don't really know about it because vegetable oil has the official seal of approval, and is widely endorsed by major health institutions.[422,423] It's known as the "heart-healthy" alternative to animal fats.

People don't really know about vegetable oil because it has the mother of all healthful-sounding branding advantages: the name *vegetable*.

You might as well call it "Jesus oil."

"Vegetable oil" evokes leafy cornucopias of colorful veggies that were somehow reduced to oils, which, like their vegetable parents, probably foster health and longevity.

But vegetable oil doesn't deserve the name *vegetable*.

And that's not an opinion. It's a fact: none of the major vegetable oils come from vegetables.

**Not a single one.**

Let me break it down.

Corn oil comes from corn. Corn is *botanically* a fruit and *popularly* a grain.[424]

Sunflower oil, safflower oil, canola oil, cottonseed oil, and sesame oil? They're all squeezed out of seeds. Seeds are not vegetables. (A "vegetable" is defined as the part of the plant *without* seeds.[425])

Soybean oil and peanut oil? They're made from legumes, which are technically a type of dry *fruit*.[426]

Even olive oil, coconut oil, and palm oil—the health oils *du jour*—all hail from botanical *fruits*.[427,428]

So no vegetables. No carrots, broccoli, asparagus, squash, or kale. No vegetables anywhere.

Especially not in cottonseed oil, which is made from cotton. Yes, *that* cotton. The one found in clothing. Cottonseed oil is the third most common food oil in the US.[429]

Further departing from the whole *vegetable* thing, most vegetable oils are highly processed. They're produced by methods more akin to refining crude oil than pressing vegetables together.

(Most, but not all. Extra-virgin olive oil is made by squeezing olives together.[430] One step. No preservatives. No chemicals. No heat. The way it's been done for 8,000 years.[431] But such wholesomeness is the rare exception with vegetable oils.)

In 1974, Canadian plant scientists bred a new type of seed for making vegetable oil: the *rapeseed*. Proud of their creation, and wanting to take the name in a different direction, they combined the words "Canada" and "ola."[432]

*Canola oil* was born.

It's the third most common food oil in the world.[433]

Making canola oil involves wholesome, artisanal methods like hexane baths, high-speed centrifuging, dousing with sodium hydroxide, bleaching with acid-activated clay, and steam-injecting at 265 °C (509 °F) in facilities that can churn out 22,000 bottles of canola oil per hour.[434,435,436]

## The Best Nutrition Study Ever

In 1995, a group of Australian scientists led by nutrition researcher Susanna Holt performed one of the most illuminating studies in the history of nutrition. They called their masterpiece, "A Satiety Index of Common Foods."[437]

Believing that different foods caused different levels of satiety (*fullness*, if you're just joining us), they figured out a way to measure the "satiety score" of a bunch of common foods.

They chose a cross section of 38 regular foods, split across six groups: *fruits, protein-rich foods, carbohydrate-rich foods, breakfast cereals, snack foods,* and *bakery products.* After an overnight fast, they had people eat 239-calorie portions of a given food, then report how full they felt. Two hours later, the subjects were offered a buffet of food and told to eat freely. (They ate freely.)

Each food had its turn.

Then the scientists crunched the numbers.

Sure enough, the more filling someone rated a food, the less food they ate at the buffet later. And the scientists were right: different foods caused vastly different satiety levels.

Each food received a satiety score.

The main finding? **Whole foods were almost universally more filling than processed foods.**

According to the scientists:

> *Simple "whole" foods such as the fruits, potatoes, steak and fish were the most satiating of all foods tested... "modern" Western diets which are based on highly palatable, low-fiber convenience foods are likely to be much less satiating than the diets of the past.*[438]

Here are the leaderboards.

(The higher the score, the more filling the food.)

## Food Satiety Scores
(the baseline is white bread, with a score of 100)

| *most* filling | score | *least* filling | score |
|---|---|---|---|
| potatoes | 323 | croissant | 47 |
| ling fish | 225 | cake | 65 |
| porridge | 209 | doughnuts | 68 |
| oranges | 202 | Mars Bars | 70 |
| apples | 197 | salted peanuts | 84 |
| whole-wheat pasta | 188 | strawberry yogurt | 88 |
| beef steak | 176 | potato chips | 91 |
| **(all whole foods)** | | **(all processed foods)** | |

The results could not be more clear.

**Whole foods are far more filling than processed foods.**

White bread was the baseline to which all foods were compared. Its score was set at 100. (A score of 200 meant a food was *twice* as filling as white bread.)

The banana was rated the least filling out of any whole food, with a score of 118—which was still 18% more filling than white bread.

The overall winner was the potato, with a score of 323. The potato obliterated every other food. Given the stigma against potatoes, this may seem surprising. But potatoes *are* vegetables,[439] after all. And like other veggies, they're high in fiber and nutrients.

Okay. So what does all this have to do with vegetable oil? Two words: *potato chips.*

Potato chips were among the *least* satiating foods (score: 91), scoring even worse than ice cream. Unlike potatoes, potato chips seemed to deserve their fattening reputation.

And what's *in* potato chips? Your basic chip has just three ingredients: potatoes, **vegetable oil**, and salt.

So what makes potato chips fattening?

According to this study, it's clearly not potatoes, which were more filling than any other food.

The thing is, in a bag of potato chips, more calories actually come from *vegetable oil* than from potatoes.[440,441]

It would be more accurate to call them "vegetable-oil chips."

Throw in a little salt, and vegetable oil takes a highly filling whole food and makes it less filling than ice cream.

## The Purest Fat

What *is* vegetable oil? At the end of the day, it's just *100%, pure fat.* There's nothing else in it. In 100 grams of vegetable oil, there are 0.0 grams of carbs, 0.0 grams of protein, and 100 grams of fat.[442] It's a thoroughbred fat.

*Calorie density* is the number of calories, per gram, that a food has. Vegetable oil is the second-most calorie-dense food in existence.

(First place: *lard.*)

Calorie density is determined by macronutrients. Every calorie in food comes from one of three sources: protein, carbs, or fat. In a gram of protein or a gram of carbs, there are four calories. In a gram of fat, there are nine calories.[443]

These numbers are rougher than widely appreciated, but they're close enough.

Protein, carbs, and fat, though, aren't the only things in food. Aside from vitamins and minerals, many whole foods also have fiber and water. Meat, for example, is around 75% water.[444]

Fiber and water take up space, but have few calories. This is good, because when food pushes against your stomach, it sends satiety signals to your brain.[445] The more space the food takes up in your stomach, the more satiety signals get sent to your brain, and the fuller you feel. Thanks to their water and fiber, whole foods take up lots of space, fill you up, and have relatively few calories.

In other words, whole foods have a *low calorie density.*

It's just the opposite with processed foods, which have little to no fiber, little to no water, and lots of calories—a *high calorie density.* This is bad.

It's bad because your stomach doesn't "speak" calories; it only speaks volume. Your stomach sends signals to your brain based on the *volume* of food inside it, not the number of calories inside it. Calories aren't "read" until they reach the small intestine, where energy (calorie) info is communicated by peptide hormones.[446]

This is bad, because it takes awhile for food to reach your small intestine. In a 2006 study of 90 healthy people, it took a median time of **over two hours** for just *half* of a meal to exit the stomach and enter the small intestine.[447]

This suggests that if you're eating processed food—even if you're eating it *slowly* and *mindfully* and all that—your stomach doesn't ever "catch up" with all those extra calories. By the time the calories register in your small intestine, the damage is already done. (You've overeaten.)

Indeed, the more calorie-dense a food is, the less filling it is.[448] Our stomachs evolved for eons getting stretched by whole foods that took up more space than modern processed foods.

This is why diets with a high calorie density are directly linked with obesity.[449] **And vegetable oil approaches the upper limits of calorie density.**

Since fat is the most energy-dense macronutrient, and fat has nine calories per gram, the highest that a food's calorie density can possibly be is *nine calories per gram*—pure fat. Pure fats like vegetable oil are the most calorie-dense foods on Earth. There's nothing more calorie-dense.

Everything edible, then, ranges from zero to nine calories per gram—from *least* to *most* calorie-dense. Fruits and vegetables are usually under *one* calorie per gram, and the numbers go up from there.

Here are the calorie densities of some common foods:

| food | calories/gram |
|---|---|
| strawberries | 0.32 |
| kale | 0.50 |
| potatoes | 0.77 |
| bananas | 0.89 |
| lean ground beef | 1.37 |
| wild-caught salmon | 1.42 |
| eggs (with yolk) | 1.43 |
| ground beef (fattiest cut) | 3.32 |
| parmesan cheese | 3.92 |
| Kit Kat bar | 5.18 |
| potato chips | 5.47 |
| butter | 7.17 |
| **vegetable oil** | **8.84** |

Sources:[450,451,452,453,454,455,456,457,458,459,460,461,462]

You heard it here first: **vegetable oil is over 20% more calorie-dense than butter.** (Butter isn't known for being light on calories.)

Whole foods generally have between zero and four calories per gram. If a food has more than four calories per gram, it's almost always processed.

(The only real exception is nuts, which have between five and seven calories per gram.[463,464,465] But unlike processed foods, nuts are high in vitamins, minerals, fiber, and protein.)

As the chart above shows, even the fattiest ground beef (the kind with 30 grams of fat in one serving) only has 3.3 calories per gram. That's the power of water and protein, which naturally limit the calorie density of whole foods.

On the other hand, **all major vegetable oils have 8.84 calories per gram**.[466,467,468,469,470,471,472,473]

(The only exception is coconut oil, at 8.62 calories per gram.[474])

In short, adding vegetable oil to food is one of the most efficient ways to raise a food's calorie density. In the process, filling food becomes *un*-filling, and slimming food becomes fattening.

But who would do such a thing?

## More Common Than Sugar

Now I can tell just by looking. For a long time, though, if I didn't know what was in a food, I would read the ingredients list.

I read thousands of ingredients lists.

I learned a lot about food.

The most important thing I learned from this odd obsession with ingredients lists?

**Vegetable oil is everywhere.**

*Everywhere.*

For starters, anything even remotely resembling a chip will have vegetable oil every single time. You could bet your life on it.

Vegetable oil is in almost every "snack"-type food—bars, crisps, sweets, bites, bits, nibs, cakes, whatever. All of them.

Vegetable oil is in most foods that come in a box, like cereal.

In fact, **most foods with more than one ingredient will have vegetable oil**.

It doesn't matter how healthy they may appear.

The word *ubiquitous* isn't enough to describe the scale of vegetable oil in the US food supply. While added sugar is mind-blowingly pervasive, vegetable oil probably has it beat.

And I don't say that lightly.

Worst of all, unlike sugar, vegetable oil is still invisible to the average person.

But why all this oil?

## The Magic Number

Like added sugar, there is only one reason that vegetable oil is added to food: to make it taste better. Vegetable oil is an *added fat*, and added fat gives food a charming taste and delightful consistency the food scientists call "mouthfeel."[475]

Our tastes evolved when calories were more scarce, so we evolved a taste for calorie-dense foods. And foods don't come any more calorie-dense than pure fat.

Here's how food companies see it:

When food has added fat, it tastes better.

↓

When food tastes better, people buy more.

↓

When people buy more, we make more money.

↓

**ADD FAT TO EVERYTHING.**

Which fat to add? Well, not only is refined vegetable oil much cheaper than butter or lard, but it's also considered "healthier" than these animal fats. So it's a real no-brainer for food companies: *add refined vegetable oil to everything*.

It's simple economics.

It's not that processed food would be that much healthier or less fattening if all the vegetable oil were replaced with butter, it's just that vegetable oil is the de facto added fat in the US food supply. If a food *has* added fat—which most processed foods do—it's almost *always* vegetable oil.

I'd estimate that a food's added fat is vegetable oil around 98% of the time.

That's just the way it is.

And just like adding sugar, adding vegetable oil has become a science. Through countless taste tests and endless trial and error, food companies have figured out exactly how much oil makes food pop.

They've learned to add oil until a food's calorie density hovers right around *five calories per gram*. That's the magic number of processed food. *Five calories per gram.*

Five calories per gram is the calorie density that best bewitches our taste buds, best beguiling us into eating more and more—and more and more (and more and more).

*Five calories per gram* is why you can't have just one.

And it's all thanks to vegetable oil.

Pringles? Five calories per gram.[476]
Lay's Potato Chips? Five calories per gram.[477]
Doritos? Five calories per gram.[478]
Cheetos? Five calories per gram.[479]
Fritos? Five calories per gram.[480]
Kit Kat bars? Five calories per gram.[481]
Butterfingers? Five calories per gram.[482]
Oreos? Five calories per gram.[483]
Ruffles Potato Chips? Five calories per gram.[484]
Tostitos? Five calories per gram.[485]
Munchos? Five calories per gram.[486]
Cheez-Its? Five calories per gram.[487]
Smartfood White Cheddar Popcorn? Five calories per gram.[488]
Goldfish? Five calories per gram.[489]
Funyuns? Five calories per gram.[490]
Baby Ruth? Five calories per gram.[491]
SunChips? Five calories per gram.[492]
Twix? Five calories per gram.[493]

Get the picture?

## A Word About Salt

In that tower of junk foods on the previous page, there are only two ingredients shared by every single food: vegetable oil and salt.

Salt gets a bad rap. There's evidence that a very high salt intake promotes heart disease.[494] (Then again, there's also evidence that a *low* salt intake promotes heart disease.[495])

When food is salted, people do tend to eat more of it. A 2016 study found that adding salt to macaroni increased calorie intake by 11%.[496]

Salt is yet another substance that food companies add to foods in precise and proven amounts to woo our taste buds, fool our satiety systems, and inadvertently foster widespread obesity.

Nevertheless, I've long felt that salt is a trivial thing to focus on—a case of missing the forest for a tree. According to the CDC, 77% of the salt in our diet comes from "processed and restaurant foods."[497]

For most of us, then, excess salt isn't coming from the kitchen salt shaker. It's coming from processed food. Rather than focusing on eating less salt, just focus on *not* eating processed food most days of the week.

Among many other things, this should solve your salt problem.

## A Culture in Denial

As a society, we are oddly delusional about vegetable oil. For instance, how many times have you been told to avoid "fried food"?

A lot of times, right?

Now, how many times have you been told to avoid *vegetable oil?*

Not a lot of times, right?

If anything, you're told to *choose* vegetable oil.

If you think about it, this is very odd, because "fried food" is almost universally fried…*in vegetable oil*. From McDonald's[498] to KFC[499] to Chipotle[500] to Olive Garden[501] to restaurants around the world, "fried" means "fried in vegetable oil."

Vegetable oil literally puts the *fry* in fried food. It's the very essence of the term. French fries, onion rings, deep-fried calamari, chicken wings, nachos, mozzarella sticks, deep-fried Oreos (where did those come from?), and many other fried foods are fattening and unhealthy…*because they're fried in vegetable oil*.

Vegetable oil is the only thing that ties them all together.

Again, it's not that frying foods in lard or butter would be so much better. It's just that, in practice, **almost all fried food is fried in vegetable oil**.

And almost no one talks about it.

It's hardly just the obvious junk foods, either. Many foods marketed as slimming and healthy have enough added vegetable oil to hit the magic number, too.

SkinnyPop Popcorn? Five calories per gram.[502]
Nature Valley Oats 'n Dark Chocolate? Five calories per gram.[503]
belVita Mixed Berry Bites? Five calories per gram.[504]
KIND Peanut Butter Breakfast Bars? Five calories per gram.[505]

Other foods with significant added vegetable oil include Whole-Grain Fig Newtons,[506] Wheat Thins,[507] Sabra Classic Hummus,[508] Lay's *Baked* Potato Chips,[509] Nature Valley Granola,[510] Nutri-Grain Bars,[511] most "100% Whole-Wheat" breads,[512] and most brands of nuts (even nuts labeled "Whole"[513]).

It's time to expand your definition of *junk food*.

## Refined Oils, Heart Disease, and Death

Aside from sky-high calorie density and ubiquity in processed food, there are other reasons to be suspicious of added vegetable oil.

First, refined vegetable oils weren't widely eaten until the early 20th century.[514] Since evolution is the foundation of nutrition, this alone should sound the warning bells. There hasn't been any time to adapt.

Second, refined vegetable oils have stratospheric amounts of something called *polyunsaturated fats*. These are fats with more than one double bond. They include *omega-6 fatty acids* (linoleic acid) and *omega-3 fatty acids* (alpha linolenic acid).

Aside from the sheer amounts, the *ratio* of these polyunsaturated fats in refined vegetable oils is equally unsettling. Most refined oils have gobs of omega-6s, and relatively few omega-3s.

Omega-6s and omega-3s are both essential; your body can't make them. They help control inflammation.[515] Omega-3s tend to be anti-inflammatory, and omega-6s tend to be pro-inflammatory. And they compete for the same enzymes.

Some scientists think the ratio of omega-6s to omega-3s in our diet is important, that we evolved eating a much lower ratio of omega-6s to omega-3s than we're eating today, and that this discrepancy has led to many inflammatory diseases.[516,517]

This theory remains rather speculative. But there are plausible mechanisms by which gobs of omega-6s from refined oils could be a problem.[518]

Three things are certain.

1. We only require small amounts of omega-6s and omega-3s.[519]

2. We are currently eating much larger amounts of omega-6s and omega-3s than we ate in the past.

3. Most of this increase is coming from refined vegetable oils.

Between 1909 and 1999, the average American's intake of

omega-3s increased by 109%. Their average intake of omega-6s increased by 223%.[520]

Similarly, a 2015 study found that the amount of omega-6s in American fat tissue increased 136% since 1955.[521]

Could all these omega-6s be a problem?

A well-conducted 2010 meta-analysis[522] of eight randomized controlled trials in humans (the strongest possible form of evidence) compared replacing saturated fat and trans fat with either high-omega-6 vegetable oils or vegetable oils with more balanced omega profiles.

This was big, because previous meta-analyses hadn't segregated vegetable oils by omega content—they'd just grouped all vegetable oils together.[523]

But this meta-analysis found that when you replaced saturated fat and trans fat with high-omega-6 vegetable oils, it "tended to increase CHD [coronary heart disease]," and "increased risk of death from all causes."[524]

That's no good.

On the other hand, replacing saturated and trans fat with vegetable oils with more balanced omegas tended to *decrease* risk of heart disease.

Vegetable oils aren't created equal, it seems.

The so-called "Israeli Paradox" is that Israeli people eat lots of omega-6s and little saturated fat, but have high rates of heart disease[525]—the opposite of what popular nutritional wisdom would suggest.

But this study suggests that Israelis get lots of heart disease *because* they eat so many omega-6s, not in spite of it—and that there's really no "paradox" at all.

The take-home message is that **vegetable oils aren't the same, and high-omega-6 vegetable oils probably cause heart disease and death.**

With this in mind, here are seven vegetable oils you should probably avoid (the ones in bold):

| OIL | total omega-6 (milligrams/ounce) | total omega-3 (milligrams/ounce) |
|---|---|---|
| safflower oil | 20,982 | 0 |
| sunflower oil | 18,397 | 0 |
| corn oil | 14,983 | 325 |
| cottonseed oil | 14,421 | 56 |
| soybean oil | 14,118 | 1,901 |
| sesame oil | 11,565 | 84 |
| peanut oil | 8,961 | 0 |
| canola oil | 5,221 | 2,559 |
| olive oil | 2,734 | 213 |
| palm oil | 2,548 | 56 |
| coconut oil | 504 | 0 |
| butter (reference) | 764 | 88 |

Sources:[526,527,528,529,530,531,532,533,534,535,536,537]

The problem with the oils at the top is that they have lots of omega-6s, and very few omega-3s (except for soybean oil).

Safflower oil has more omega-6s than any other food,[538] and is commonly added to processed foods.

Shockingly, safflower oil has *zero* omega-3s.

Sunflower oil is the third-highest food source of omega-6s on Earth.[539] It's also commonly added to processed foods.

It also has *zero* omega-3s.

Talk about screwing up omega ratios.

The rest of the refined oils aren't much better. Corn oil is the seventh-highest omega-6 food, cottonseed oil the tenth, and soybean oil the eleventh (this is out of *thousands* of foods).[540]

And all these oils are commonly added to processed foods.

If you just see "vegetable oil" on an ingredients list, it usually means soybean oil.[541] As the above chart shows, while not the worst oil, soybean oil is still problematic.

Is it a coincidence that the more benign oils at the bottom of the chart are much less processed than the oils at the top? Food for thought.

Oh, one last thing.

The fat composition of our cell membranes, from red blood cells to neurons, is a reflection of the fats in our diet.[542,543] Some scientists believe that these membrane fats, particularly the *omega* membrane fats, are a major determinant of our metabolic rate.[544] There's also evidence that dietary imbalances of fatty acids can lead to depression,[545,546] aggression,[547] bipolar disorder,[548] and suicide.[549]

There are many unknowns here, but it's probably not ideal to eat massive, evolutionarily novel amounts of omega-6s.

In other words, it's probably not ideal to include refined vegetable oils in your regular diet.

## "Healthy Fats" in Perspective

Vegetable oils—*all* vegetable oils—have an extremely high calorie density. Replacing the safflower oil in processed foods with coconut oil may be better for our hearts, but it's not the solution to anyone's weight problem.

This is despite the fact that coconut oil is rich in medium-chain triglycerides, which have been shown to increase calorie expenditure and reduce visceral fat compared to other fats.[550,551]

But in the context of processed food, all bets are off.

For example, Bugles are made with coconut oil.

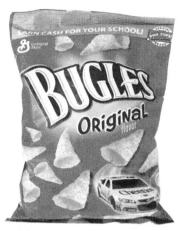

**INGREDIENTS: Degermed Yellow Cornmeal, Coconut Oil, Sugar, Salt,** baking soda, BHT.[552]

Bugles are the only example I've ever seen of a popular processed food made with coconut oil. Still, Bugles are a *processed food*. Combining coconut oil with processed corn, sugar, salt, and a preservative does *not* make for a slimming, healthy whole food.

On the other hand, using a little canola oil to grease your pan of whole foods at home is **not a big deal**. (Despite being highly processed, canola oil has a good omega ratio compared to other refined oils.)

The point is to be aware of a huge problem with processed food (added vegetable oil), not to expunge all traces of vegetable oil from your home while you gleefully bathe your food in butter and coconut oil.

While I normally dislike the word *moderation*, when it comes to added fats of *any* kind (including coconut oil, extra-virgin olive oil, and grass-fed butter), for those of us trying to lose weight, moderation is in order.

Keep that calorie density low.

Between 1980 and 2010, US intake of added fat (mostly vegetable oil) increased by 28%.[553] The trend lines for added-fat intake and obesity during that time are eerily similar:

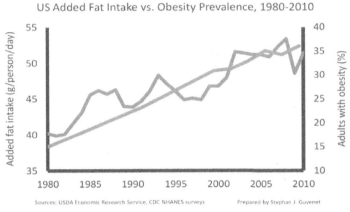

US Added Fat Intake vs. Obesity Prevalence, 1980-2010

Sources: USDA Economic Research Service, CDC NHANES surveys        Prepared by Stephan J. Guyenet

Source: Stephan Guyenet, WholeHealthSource.[554]

## Take-Home

Added fat is as fattening and widespread as added sugar. Unlike added sugar, added fat is easy to spot on ingredients lists—it almost always ends with *oil*.

Anytime you see *oil*, remember why it's there.

To make that food taste better.

So you'll eat more of it.

# 15

# WHITE FLOUR SHOWER

Can we ever forget this?

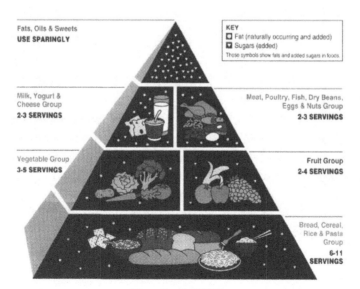

Photo Credit: USDA

The USDA Food Pyramid stood from 1992 to 2005.[555] It helped shape the nutritional beliefs of hundreds of millions of people. For more than a decade, we saw *Bread, Cereal, Rice, & Pasta* sprawled across the most valuable nutrition real estate on Earth: the base of the Food Pyramid.

But from the very beginning, the Pyramid had prominent critics.[556]

The logic of the thing seemed to be that the foods got healthier as you went down. At the very top were *Fats, Oils & Sweets.* These got the skull-and-crossbones, **USE SPARINGLY** treatment.

Below them was a healthier (or perhaps less *un*healthy) category: a hodgepodge of animal foods, beans, and nuts. We were semi-scolded to stick to just *2-3 Servings* of these guys per day.

Below that level was clear-cut Health Land: fruits and vegetables. Surely we couldn't go wrong here. But since vegetables (*3-5 Servings*) commanded a slightly larger range than fruit (*2-4 Servings*), veggies appeared to be the slightly healthier plant.

But even they couldn't hold a candle to what lay beneath: the *6-11 Servings* of *Bread, Cereal, Rice, & Pasta* at the broad base of the Pyramid.

*11 servings.* That's bigger than the small end of every other food group in the Pyramid's range, *combined.*

Based on the Food Pyramid, a sensible person might easily conclude that grains are the healthiest food on Earth.

And not just *whole* grains. The Pyramid didn't lift a finger to distinguish between whole and refined grains. A young child, a Martian, or even an unsuspecting adult may have reasonably concluded that *refined* grains were among the healthiest foods on Earth.

## MyPlate

Apparently the Pyramid was built on shifting sands. In 2011, the USDA retracted the Pyramid and introduced a brand-new structure: *MyPlate*. It sang a slightly different tune.

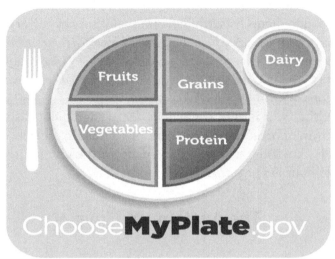

Photo Credit: USDA

On the more intuitive *Plate*, all food groups have their territory. The mighty Kingdom of Grains was invaded by vegetables, which now hold a *slight* size advantage (though this may be an optical illusion). Still, *Grains* rule a vast territory—clearly bigger than *Fruits*, *Dairy*, or the nebulous *Protein*.

And still, there isn't the faintest whisper of "whole," "refined," or any trace of dividing line. Just *Grains*.

As of this writing, this plate remains the USDA's official diet advice. Let's learn more about the refined grains our institutions are so soft on.

## White Flour in the Wild

It's not unusual for a person to start their day with a bowl of cereal or a bagel, eat a sandwich for lunch, and have some pasta for dinner. Not unusual at all.

This rather usual person just ate white flour at every meal. (Not counting the cookie for dessert.)

And this is partly why it's not unusual for a person to be overweight. Not unusual at all.

On ingredients lists, white flour usually goes by *wheat flour*, *enriched flour*, *bleached flour*, or *enriched bleached flour*. It's basically any *flour* except *whole-wheat flour*. ("Wheat flour" is white flour.[557]) *Corn starch* and *degermed corn meal* are the corn versions of white flour. (Avoid them, too.)

White flour is also a staple *outside* of ingredients lists, in the form of bread, pasta, crackers, pizza dough, pretzels, and bagels. Anything at a bakery is made with white flour, and white flour is in *countless* snack foods.

## The Anatomy of Flour

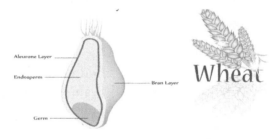

*The parts of a whole grain.*
Photo Credit: Tefi/Shutterstock.com

There are three parts to a whole grain. The *bran* is the outer protective shell, the *germ* is the seed, and the *endosperm* is the starch that the seed uses for energy to grow.

Refined grains—like white flour—are pure endosperm.

The endosperm is low in nutrients compared to the bran and the germ. It's basically just starch.

For example, the *aleurone layer* is a thin coat surrounding the endosperm. It has *25 times* the mineral content of the endosperm.[558] But along with the bran and the germ, the aleurone layer is removed in the process of making white flour. In refining whole wheat into white flour, here's how much the following nutrients are *reduced*:

| NUTRIENT | REDUCTION |
|---|---|
| folate | 41% |
| selenium | 45% |
| calcium | 56% |
| copper | 65% |
| iron | 67% |
| phosphorus | 70% |
| potassium | 71% |
| zinc | 73% |
| niacin | 75% |
| riboflavin | 76% |
| thiamin | 76% |
| manganese | 83% |
| magnesium | 84% |
| vitamin K | 84% |
| vitamin B6 | 89% |
| vitamin E | 92% |

Source:[559]

It's a bloodbath. In a vampiric transformation, nutrient-rich whole wheat is reborn as nutrient-poor *white flour*—and often bleached a ghostly white with chemicals like benzoyl peroxide.[560]

Why go through all this trouble to suck out nutrients? Well, fitting the vampire theme, it's partly done to give grains a nearly *immortal* shelf life. The bran and germ have fats that cause whole-grain flour to spoil rather quickly. So they're sucked out to extend shelf life—and profits.

## "Enriched"?

Before 1870, the only widely available wheat flour was stone-ground, whole-wheat flour.[561] Entire populations of poor people subsisted almost exclusively on whole-wheat bread made from stone-ground, whole-wheat flour.

Then, in 1870, new milling technology replaced the old stone grinders, and whole-wheat bread was replaced with... *white bread.*

For the poor, white bread became the new staple.

Very quickly, diseases like pellagra became widespread.[562,563]

Pellagra is caused by a deficiency in niacin, a B-vitamin that's high in whole-wheat flour and low in white flour. Pellagra causes the four *D*s—diarrhea, dementia, dermatitis, and death.

In the 1940s, as nutritional knowledge grew, governments began to require that white flour be fortified with B-vitamins and iron. This proved to be effective, eradicating diseases like pellagra.[564] White flour is still fortified or "enriched" with these synthetic vitamins today.

Problem solved? That's questionable. On the one hand, enriched white flour is certainly preferable to un-enriched white flour if you're forced to live on bread.

But this rather puny merit doesn't make it healthy.

Compared to whole wheat, even *after* enrichment, white flour is still low in magnesium, phosphorus, potassium, zinc, copper, manganese, and selenium.[565,566]

And this is *assuming* that artificial vitamins are just as healthy as natural vitamins. Enrichment is, more or less, the same as crushing up a vitamin pill and sprinkling it on food.

Eating isolated, artificially concentrated, lab-synthesized

vitamins is almost certainly not the same as eating the natural vitamins found in food. Natural vitamins have natural chemical contexts that probably have important synergistic, activating effects on the vitamins—effects that are lost in vitamin pills and enriched foods.

A 2013 editorial review in *Annals of Internal Medicine* was titled "Enough is Enough: Stop Wasting Money on Vitamin and Mineral Supplements."[567] This review was conducted by five MDs who analyzed 27 controlled vitamin trials with over 400,000 participants.

They concluded: "There was no clear evidence of a beneficial effect of supplements on all-cause mortality, cardiovascular disease, or cancer."[568]

In other words, **vitamin and mineral supplements did nothing to reduce cancer, heart disease, or death**.

They went on:

> *Evidence involving tens of thousands of people randomly assigned in many clinical trials shows that β-carotene, vitamin E, and possibly high doses of vitamin A supplements increase mortality and antioxidants, folic acid and B vitamins, and multivitamin supplements have no clear benefit.*[569]

Taking vitamins was not only worthless, but possibly harmful. They continued:

> *The case is closed—supplementing the diet of well-nourished adults with (most) mineral or vitamin supplements has no clear benefit and might even be harmful. These vitamins should not be used for chronic disease prevention. Enough is enough.*

Americans spent $28 billion on dietary supplements in 2010.[570]

Other than preventing gross deficiency in malnourished populations, there is no clear evidence that the synthetic vitamins found in vitamin pills, supplements, and enriched foods are doing anything healthy.

## The Evidence Against Refined Grains

Refined grains like white flour are not associated with the same heart-healthy effects as whole grains.[571] A 2017 meta-analysis of prospective studies found that refined grains had *none* of the death-preventing benefits of whole grains (which were significant).[572]

Another 2017 meta-analysis of prospective cohort studies found that refined grains were associated with diabetes.[573]

White flour has significantly less protein than whole-wheat flour, and only about a quarter of the fiber.[574,575] In the satiety study we saw before, the satiating power of every food was compared to white bread, which served as the baseline. (White bread is made from white flour.) A total of 16 whole foods were tested, and *every single one*, including whole-grain bread and whole-grain pasta, was significantly more filling than white bread.[576]

Popcorn was rated 54% more filling than white bread. Even cookies, jelly beans, and french fries were more filling than white bread.

This lack of filling-ness is why refined grains like white bread have been independently associated with weight gain.[577] In a prospective cohort study of 74,091 women, eating more whole grains was tied to weight loss, while eating more refined grains was tied to weight gain.[578]

Along the same lines, a 2017 randomized controlled trial found that refined grains caused a smaller increase in metabolic rate (the number of calories your body burns) than whole grains.[579]

## Why Governments Love Grains

Here is the official advice on grains from the USDA:

*Most Americans consume enough grains, but few are whole grains. At least half of all the grains eaten should be whole grains.*[580]

This advice seems reasonable, and dietitians echo it almost verbatim. But let's break it down.

*At least half of all the grains eaten should be whole grains.*

This statement implies that eating grains is a foregone conclusion, and that eating *refined* grains is nearly unavoidable—like death and taxes. It might as well say, "We know you're going to eat refined grains, but just TRY to make sure half your grains are whole."

Not eating refined grains in your regular diet doesn't take some kind of Spartan self-denial. It's actually pretty doable.

And it's much healthier.

According to official US nutrition advice, though, you can eat large amounts of refined grains on a regular basis. After all, if you eat lots of grains, and half of them are refined, you're still following the official advice to a *T*.

But that doesn't mean you're doing good. No competent nutritionist would give refined grains that big of a pass. They'd be far more likely to lump them into the old **USE SPARINGLY** doghouse at the top of the Food Pyramid.

So why does our government look the other way on refined grains?

A big part of the reason government institutions tell us to eat grains, both whole and refined, has nothing to do with health science. And I'm not talking about powerful corporate interests, either. There's something even more important at stake: *national food security*.

It's not easy overseeing the food supply of hundreds of millions of people. And the most important food issue to big governments isn't that their people are eating as healthy as possible. Instead, the most important food issue to big governments is that their people aren't starving to death.

To their credit, governments want food supplies to be as stable as possible to prevent the chronic undernourishment experienced by 795 million people worldwide.[581]

Lest we think hunger problems are unique to Africa, there were 49 million Americans living in food-insecure households in 2013—over 15% of the population.[582,583] And with our population growing by one every 15 seconds,[584] this situation isn't likely to improve anytime soon.

Why does this matter? Because grains, *especially* refined grains, are uniquely suited to feed the masses and prevent starvation.

Healthy whole foods like fruits, vegetables, dairy products, and meat have to be refrigerated. Refined grains don't.

Refined grains can also be stored for much longer periods than whole foods (including whole grains[585]) without spoiling.

Furthermore, refined grains are much cheaper than whole foods. And unlike added sugar and vegetable oil, refined grains are actually somewhat capable of sustaining human life.

For reasons like these, grains make up a whopping 45% of all the calories eaten in the world.[586] (The combined total of produce, meat, dairy, and eggs is only 28%.)

There's simply no way to feed everyone on this planet without grains—including refined grains.

Because of this, *regardless of health science*, most governments won't put forth a clear message to avoid refined grains. Their hands are tied. They need their people eating refined grains if they want to feed everyone.

The point is, a food's healthiness is just *one* factor that goes into official dietary guidelines. Other factors like availability, affordability, geographical context, and cultural context are all explicitly factored into official dietary guidelines,[587] which are written with population-wide practicalities in mind—like preventing starvation, not optimizing your health. **Dietary guidelines aren't written to optimize your health.** So take them with a grain of salt. (And for an example of *good* government dietary guidelines, read Brazil's.[588])

## Take-Home

No one is adapted to white flour. Like added sugar and vegetable oil, white flour is ubiquitous today, but has only been widely eaten for under 200 years.

On ingredients lists, white flour usually goes by *wheat flour*, *enriched flour*, *bleached flour*, and *enriched bleached flour*. Any *flour* not preceded by *whole* is white flour. (And if whole-grain flour is followed by other ingredients, it's a processed food.) Read ingredients lists.

> **processed food** *n* : *a food with an ingredients list longer than one item*

*Outside* ingredients lists, white flour looks like this:

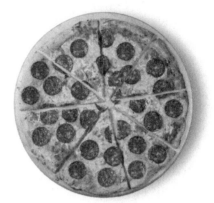

Photo Credit: adidads4747/Shutterstock.com

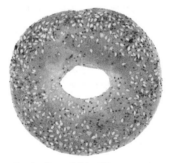

Photo Credit: DenisMArt/Shutterstock.com

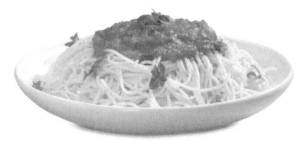

Photo Credit: dinceras/istockphoto.com

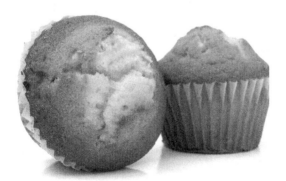

Photo Credit: Hong Vo/Shutterstock.com

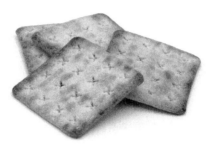

Photo Credit: tonephoto/Shutterstock.com

I know, I know. These are some of my favorite foods.
But don't worry.
You only have to give them up *most* days.

# 16

# THE PROBLEM WITH PROCESSED MEAT

Many meats are wrongfully accused. We'll get to them later. But *processed meat*—meat that has been modified to enhance its taste or shelf-life, usually by salting, smoking, or curing—deserves its awful reputation.

A 2013 study of meat intake in 448,568 people concluded that processed meat causes 3.3% of all deaths.[589] In fact, processed meat is consistently associated with worse health outcomes than *any other food*.[590,591] The associations between processed meat and heart disease, cancer, and death are consistent and strong.[592,593]

Confounding variables be damned: it's flat-out irresponsible to ignore the association data on processed meat.

## Salted to the Max

The main problem with processed meats is that they're chock-full of salt. Reasonable amounts of ham, bologna, salami, sausage, cold cuts, hot dogs, and bacon (all processed meats) tend to have very large amounts of salt.

Here's the salt content in 100 grams (around 200-400 calories) of the following processed meats.

| processed meat | sodium content |
| --- | --- |
| salami | **60%** |
| bologna | **45%** |
| ham | **63%** |
| bacon | **35%** |
| hot dog | **48%** |

*(% daily reference value)*

Sources:[594,595,596,597,598]

Eat these foods until you're full, and you'll eat huge amounts of salt.

Using your salt-shaker is one thing, but regularly eating heavily salted meats is probably a bad idea. Aside from potentially causing heart problems,[599] all this added salt makes food more palatable, and more likely to be overeaten.[600]

Especially when you consider the next factor.

## Protein Deficient

Protein is the most filling macronutrient.[601] Gram for gram, calorie for calorie, protein fills you up more than fat or carbs. This is why it's good to eat high-protein foods when you're trying to lose weight—you'll be fuller on fewer calories, so you'll probably eat less.

But processed meats are lower in protein and higher in fat than unprocessed meats. Check it out.

| meat | protein | fat |
|------|---------|-----|
| chicken breast | 21 grams | 9 grams |
| bologna | 10 grams | **28 grams** |
| bacon | 12 grams | **45 grams** |
| hot dog | 11 grams | **30 grams** |

*per 100 g.* Sources:[602,603,604,605]

Bologna, bacon, and hot dogs have less than *half* the protein and more than *triple* the fat of chicken breast. And that's chicken breast *with the skin*, not boneless-skinless. (You don't have to be an ascetic monk.)

When you combine more fat, less protein, and gobs of salt, you get a food that's highly likely to be overeaten.

## Nitrite

Another issue with processed meats is *nitrite*. Nitrite is a preservative added to processed meat to kill bacteria and enhance color. Every cured meat has nitrite.[606]

While nitrite isn't harmful by itself, under certain conditions it can produce *nitrosamines*, which *are* harmful. These are some of the major carcinogens in tobacco smoke.[607]

Conditions that favor nitrosamine formation include high heat, the acidic conditions of the stomach, amino acids, and heme iron[608]—all of which are present in the production and consumption of processed meats.

Nitrosamines are believed to be one of the reasons eating processed meat is associated with several cancers.[609,610]

## Partners in Crime

We haven't even mentioned the *worst* processed meats. For instance, Panda Express is America's largest Chinese-food chain.

Here's how their "orange chicken" is made:

> *Preparation of the dish begins in the factory, where the meat is processed, battered, fried, and frozen… oil and salt are added as well… More salt and spices are added before the battered chicken nuggets are prebrowned in soybean oil, frozen, then shipped out to Panda Express outlets around the country. At the restaurants, the meat is deep-fried in oil for at least five minutes just before it's served. The accompanying chili sauce strikes all three points of the food consultant's compass, with sugar, salt, and soybean oil complementing the vinegar and spices.*[611]

-David Kessler, *The End of Overeating* (2010)

Such processing isn't uncommon with processed meats.

Buffalo wings are commonly fried in refined vegetable oil at the production plant before they're shipped out to restaurants, where they're fried in refined vegetable oil *again* before serving.[612]

Chili's "Margarita Grilled Chicken" sounds like a reasonably healthy choice. But this chicken was processed with a sugar-and-salt marinade that not only *coats* the chicken, but was actually sucked *into* the chicken by a big machine that looks like a cement mixer.[613]

Another common trick to get these sugar-salt marinades into restaurant meat is *needle injection*, in which hundreds of tiny needles pierce and tenderize the meat.[614] The result is a consistency closer to baby food than actual *meat*—a super-soft texture that's abnormally easy to chew and swallow, and abnormally tasty. (Think of restaurant chicken versus home-prepared chicken.)

This is why it's best to avoid restaurants most days of the

week. It's very hard to tell how restaurant food was prepared. And restaurants have every incentive to make their food as tasty as possible.

(Even restaurants with the healthiest intentions.)

In general, what we call "meat" is often breaded (*white-floured*), fried in oil, and slathered in sugar and salt.

Basically all commercial meat sauces have sugar, salt, or both. I'm not aware of any exceptions here. For example, Frank's RedHot has salt.[615] Ketchup, A1 Steak Sauce, and Sweet Baby Ray's have sugar *and* salt.[616,617,618]

On top of all this, meat may be served in a bun or roll, like hamburgers and hot dogs are. Buns and rolls are made of white flour, added sugar, *and* refined vegetable oil.[619,620] (All three.)

Such factors radically shift the macronutrient profile of this "meat." Real meat has zero carbs; it's only made of protein and fat. But "meats" like General Tso's chicken, Chicken McNuggets, and Arby's chicken fingers actually have more grams of *carbs* than protein.[621,622,623]

And these carbs come from the worst possible sources: white flour and sugar.

And they come with loads of salt.

## Take-Home

Processed meat is overly salted, relatively low in protein, relatively high in fat, and textured in an unnatural way. Processed meat is bad on its own, and it's often doused with sugar, flour, and oil to create a fattening monster.

# 17

# THE FAT FOUR: RECAP

You made it. Long ago, we set out to describe the only four foods that are universally bad and fattening for everyone… *The Fat Four*:

## 1. added sugar
## 2. added oil
## 3. white flour
## 4. processed meat

Foods made from the Fat Four taste great, but we've seen how they make us fat and sick. Cutting them from our regular diet helps us get skinny and healthy.

The easiest way to cut them from our regular diet is to avoid foods with more than one ingredient (*processed foods*).

# The Five Golden Weight-Loss Habits

1. Cut out all sugary drinks.

2. Only eat whole foods most days.

**processed food** *n* : *a food with an ingredients list longer than one item*

Until now, it has been mostly bad news.
*Don't eat this.*
*Avoid that.*
It had to be this way. The main reason so many people are overweight is because they regularly eat processed food and drink sugary drinks. Getting in the habit of eliminating processed food and sugary drinks from your regular diet is the alpha and omega of long-term weight loss.

On the flip side, as we'll see, the evidence tells us that people can be slim and healthy on a huge variety of diets—as long as they're made of whole foods.

If your diet is mostly whole foods, you have a good diet. If you regularly eat processed foods, you have a bad diet. Period.

**A good diet is mostly about what you *don't* regularly eat.**

Ultimately, it's about making a choice. What's more important to you: eating processed food every day, or being slim?

For most of us, it's that simple.

Now it's time for the good news.

# 18

# THRIFTY GENES?

The obesity epidemic is often blamed on "thrifty genes." According to this theory, we evolved in a food-scarce environment. When food was actually plentiful, the theory goes, it paid to eat as much as possible, and gain lots of fat.

This fat allegedly helped save us during future famines—famines which no longer come.

Hence, modern obesity.

This theory is often presented as if it were a fact.

But the thrifty-gene hypothesis is directly contradicted by the people of Kitava. The Kitavans are a Melanesian island people who were studied by a team of researchers in the early 1990s. At the time, the Kitavan population numbered about 2300 people.

Interestingly, in this entire population, obesity was nonexistent. No one was fat. Instead, the Kitavans were quite skinny, with average middle-aged BMIs of 18 for women, and 20 for men.[624]

("Overweight" is 25+.)

What did the Kitavans eat? Their diet mostly consisted of fruit and root vegetables.

And here's the thing. According to Staffan Lindeberg, MD, PhD, the lead scientist studying the Kitavans:

> *It is obvious from our investigations that lack of food is an unknown concept, and that the surplus of fruits and vegetables regularly rots or is eaten by dogs.*[625]

The Kitavans, then, had plenty of food. They didn't live in food scarcity. They didn't endure periodic famines that kept them lean. They regularly threw food away.

Nor were the Kitavans terribly active. Based on their average daily calorie expenditure (which was 1.7 times their basal metabolic rate) the Kitvans only fell into the "moderately active" category.[626]

So the Kitavans were neither short on food nor long on exercise.

*And none of them were fat.*

The reason the Kitavans were skinny and we are fat wasn't due to food *quantity*, as the thrifty-gene hypothesis suggests. The Kitavans had all the fruit and root vegetables they wanted.

We have all the processed food we want.

What causes obesity isn't food *quantity*, but food *quality*.

## Hungry Hunter-Gatherers?

It's commonly thought that hunter-gatherers—and by extension, early humans—are in a constant struggle to get enough food. Hunter-gatherers are often depicted as running around all day like chickens with their heads cut off in a desperate and nearly futile attempt to find enough calories to stay alive.

But despite this widespread and rather grim belief, evidence indicates that hunter-gatherers don't actually experience more food shortages than agriculturalists.[627]

They generally have enough to eat.

And critically, this goes for *modern* hunter-gatherers, who have been relegated to marginal environments by encroaching civilization.

*Ancient* hunter-gatherers—the ones that helped shape our genes—likely enjoyed much more food-rich and bountiful environments than their modern kin.

Nevertheless, modern hunter-gatherers only spend about two to three hours a day actively procuring food.[628] For them, getting enough to eat is only a part-time job.

(And as we saw with the Hadza, hunter-gatherers don't necessarily burn more calories than we do, in absolute terms, because we burn more calories at rest.[629])

But most egregiously, perhaps, the thrifty-gene hypothesis sells ancient humans short. In our evolutionary niche, we were apex predators who could make flint-tipped spears, control fire, and were equally capable of subsisting on plants.

We were one of the smartest species alive, with profound environmental knowledge accumulated over hundreds of generations, and much of our collective brainpower devoted to figuring out the most efficient ways to hunt and gather.

Getting enough food was unlikely to have been a regular problem.

## A Theory Unraveled

The thrifty-gene hypothesis completely fails to explain the recent obesity explosion. Widespread obesity really only took off in the late 1970s.[630] But in countries like the United States, it's not like food was scarce in the 1950s and 1960s.

If our genes were really so thrifty, obesity should have exploded as soon as the Industrial Revolution stabilized national food supplies, which happened long before the 1970s.

On a more basic biological level, the thrifty-gene hypothesis is simply implausible. It isn't plausible that humans and other species wouldn't have an innate weight-regulating mechanism to keep their weights in a stable range when food was plentiful.

A species that stuffed itself until it got fat and slow at the first sign of surplus would have been at a major evolutionary disadvantage to one that maintained a lean and healthy weight during times of plenty—and would have gone extinct.

## Eat Until You're Full

To purposely eat less than you want is dreary and unnatural. Eating until you're full is a far more enjoyable, practical, and sustainable way to go through life.

One of the core premises of this book is that if you're eating whole foods, you can eat until you're full, and lose weight.

(Or at the very least, stop gaining weight.)

It's not *food* abundance, but *processed*-food abundance that throws a wrench in our weight-regulating mechanism and makes us fat.

As we'll see, you can eat just about any whole food with impunity.

# 19

# IF DEFENSE OF FAT AND CARBS

First we were taught to fear fat. It kind of made sense, given the name. *Fat* must be fattening, right?

Recently, the tide has turned. *Carbs* are now the fattening, evil macronutrient *du jour*. Carbs are the new fat.

But condemning either fat or carbs is preposterous.

Discounting alcohol (*who can?*), there are only three major calorie sources: fat, protein, and carbs.

Protein is not primarily used for energy.[631]

That leaves only two major energy sources: fat and carbs.

Is it wise to indict one of *two* major energy sources?

## Diets

A 2014 meta-analysis of 48 randomized diet trials concluded:

> *Significant weight loss was observed with any low-carbohydrate or low-fat diet. Weight loss*

*differences between individual named diets were small. This supports the practice of recommending any diet that a patient will adhere to in order to lose weight.*[632]

Both low-fat and low-carb diets can work.

Since there are only *two* major energy sources, any diet that severely restricts either one is likely to be effective. (Though low-carb diets may be more effective than low-fat diets.[633,634])

But while some people can make low-carb or low-fat dieting a lifestyle, for most of us, they're just a short-term thing.

And just because low-fat and low-carb diets *work*, that doesn't make fat or carbs inherently fattening.

In one illuminating study, patients were kept in hospital wards and fed liquid meals of varying amounts of fat, carbs, and protein. Each day, their calorie intake and body weight were measured precisely.

Protein was kept at a flat 15% of total calories, while fat and carbs were varied over huge ranges. Fat was dialed from 0% to 70% of total calories, and carbohydrate was dialed from 15% to 85% of total calories, with various percentages in between.[635]

These diets lasted an average of 32 days.

The main finding? Regardless of the amount of fat or carbs in the patients' diets, **no differences in body weight were found between the diets.**

The only number that mattered? Total calories.

## In Defense of Fat

The Maasai are a cattle-herding African tribe who subsist almost entirely on meat and milk. They eat lots of fat, and lots of saturated fat. Their diet is 66% fat.[636]

This is extraordinarily high. It's roughly *double* the average American's fat intake.[637]

Are the Maasai fat?

If anything, the Maasai are underweight.[638]

Similarly, the Arctic-dwelling Inuit were forced to subsist mostly on aquatic animal food before contact with the industrialized world. Their diet was necessarily high in fat.

Were the Inuit fat? Only four percent of Inuit men were overweight as late as the 1960s.[639]

Along the same lines, modern hunter-gatherers generally eat as much or more fat than Westerners.[640]

They rarely have any sort of weight problems.

This ethnographic evidence indicates that whole-food fat is *not* inherently fattening. While it doesn't mean that slathering your food with butter will help you lose weight, it does indicate that even large amounts of fat in the context of protein-rich whole foods can be compatible with leanness.

In 1998, superstar Harvard nutrition researcher Walter Willett published a review of many nutrition studies in the *American Journal of Clinical Nutrition*. He concluded:

> *Diets high in fat are not the primary cause of the high prevalence of excess body fat in our society, nor are reductions in dietary fat a solution.*[641]

Two decades later, Willett's opinion hasn't changed.[642]

## Low-Fat Diets

Despite popular belief in the low-carb community, low-fat dieting was based on real, legitimate science.

Many controlled trials have found that if people eat as much as they want, they'll eat more—and weigh more—on diets high in fat than diets high in carbs.[643,644,645,646,647,648,649]

(At least in the short term.)

So the low-fat thing wasn't pulled out of thin air.

But there are major caveats. The studies supporting the idea that high-fat diets are fattening generally used processed foods.[650,651,652,653,654] In many of these studies, the fat used to make the diets "high-fat" was vegetable oil.[655,656,657]

Several of these trials featured scones, muffins, and puddings.

Diets with "high-fat" foods like those tell us little about the fat in meat, dairy products, and nuts—the kind ensconced in protein (the most filling macronutrient).

But in typical reductionist fashion, these trials were used as evidence to indict *all* fat. Food companies responded, sucking the fat out of foods (even whole foods), adding lots of sugar, and branding them "low-fat."

To say the least, this didn't stop the obesity epidemic.

In fact, studies have shown that eating foods labeled "low fat" actually causes people to eat more total calories.[658] People may think low-fat foods are healthier, so they have a license to eat more. But "low fat" usually just means "high sugar."

Which means "fattening."

Still, the evidence supporting low-fat diets does show that *added* fat is quite fattening. Many people fixate on refined carbs, oblivious to the dangers of added fat. As we've seen, between 1980 and 2010, soaring obesity rates increased in lockstep with increasing intake of added fat.

Due to its higher calorie density, added fat may be even more fattening than added sugar. (Check ingredients lists for any "oil.") Many processed foods combine added fat *and* refined carbs—the perfect storm for weight gain and obesity.

## In Defense of Carbs

Fruit is almost entirely carbohydrate—mostly sugar. Due to its high sugar content, many nutrition authorities have told us to avoid eating too much fruit. This is full-blown reductionist thinking—"*all fructose bad.*" The idea that fruit is contributing to obesity is incompatible with the theory of evolution, as well as a good deal of scientific evidence.

In fact, it's downright absurd.

Of all the foods we eat today, the most ancient is probably fruit. We've been eating fruit for around 60 million years.[659]

Talk about being adapted to a food.

Fruit has fiber and vitamins, and there isn't a shred of evidence that eating fruit causes weight gain, obesity, or diabetes.

In fact, it's just the opposite. Eating more fruit *reduces* the likelihood of obesity[660] and diabetes,[661] and fruit is very filling.[662]

Despite being perceived as slightly less healthy than vegetables, eating fruit is associated with just as much of a reduction in heart-disease risk and all-cause mortality as eating vegetables.[663]

In the context of fruit, at least, sugar is not fattening. (Note: juice is not fruit.)

So eat as much fruit as your heart desires, any time it desires it. This goes for *any* fruit: watermelon, pineapple, whatever.

There isn't a shred of convincing evidence to do anything else.

Whatever differences may exist between fruits are trivial compared to the difference between any fruit and processed foods.

Aside from fruit, humans may have been eating starch-rich *tubers* as a staple food for over a million years. Some eminent anthropologists believe tubers were so important to our evolutionary success that it was actually cooking *tubers*—not meat—that was the main impetus for controlling fire.[664]

(Potatoes are tubers.)

Tubers are very high in carbs. But despite eating lots of tubers since forever, widespread human obesity is a very recent problem.

But enough theory. We have direct evidence of entire

human societies eating sky-high-carb diets year-round, and being almost universally skinny and healthy.

## The Kitavans

The skinny Kitavans we met last chapter ate a diet of around 69% *carbs*[665]—again, mainly from tubers and fruit.

Were the Kitavans skinny-fat? Did their feathery weights belie some sort of carb-induced health problems?

The evidence suggests a hard *no*.

In Kitava, heart disease and stroke were virtually nonexistent.[666] This is despite over 75% of Kitavans being daily smokers.[667]

You really can't explain the Kitavans away. They ate tons of carbs every day, weren't terribly active, and were thin as rails.

And before you can say "genes," there *were* two cases of abdominal obesity seen in Kitava. Only two. Both bulging bellies belonged to Kitavan men who were only *visiting* Kitava during the study, and were actually living abroad—and eating a processed, "modern" diet.[668]

This suggests that it's the traditional Kitavan diet—*not* great genes—that's the secret sauce.

## The Hadza

We met the Hadza awhile back. They're hunter-gatherers in Tanzania. Similar to the Kitavans, about 68% of the Hadza diet is carbs. Remarkably, about 50% of their diet is *sugar* (mainly from honey and fruit).[669]

Talk about an atomic fructose bomb—every day, for life.

But similar to the Kitavans, the average Hadza BMI is just over 20.[670]

And as we saw, the Hadza aren't lean because they're "burning off" all those carbs.

## The Murapin

The Murapin of Papa New Guinea were a community of farmers and pig-herders who were studied in the 1960s and '70s. This is not a misprint: the average Murapin's diet was *94.6%* carbs, mostly from sweet potatoes.[671]

This amount of carbs is almost sickening. The average Murapin man ate 543 grams of carbs a day—a year-round carbicide. If carbs were the *least* bit fattening, the Murapin would have been morbidly obese.

Were they? At ages 20-29, Murapin men weighed an average of 132 pounds, while Murapin women weighed 112 pounds. And unlike us, their weights *declined* with age.[672]

Heart disease was rare among the Murapin, and diabetes was nonexistent.[673] Murapin men ate an average of 2300 calories a day,[674] which is fairly reasonable for a 132-pound man.[675]

It's not like they were starving or something.

And there you have it. Three living, breathing human populations who ate cartoon amounts of carbs, were thin as rails, and healthy as horses.

Despite what many people say about carbs, most epidemiological studies show that the higher the proportion of carbs in someone's diet, the *less* they weigh.[676,677]

This doesn't prove that eating more carbs will make you thin. But it does indicate that carbs don't inherently make people fat.

## Keto?

Ketogenic ("keto") diets are currently quite popular. Keto diets are high in fat and very low in carbs, and they seem to work for many people.[678] The name derives from *ketosis*, a state that can happen on very-low-carbohydrate diets where the body switches to burning mostly fat for energy.[679]

Burning fat may sound like a sure-fire way to lose fat, but it really isn't. Just because you're *burning* fat for energy doesn't mean you're *losing* fat; the fat could just as easily be coming from your diet rather than the fat on your body. People confuse these two. Unless you're in a calorie deficit, you won't lose any fat—even if you're in ketosis. Indeed, a strictly controlled 2006 trial found that ketosis had "no metabolic advantage" over a non-ketogenic, low-carb diet.[680] A 2016 trial found that, compared with a high-carb diet with equal calories, a ketogenic diet was "not accompanied by increased body fat loss."[681]

Studies *have* found that ketogenic diets lead to less hunger,[682] which can certainly lead to fat loss over time. Most importantly, perhaps, nearly every junk food has carbs. When you eliminate all carbohydrates, you eliminate all processed junk food. And it's this elimination of processed junk food, *not* the alleged metabolic magic of ketosis, that's the main reason for keto's success.

## Take-Home

The Maasai weren't eating *fat*, they were eating meat and drinking milk. The Murapin weren't eating *carbs*, they were eating sweet potatoes. The Hadza weren't eating *sugar*, they were eating fruit and honey.

The Kitavans weren't eating *starch*, they were eating tubers.

Natural whole foods like these—the kind we've been eating for millions of years—aren't fattening.

*Carbs aren't fattening.*

*Fat isn't fattening.*

**Don't worry about fat or carbs.**

Instead, worry about *processed* fat (vegetable oil) and *processed* carbs (white flour and added sugar) in *processed* food (food with more than one ingredient).

Those are the only fat and carbs to worry about.

# 20

# IN DEFENSE OF WHOLE GRAINS

## Grains and Evolution

Evolution is the foundation of nutrition, and we've evolved a lot in the last 10,000 years. (See "Paleo Fantasies.")

But we seem to have been eating grains since long before then. In 2009, evidence emerged that humans were processing grains with primitive tools as long as 105,000 years ago.[683]

You could counter that grains were probably still an inconsistent and trivial food source until widespread agriculture, but that's just speculation. We simply don't know the extent that people ate grains (which have to be threshed and winnowed before you can eat them[684]) during the Paleolithic Era.

And considering that the alleged start-date for grain-eating was recently pushed back roughly *ten*-fold, it seems highly dubious to make grain claims based on assumptions about what our distant ancestors ate.

## Fossil Evidence

One thing seems certain: being a farmer at the dawn of agriculture was a miserable time to be alive. Humans went from eating a varied, nutrient-rich diet to eating a diet based on one or two grains. Compared with their ancestors, early farmers had more nutrient deficiencies, more infectious diseases, more dental diseases, and more skull deformities.[685]

We see this in the fossil record. Early farmers were strikingly shorter than hunter-gatherers.[686]

(Stunted growth is a sign of malnourishment.)

In fact, humans have only recently recovered their height from cavemen days. In 3000 BC, the average man was 5-foot 3.[687] In ancient Rome, he stood around 5-foot 5.[688]

Today, he stands about 5-foot 9.

Crowding and lifestyle changes likely played a role, but the primary suspect behind the nasty changes following the transition to agriculture is *diet*.

If anything, though, the health problems of early farmers indicate a strong selective pressure to *tolerate* grain-based diets. People who couldn't thrive on grains were more likely to die, while people who did well on grains were more likely to live—and pass on their genes.

And the gene pool adapted. Grain-based diets may not have been ideal for the first farmers, but selection and adaptation eventually made grains a lot healthier for their descendants.

The problem is, not everyone descends from farmers.

Today, grains seem to be healthy for a great number of people—but not everyone. The selective pressure for grains wasn't uniform, and different populations have been eating different grains to very different extents ever since the dawn of agriculture.

Some populations hardly ate grains at all. The Saharawi of North Africa have only been eating wheat as a staple for the last century. Their rate of Celiac Disease—a disease of intolerance to certain grains—is six times the global average.[689]

As we saw, Navajo Indians only started farming about 1,000 years ago, and are 250% more likely to get diabetes than people of European descent. Australian Aborigines never really started farming at all, and they're 400% more likely to get diabetes than other Australians.[690]

Most diabetes is characterized by abnormally high blood sugar, and these pronounced population differences in diabetes rates may reflect relatively poor adaptation to the blood-sugar spikes following digestion of the starch in grains.

Blanket advice to base your diet on grains is probably misguided.

## Issues with Grains

Grains are high in something called *phytic acid*, which interferes with mineral absorption.[691] Phytic acid can disrupt minerals from being absorbed in both the grains themselves and *other* foods present in the GI tract at the same time.[692] Mineral deficiencies are very common. Around two billion people suffer from iron deficiency.[693]

For thousands of years, people fermented bread in ways that significantly reduced phytic acid.[694,695] Some whole grains are still prepared in such traditional ways today, but most aren't. This can be a problem if your diet is based on industrial whole wheat, which is already lower in minerals than it used to be.[696]

Wheat, in particular, has been embroiled in controversy. Despite being endorsed by heavy-hitting health institutions like the CDC and AHA,[697,698] best-selling books blame a host of health problems on wheat.

While these concerns are overblown, they have some points. Gluten is the major protein in wheat. Gluten helps bread rise.

It also causes a host of problems in the one percent of all people with Celiac Disease, as well as the estimated six to seven percent of all people with gluten sensitivity.[699]

Gluten sensitivity is real. It can cause digestive problems, fatigue, rashes, headaches, and neurological problems.[700,701]

If you have digestive issues or other mysterious ailments, it may be worth going gluten-free for a month to see if you feel better.

But for the vast majority of us, gluten is probably nothing to worry about. And whether you're sensitive to gluten or not, a "gluten free" label certainly doesn't make a food healthy.

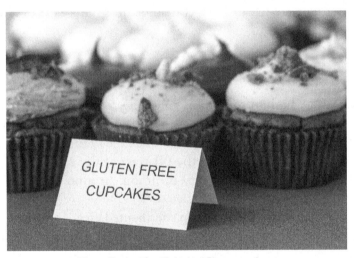

Photo Credit: Teri Virbickis/ Shutterstock.com

## Pulverized Flour Dust

A bigger issue with wheat, and flour-based grains in general, is the way flour is made. Until 1870, basically all wheat flour was ground between two big stones. Today, the vast majority of whole-grain flours are mechanically pulverized at high temperatures into ultra-fine powders made of much smaller particles than the particles in stone-ground flours of old.[702]

When all the work of chewing and breaking down a food is already done for you, the food isn't as filling. That's partly why liquid calories are less filling than solid ones, and why whole foods are more filling than processed foods.

Most commercial whole-grain flours are hyper-pulverized, and studies have shown that pulverized whole-grain flours are less filling[703] and cause greater insulin spikes than traditional, coarse whole-grain flours.[704,705]

The difference in calorie density between modern whole-grain flour and white flour is only about seven percent.[706] This may explain why a 2017 randomized trial found that whole-grain bread didn't lead to significantly better health outcomes than white bread.[707]

While whole-grain flours are *technically* whole foods, they're more processed than rice, oats, corn, and quinoa. These other grains are digested more slowly, are more filling, and are probably better for weight loss.

And of course, all of this applies to *actual* whole grains. The "whole grain" label is pervasive, deceptive, and shameless.

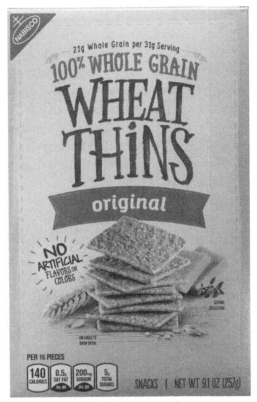

Photo Credit: Shutterstock.com

**INGREDIENTS**: Whole Grain Wheat Flour, **Soybean Oil**,
**Sugar**, **Cornstarch**, **Malt Syrup** (from Corn, and Barley), **Salt**,
**Refiner's Syrup**, Leavening (Calcium Phosphate and Baking
Soda), Vegetable Color (Turmeric Oleoresin, Annatto Extract).[708]

Is "Thins" a reference to the thin wafers? Or is it a subtle hint
that they'll make *us* thin? This double-entendre wasn't lost
on the marketing Michelangelo who came up with "Wheat
Thins."

The first ingredient in Wheat Thins is whole-wheat flour.

The next six ingredients are refined vegetable oil, added
sugar, white flour, added sugar, salt, and added sugar.

In that order.

In general, package claims like "Made with 100% Whole Grains" are absolutely meaningless. The first ingredient may be a whole grain, but it's often followed by added sugar and oil. This goes double for any kind of bread. (It's very rare to find a *true* whole-grain bread.) *Read ingredients lists.*

## Rice

What about rice? In a 2013 meta-analysis of randomized controlled trials involving whole grains and weight loss, brown rice was the only grain that decreased bodyweight compared with a control.[709] The fossil record indicates that early farmers transitioning to a diet based on rice may have had fewer health problems than farmers transitioning to other grains.[710]

Rice doesn't have gluten, after all.

*White* rice is relatively low in nutrients, but it's also low in anti-nutrients like phytic acid.[711] In the satiety study, white rice was rated 38% more filling than white bread.[712] In China, white rice has long been a staple food,[713] and Chinese people have been characteristically lean.

Still, eating lots of white rice may not be ideal. A 2012 meta-analysis of association studies found that people who ate more white rice got more diabetes.[714]

White rice has much less fiber than brown rice.[715,716]

At the end of the day, white rice is still a refined grain. (Though it's almost certainly better than white flour.)

## Grain Studies

Whole grains are generally associated with a slew of positive things—like less heart disease, lower diabetes risk, less weight gain, and lower odds of death.[717,718] There are many confounding variables here,[719,720] but this data indicates that whole grains are compatible with good health, and are probably much healthier than some people claim.

While most randomized controlled trials on grains have been short-term and had relatively few subjects, these trials do seem to indicate that whole grains have beneficial health effects for many people,[721] including less weight gain[722] and lowered body fat.[723]

(At least compared to refined grains, anyway.)

## Are Grains Optimal?

*Blue Zones* are populations of the longest-lived people on Earth. And Blue Zone populations tend to eat grains.[724] There are many other factors at play here, but this tells us that grains are compatible with a very long life.

On the other hand, scientists have studied many populations that effectively *never* ate grains, many of whom were in superb health.[725,726]

So we don't *need* grains to be healthy.

At the end of the day, whole grains are like any other whole food: generally healthy, but not essential.

## Take-Home

If you lived through the Food Pyramid, it's important to realize that grains aren't a requirement for human health. There is nothing uniquely essential about whole grains (let alone refined grains). There is no vitamin or mineral in grains that you can't get from other foods, usually in higher amounts.[727]

Compared to other whole foods, flour-based whole grains like bread are generally subpar, due to the dust-like particle size of the flour.

And there's lots of junk food masquerading as "whole-grain."

*Read ingredients lists.*

Still, an objective look at the science tells us that whole grains like oats, corn, quinoa, and brown rice are full-blown health foods.

(For most people, anyway.)

# 21

# IN DEFENSE OF NUTS

Nuts are an ancient, high-fat whole food. Traditional weight-loss rhetoric is anti-nut, with the standard advice being to consume nuts very moderately or to outright avoid them.

As we've seen, though, there is nothing inherently fattening about fat. It's one of only two basic energy sources.

Nuts are often declared "high" in calories. But this is thinking about it all wrong. We all eat thousands and thousands of calories each week. These calories *have* to come from somewhere. What's important is the *quality* of calories you're eating. If you eat high-quality whole foods like nuts—which are filling,[728] and have fiber, protein, and lots of minerals[729,730]—this will naturally restrain the *quantity* of calories you eat.

Far from making us fat and unhealthy, eating more nuts is associated with both weighing less[731] and dying less.[732] And clinical trials show that nuts don't lead to weight gain. In fact, they show that nuts lead to slight weight *loss*.[733]

In a 2011 study of 120,877 Americans, eating nuts was associated with more weight loss than eating fruits, vegetables, or whole grains over a period of four years.[734]

But there's a major caveat. If nuts have added vegetable

oil—*which most do,* even if the front packaging says something
like "Whole Cashews"—**they're no longer a whole food, and
all bets are off.**
*Read ingredients lists.*
Nuts have enough natural fat. They don't need any extra
fat added on top.
But as long as there is only one ingredient, go nuts.

## A Fruit-and-Nut Diet

In a very unique study done in 1971, nine Africans were
placed on a diet of nothing but fruit and nuts for six months.
(This is the type of study that would never happen today.)
Over the course of the study, the Africans initially lost weight,
after which, according to the authors, there was a "tendency
for the weights to level off more or less at the 'theoretically
ideal' weight for the subject."[735]
The Africans reported feeling good during the diet.
For someone's weight to level off at their "theoretically ideal"
weight is very, *very* good. This study suggests that humans are
adapted to eating fruit and nuts, and that these foods will help
us reach a healthier body weight.

# 22

# IN DEFENSE OF
# WHITE POTATOES

No edible plant has a more foul reputation than the white potato. Scorned, uttered in the same breath as pizza and candy, nearly banned from school cafeterias,[736] the hapless white potato is a perennial fixture in Pop Nutrition's dog house.

Somewhere along the way, people forgot that white potatoes are whole foods. And that they're *vegetables.* That's right: despite the "starch" label, white potatoes are, botanically, vegetables.[737] They have all the trappings of a vegetable: white potatoes are nutrient-dense, fiber-rich, and antioxidant-packed.[738]

Hat in hand, the humble white potato offers us significant amounts of fiber, vitamin C, vitamin B-6, niacin, thiamin, folate, phosphorus, magnesium, copper, iron, manganese, and potassium.[739] (Per gram, baked potatoes have 54% more potassium than bananas.[740,741])

How did things get so bad for the spud?

## The Glycemic Index

The *glycemic index* (GI) attempts to describe the complex chemical tango between food and blood sugar with a single number. The higher a food's glycemic index, the faster it causes blood sugar to rise.

Apparently, foods with a high glycemic index are bad. Since white potatoes have a very high glycemic index, they must be bad, too, the thinking goes.

But a food's glycemic index is actually a very crude average. There's huge variability in glycemic index numbers between studies,[742] and even more variability in the blood-sugar responses of different people *to identical meals.*[743]

One person's blood-sugar roller coaster is another's lazy river.

In any case, high-glycemic foods usually aren't eaten alone. High-GI carbs are often eaten with fat and protein, which significantly blunt the blood-sugar spike.[744]

And we have evidence of entire societies eating almost nothing *but* high-GI carbs for their entire lives and being healthy and thin, with no obesity and no diabetes.

Like the Murapin, who ate almost nothing but sweet potatoes—which have a high glycemic index and an even higher glycemic load.[745] As we saw, though, the Murapin experienced no heart disease, diabetes, or obesity.

Similarly, the extremely healthy Kitavans ate a lot of high-GI carbs.[746,747] Clearly, high-GI carbs don't inherently make people unhealthy and fat.

If there's any merit to the glycemic index, it's that most of the highest-GI foods are junk foods (like bagels, pizza, and fruit-roll-ups). So it isn't surprising that, on average, people with high-GI diets tend to get more diabetes,[748] or that low-GI diets lead to fairly good outcomes.[749]

But these benefits come from people *eating less junk food*, not fewer sweet potatoes. Overall, the glycemic index is a poor measure of nutritional value. M&M's, ice cream, Snickers bars, and even soda, for instance, have much lower glycemic indices than white potatoes.[750]

If you think that makes these foods healthier than potatoes, I have a bridge to sell you.

A 2016 meta-analysis of 19 randomized controlled trials found that low-GI diets don't cause significantly more weight loss than high-GI diets.[751] Some trials even found that *high*-GI diets cause more weight loss.[752]

A 2013 review of trials where dieters were actually *provided* with the foods they ate—and not simply given guidelines— didn't find any significant benefit of low-GI diets over high-GI diets for various big health markers.[753] Two of the trials even found better blood-sugar results from *high*-GI diets.

But forget the word *glycemic*.

We're talking about potatoes.

A 2016 review of 13 potato studies found that:

> *The identified studies do not provide convinc-*
> *ing evidence to suggest an association between*
> *intake of potatoes and risks of obesity, T2D* [dia-
> betes], *or CVD* [heart disease].[754]

It seems that the high glycemic index of potatoes is nothing to worry about.

However, this review did find that "french fries may be associated with increased risks of obesity and T2D [diabetes]."

And that brings up an important point.

## The Bad Company of Potatoes

A lot of the rotten reputation of potatoes is due to guilt by association. Through no fault of their own, potatoes go great with fat, and have a perfect texture for frying. More than any other plant, white potatoes are smothered with butter, bacon, and salt, and fried in vegetable oil.

This is highly fattening.

Nothing better illustrates the Bambi innocence of white potatoes and the Cruella guilt of added fat than the satiety study from before. Out of 38 common foods—like fruit, beans, lentils, brown rice, porridge, steak, eggs, and fish—the white potato crushed every other food in its ability to instill fullness. The white potato beat the 2nd-place food (ling fish) by 44%.

But potato *chips* were among the least satiating foods in the entire study, scoring even worse than ice cream.[755] Again, a better name for potato chips would be *vegetable-oil* chips. (Most of their calories come from vegetable oil.)

Similarly, "mashed potatoes" usually includes butter and white-flour-laden gravy. But mashed potatoes, potato chips, and french fries are often simply counted as "potatoes" in nutrition studies that happen to show bad things about "potatoes."[756,757]

Potatoes are much better than the company they keep.

## Hot Potatoes

What would happen if you ate tons of potatoes every day for a long time? We have that data.

In a 1927 study, a 142-pound man and a 140-pound woman were put on a diet of potatoes—and allowed to eat freely—for 167 days.[758]

They ended the study at 135 and 136 pounds, respectively—with no ill health effects. The scientists remarked that "digestion was excellent throughout the experiment and both subjects felt very well."

Remarkably, neither of the subjects lost any muscle, even though potatoes were their sole source of protein—and even though the man was very active.

In a study of 77 Peruvian men whose regular diet was mostly

(74%) white potatoes, average body-fat percentage fell in the "fitness" range, according to body-fat charts.[759,760,761]

And these men were eating an average of 3,170 calories a day, so you can't say they were starving or food-insecure or something. In 2010, the director of the Washington State Potato Association went on a 60-day potato diet, during which he ate nothing but white potatoes (20 per day, apparently) to protest his government's restriction of potatoes in school lunches.[762]

He lost 21 pounds, and saw massive drops in his cholesterol, triglycerides, and blood sugar.[763]

Similarly, an Australian blogger claims to have eaten nothing but potatoes for a year and lost 117 pounds.[764] I've encountered several similar stories.

## The Greenest Food on Earth

Unlike green vegetables, which are more like natural vitamins than actual *foods*, the white potato is almost single-handedly capable of sustaining human life.

And that's exactly what it's done.

White potatoes have been the nutritional backbone of entire civilizations, from the Incas[765] to the Irish[766] to the Russians.[767] Potatoes helped underpin the Industrial Revolution in England,[768] with Frederick Engels once comparing potatoes to iron for their "historically revolutionary role."[769]

In *The Wealth of Nations*, Adam Smith, the father of economics, remarked:

> *No food* [but the potato] *can afford a more decisive proof of its nourishing quality, or of its being peculiarly suitable to the health of the human constitution.*[770]

The white potato is the most productive, highest-yielding

food crop in the world.[771] Per acre, potatoes produce considerably more calories than grains.[772]

According to *The Economist*, the white potato:

> *provides more calories, more quickly, using less land and in a wider range of climates than any other plant.*[773]

In a time of great environmental concern and pervasive poverty, this makes white potatoes the greenest food on Earth. The most environment-friendly food choice you can possibly make is to base your diet on white potatoes.

## Take-Home

Where I live, a five-pound bag of potatoes costs two dollars. When you combine this extreme affordability with extreme eco-friendliness, great taste, phenomenal nutritional value, and a time-tested and crucial role in human civilization, you can make a strong case that, far from being fattening and unhealthy, white potatoes are among the best foods on earth.

Your calories have to come from somewhere.

Shouldn't they come from a vegetable?

# 23

# IN DEFENSE OF CHOLESTEROL

You really can't trust official nutrition advice. Case in point: cholesterol. We can learn a lot from cholesterol.

They scolded us about cholesterol for decades. How it was bad to eat because it would clog our arteries. But if you pored over your copy of the USDA's *2015 Dietary Guidelines*—specifically, the science part—you stumbled on this gem:

> *Previously, the Dietary Guidelines for Americans recommended that cholesterol intake be limited to no more than 300 mg/day. The 2015 DGAC will not bring forward this recommendation because available evidence shows no appreciable relationship between consumption of dietary cholesterol and serum cholesterol, consistent with the conclusions of the AHA/ACC Report.* **Cholesterol is not a nutrient of concern for overconsumption.**[774]

(Emphasis mine.)

This is the most official cholesterol advice in the United States. It's *health.gov.*

Translation:

> *Remember how we always told you to cut down on cholesterol? We're not saying that anymore. Science says there's actually no link between the cholesterol you eat and the cholesterol in your blood. As far as we know, you could eat ten egg yolks a day for 20 years without any heart trouble.*

Ten egg yolks a day is no exaggeration. That's what "not a nutrient of concern for overconsumption" and "no appreciable relationship" really mean.

These phrases don't mean that the previous advice to limit cholesterol was sort of on the right track. They don't mean it's best to stick to one egg a day—*moderation* and such.

They don't mean the truth is somewhere in the middle.

Instead, they mean that if you were to eat ten eggs a day for the next 20 years, the top nutrition scientists in the US don't have hard evidence that something bad would happen to you.

This recent shift in official cholesterol thought was a long time coming. We were years behind European countries, as well as India.[775] In hindsight, it should have happened long ago.

If food cholesterol were bad for your heart, then eggs would absolutely and unequivocally be bad for your heart. There is no escaping this logic. One medium egg has a whopping 62% of the Daily Value for cholesterol.[776] And eggs are by far the biggest source of cholesterol in the US diet.[777]

But a 2016 meta-analysis of prospective cohort studies found "no clear dose-response trends" between egg consumption and heart-disease risk.[778] (Eating more eggs *was* associated with a 12% lower risk of stroke.)

Similarly, a 2013 meta-analysis found "no significant association between egg consumption and risk of coronary heart disease or stroke."[779]

Another 2013 meta-analysis found that eating more eggs was "not associated with an increased risk of overall CVD [cardiovascular disease], IHD [ischemic heart disease], stroke, or mortality."[780]

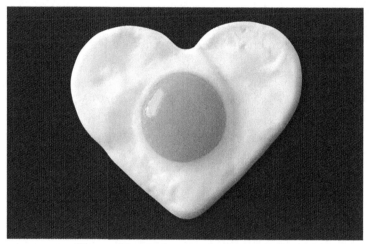

*Clear evidence of an egg-heart association.*
Photo Credit: Marcel Mondocko/Shutterstock.com

You get it:

Eggs are loaded with cholesterol.

↓

Eating more eggs does not cause heart disease.

↓

**Cholesterol does not cause heart disease.**

This kind of ironclad logic led to clear-cut statements by the USDA in the *Scientific Report of the 2015 Dietary Guidelines* that cholesterol is "not a nutrient of concern for overconsumption" and that eating cholesterol has "no appreciable relationship" with blood cholesterol levels.

The matter is settled, scientifically.

But if you read the actual *Dietary Guidelines for Americans: 2015-2020* (which are supposedly based on that *Scientific Report*) you heard a much different tune—a tune of stale myths and stodgy bureaucracy, not modern science.

Let's break down the latest cholesterol advice from *Dietary Guidelines.*[781]

> *The Key Recommendation from the 2010 Dietary Guidelines to limit consumption of dietary cholesterol to 300 mg per day is not included in the 2015 edition...*

So far, so good.

> *...but this change does not suggest that dietary cholesterol is no longer important to consider when building healthy eating patterns.*

Translation:

> *While this is precisely what the removal of the cholesterol cap suggests, we can't just say "we were completely wrong for the past 35 years."*

They go on:

> *As recommended by the IOM,[24] individuals should eat as little dietary cholesterol as possible while consuming a healthy eating pattern.*

Translation:

> *We want this to sound legit, so we'll cite these random IOM guidelines from 2002.*[782] *Hopefully no one checks that reference.*

And finally:

> *In general, foods that are higher in dietary cholesterol, such as fatty meats and high-fat dairy products, are also higher in saturated fats.*

Translation:

> *Despite strong and steadily mounting evidence to the contrary, we're still saying saturated fat is bad—which seems like a decent ad hoc hypothesis for avoiding cholesterol.*

## Egg Nutrients

Like most whole foods, eggs are full of nutrients. But traditional nutrition advice has us ditching the yolk for fear of cholesterol, and only eating the egg white.

The thing is, the vast majority of an egg's nutrients are in the yolk. Let's see the Percent Daily Values for the nutrients in an egg white versus an egg yolk, with the winner in bold:

| nutrient | egg white | egg yolk |
|----------|-----------|----------|
| vitamin A | 0% | 5% |
| vitamin D | 0% | 5% |
| vitamin E | 0% | 2% |
| thiamin | 0% | 2% |
| riboflavin | **9%** | 5% |
| vitamin B6 | 0% | 3% |
| folate | 0% | 6% |
| vitamin B12 | 0% | 6% |
| vitamin B5 | 1% | 5% |
| choline | 0.4mg | **116mg** |
| calcium | 0% | 2% |
| iron | 0% | 3% |
| magnesium | **1%** | 0% |
| phosphorus | 0% | 7% |
| potassium | **2%** | 1% |
| zinc | 0% | 3% |
| copper | 0% | 1% |
| selenium | 9% | **14%** |

Sources:[783,784]

Egg whites are relatively barren. Almost all the nutrients are in the yolk, which beats the egg white in almost every category. The yolk has great stuff like vitamin A, vitamin D (rare in food), and choline—three nutrients Americans don't get enough of.[785,786]

Choline isn't a pop-culture nutrient yet, but it plays important metabolic and neural roles in the body. Choline was crowned an "essential nutrient" by the Institute of Medicine in 1998, and choline deficiency is implicated in liver disease and heart disease, and may play a role in neurological disorders.[787]

Egg yolks are the best source of choline out of any food on Earth.[788] (The yolk has 290 times as much choline as the white.[789,790])

## Eggs in Your Basket

Eggs aren't just highly nutritious and not bad for your heart. Eggs are also one of the cheapest sources of high-quality animal protein out there. I once bought 60 eggs at Walmart for $3.78. They weren't pasture-raised or anything, but there's no sense in letting the perfect be the enemy of the good.

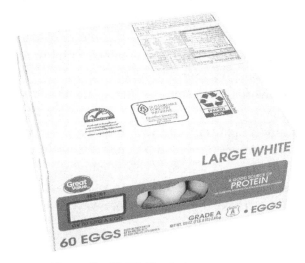

*60 eggs for $3.78. That's six cents an egg.*

A large egg only has 72 calories.[791] For the sake of argument, let's say you're counting calories to lose weight, and eating 1500 calories a day.

And let's say you split your calories into three meals, of 500 calories each.

500 calories isn't much. But one of your 500-calorie meals could hypothetically be *seven* large eggs (504 calories). Does that sound like depriving yourself?

Eggs are filling, which makes them *slimming*. Studies have shown that eggs are more slimming than bagels,[792] for instance. But by condemning cholesterol, authorities condemned eggs, which helped pave the way for bagels, cereal, pop-tarts, Eggo waffles, breakfast bars, and other "low-cholesterol," flour-based junk foods to invade breakfast.

## Cholesterol: As Natural as Water

Far from being a dose-dependent heart toxin, cholesterol is naturally found in the cell membrane of every cell in your body—right next to saturated fat.[793] Cholesterol controls the fluidity of cell membranes, and is an essential precursor to steroid hormones, vitamin D, and bile acids.[794]

In other words, cholesterol is utterly essential to life—so much so that our bodies *make* lots of it every day. That's right. Only around a quarter of all the cholesterol in the average person's body comes from food. The rest is made by the liver.[795]

If you eat more cholesterol, guess what happens? Your liver makes less cholesterol that day.[796] It's a simple, harmless bio-feedback loop. (Like if you drink more water, you pee more.)

## Take-Home

*"Cholesterol is not a nutrient of concern for overconsumption."*

# 24

# IN DEFENSE OF SATURATED FAT

*Fat* was bad enough. Apparently it was fattening. But *saturated* fat was an especially villainous *kind* of fat—an artery-clogging, heart-wrecking disaster.

The worst of the worst.

This epic stigma against saturated fat still exists today. For many people, saturated fat will be forever tainted, regardless of what the latest science may show.

But here goes nothing.

## Utterly Natural

Saturated fat is as natural as things get. Of the 10 billion fatty acids surrounding every one of your cells, the most common type are *phospholipids*. Phospholipids are the basic structural unit of cell membranes. Most phospholipids have a tail made of **saturated fat**.[797] Far from being a dangerous *external* substance, then, saturated fat is an *internal* substance that's a crucial part of our most basic biological unit: the cell. It doesn't get more natural than that.

Well, maybe it does. Human breast milk is high in saturated fat. Around half the fat in breast milk is saturated.[798]

Are moms trying to give their babies heart disease?

## How "Saturated" Became "Bad"

The idea that saturated fat causes heart disease took hold with the Seven Countries Study, a long-term association study published in 1970.[799] This study found that people living in countries that ate more saturated fat had higher blood cholesterol, and got more heart disease.

At first glance, this may seem like solid evidence.

But there were flies in the ointment.

First, the Seven Countries Study only included middle-aged men. This makes it faulty to generalize its results to everyone.

Second, the study had methodological flaws. Foods like cake and ice cream, which are full of added sugar (which is heavily associated with heart disease[800]) were simply counted as "saturated fats."[801]

Third, there were huge discrepancies in the data. For instance, the Greek islands of Corfu and Crete ate the same amount of saturated fat. But the island of Corfu had *16 times* the rate of heart-disease mortality as the island of Crete.[802]

There were clearly other important factors at play.

Finally, the study merely showed a correlation. It wasn't a randomized controlled trial.

Nevertheless, the lead author of the Seven Countries Study, Ancel Keys, was convinced that saturated fat causes heart disease.

Keys was a respected scientist and gifted evangelist who rose to great power in the nutrition world, serving on the board of the American Heart Association and even appearing on the cover of *Time*.[803,804]

In the 21st century, Key's Seven Countries Study is still cited as evidence that saturated fat causes heart disease.[805]

## Cholesterol Fallacies

The bulk of the argument against saturated fat is that it raises LDL cholesterol ("bad" cholesterol).[806] According to this theory, the more saturated fat you eat, the higher your LDL cholesterol will be—and the more likely you'll get heart disease.

This is often presented as if it were a fact.

But as our knowledge of blood cholesterol has expanded, this theory has completely fallen apart.

It turns out that not only are there different types of cholesterol (HDL, LDL), but there are different *subtypes* of these types: there is "good" LDL and "bad" LDL.

Only bad LDL, which is known as "small, dense LDL," is implicated in heart disease.[807,808]

**And saturated fat doesn't raise bad LDL.**[809,810]

Instead, saturated fat raises *good* LDL.[811]

This good type of LDL, which is known as "big, fluffy LDL," is benign. It is not implicated in heart disease.[812]

So while saturated fat *does* raise LDL, it only raises the good kind. And not only that, but it is also well known that saturated fat raises HDL ("good" cholesterol).[813,814] Raising HDL is a very healthy thing. You want high HDL. No one disputes this.

Yet the known fact that saturated fat raises HDL is systematically ignored by dietary guidelines,[815] which also ignore other strong evidence in favor of saturated fat.

In 2003, a meta-analysis of 60 controlled trials concluded

that replacing carbohydrates with saturated fat doesn't have negative effects on blood cholesterol.[816]

And when you look at people in the real world who actually eat a lot of saturated fat, they don't have higher cholesterol than normal.

Let's travel back to a time when people weren't afraid to eat saturated fat. In a telling 1963 study, 99 British men were asked to weigh and record everything they ate.[817] Throughout this time, their blood cholesterol was routinely measured. The men's intake of animal fat—which is high in saturated fat—ranged from 55 to 173 grams per day (a very wide range). The men's blood cholesterol also ranged widely, from 154 to 324 mg/100 ml.

The main finding? The men who ate the most animal fat were no more likely to have high cholesterol than the men who ate the least.[818] In other words, there was no correlation between saturated fat intake and blood cholesterol.

Similarly, a 1976 study of the typical diets and blood cholesterol levels of 2,039 people concluded that saturated fat intake is unrelated to blood cholesterol.[819]

## Nail in the Coffin

Forget about cholesterol. The only reason we even care about blood cholesterol is because it allegedly predicts *heart disease*, right?

So why not skip the middleman—*cholesterol*—and go straight to the source: What's the relationship between saturated fat intake and heart disease?

A 2009 systematic review of 146 prospective cohort studies and 43 randomized controlled trials from 1950 to 2007 found no convincing evidence of a relationship between coronary heart disease and intake of total fat, saturated fat, meat, milk, or eggs.[820]

A 2010 meta-analysis of 21 prospective cohort studies including 347,747 subjects (11,006 of whom developed heart disease) found that eating more saturated fat was "not associated with an elevated risk of CHD [coronary heart disease], stroke, or CVD [cardiovascular disease]."[821]

A rigorous 2011 meta-analysis of randomized controlled trials found that reducing saturated fat had no effect on heart-disease mortality or all-cause mortality.[822] (They found that replacing saturated fat with polyunsaturated fat was beneficial, but replacing saturated fat with carbs was "not clearly protective of cardiovascular events.")

A 2017 meta-analysis of 11 randomized controlled trials on the effect of replacing saturated fat with n-6 polyunsaturated fats found that reducing saturated fat was "unlikely to reduce CHD [coronary heart disease] events, CHD mortality, or total mortality."[823]

According to a 2012 review in the journal *Nutrition*:

> *Results and conclusions about saturated fat intake in relation to cardiovascular disease, from leading advisory committees, do not reflect the available scientific literature.*[824]

A 2013 editorial by an influential cardiologist in *The British Medical Journal* was titled "Saturated Fat Is Not the Major Issue: Let's Bust the Myth of Its Role in Heart Disease."[825]

In 2014, a group of four MD-PhDs and ten other scientists performed a meta-analysis of 32 observational studies and 27 randomized controlled trials. They concluded:

> *Current evidence does not clearly support cardiovascular guidelines that encourage high consumption of polyunsaturated fatty acids and low consumption of total saturated fats.*[826]

To sum up, there seems to be no relationship between saturated fat intake and heart disease. Instead, we have the "French Paradox," which is the observation that French people eat lots of cholesterol and saturated fat, but get relatively little heart disease.[827]

Indeed, this would be quite the paradox if saturated fat and cholesterol caused heart disease.

But it's not a paradox. They don't.

## Saturated Fat: Heart-Healthy?

Given the titanic and decades-long stigma against saturated fat, its lack of correlation with heart disease is somewhat surprising.

People who eat lots of saturated fat are people who ignore official diet advice. While some of them may be otherwise healthy people who pored over the primary nutrition literature and decided the official advice on saturated fat was incorrect, most of them are probably not very concerned with eating healthy.

Oftentimes, people who aren't terribly concerned with *eating* healthy aren't terribly concerned with *being* healthy. Indeed, eating more saturated fat has been correlated with smoking,[828] eating fewer fruits and vegetables,[829] eating trans fats,[830] and exercising less.[831]

And those are just the known healthy behaviors that studies can easily track. People who eat lots of saturated fat are probably also less likely to meditate, manage stress, follow their doctor's advice, or do any number of healthy behaviors that studies can't fully account for.

But even with this dark confounding storm cloud over its head, saturated fat *still* isn't correlated with heart disease. It may be that saturated fat is slightly *protective* against heart disease. Who knows?

A 2010 Japanese study followed 58,453 men for 14 years.[832] Not only did the men who ate the most saturated fat have a slightly lower risk of heart disease, they also had the lowest risk of stroke out of all the men in the study. Stroke is the leading cause of death in Japan.[833] Saturated fat may not only be harmless, but healthy. But that's just speculation. The safest conclusion is that saturated fat is harmless.

## Saturated Fat and Obesity

From 1970 to 2000, US obesity levels increased by 213%.[834] If saturated fat played an important role here, we'd expect that our saturated fat intake would have increased over that time. Instead, it significantly *decreased*—by 19% in men, and 15% in women.[835]

## Take-Home

Saturated fat is harmless. It doesn't cause heart disease. Just like cholesterol before it, saturated fat will soon officially be labeled *"not a nutrient of concern for overconsumption."*

# 25

# IN DEFENSE OF MEAT

If cholesterol and saturated fat are harmless, most of the argument for avoiding meat goes out the door. This argument was already shaky, though. It contradicts the theory of evolution.

## Meat and Evolution

We are primates. Primates have probably been eating insects for the entire duration of their 66 million years on Earth.[836] Critically, insects are not plants. This means that vegan diets—diets with no animal food—have never been a natural state of affairs.

Take chimpanzees. They're our closest living relatives. Like humans, chimps are particularly violent. If a band of male chimps sees a lone male from another group, their first instinct is to kill him.[837] While chimps mostly eat fruit, they're known to spend hours "fishing" for termites and ants.[838]

And chimps eat meat. Some chimps kill and eat over 150 animals per year in the wild (monkeys, antelope, wild pigs, etc.).[839]

But it seems that humans are even more adapted to eating meat than chimps are. Chimps (and gorillas, orangutans, etc.) have large intestines roughly *triple* the size of ours.[840] Such big, complicated guts are a hallmark of herbivores that eat a lot of bulky plant fiber—like leaves—that we can't digest. On the other hand, carnivores and omnivores tend to have shorter, simpler guts.[841] Humans have smaller, shorter guts than chimps, with relatively bigger small intestines.[842] These differences indicate that we're adapted to a more calorie-dense diet than chimps are—one with less raw plant food and, in all likelihood, more meat.

Take Neanderthals. They're our closest genetic relative, living or extinct.[843] Neanderthals only diverged from us 600,000 years ago.[844] They shared 99.7% of our DNA.[845] In fact, early humans interbred with Neanderthals. Between one and four percent of our DNA is actually *Neanderthal* DNA.[846]

What did Neanderthals eat? According to the protein residues on their bones, they had a diet similar to that of wolves, lions, and hyenas.[847] (For obscure reasons, the same type of analysis isn't feasible with early human bones.[848])

But major meat eating in our lineage started long before Neanderthals. At least 2.6 million years ago, our ancestors began eating meat to an unprecedented extent.[849] Around this time, we began breaking bones, using sharp stone flakes to cut meat from bones, and butchering elephants and other animals that were larger than any we'd eaten before (or that any other primates eat today).[850]

We have no way of knowing the precise proportion that meat took up in the diets of early humans, but we know that meat was definitely on the menu—and to an extent like never before.

This was a big change. It's believed that our big brains and tool usage (the two main drivers of humanity's supreme ascendance) were intimately tied to increased meat eating.[851]

Indeed, the earliest archaeological evidence of clear human behavior includes animal bones and stone flakes.[852]

It makes intuitive sense that blossoming carnivory might have led to a prehistoric intellectual renaissance. Hunting fast animals with spears, strategy, and teamwork takes far more cooperative brainpower than looking for bananas.

This brainpower led to the control of fire. Fire meant *cooking*, and cooking was the prime mover in the high-quality, calorie-dense diets that remodeled our guts. Aside from killing harmful pathogens, cooking makes it easier to digest starch, protein, and meat.[853]

We've been able to control fire for at least 780,000 years.[854] We were probably cooking meat the entire time.

## Just a *Little* Meat?

The rise of humans directly coincided with the mass extinction of large mammalian species.[855] North America lost 35 genera (the level *above* a species) of large mammals between 10,000 and 12,000 years ago[856]—right around the time humans began spreading across the Americas.

This was not a coincidence. Humans probably hunted most of these animals to extinction. And hunting lots of big, lumbering animals to extinction isn't indicative of a species adapted to eating only occasional, petite amounts of lean meat.

An analysis of 229 modern hunter-gatherer tribes found that 73% of them got more than half their calories from animal food.[857] A more systematic analysis of the diets of 10 hunter-gatherer tribes confirmed that most of their calories come from meat.[858]

Meat, then, makes up the majority of the modern hunter-gatherer diet. From this, it seems safe to conclude that meat probably made up a decent proportion of *ancient* hunter-gatherers' diets, too.

Which means that most people today are probably adapted to eating a decent amount of meat.

## Meat in History

While the human diet became a lot more grain-focused after the start of agriculture, we never lost interest in meat. Except for the occasional religious reasons, assuming that meat was available, there isn't a single example in recorded history of a large human population who naturally ate a meatless diet.

If meat was available, people ate it. Eating meat has been utterly pervasive throughout recorded history, and is utterly pervasive today. In fact, meat is an index of a country's economic development. The more developed a country is, the more meat they eat.[859] The only countries that *don't* eat a lot of meat are the ones who can't afford to.

For better or worse, eating meat is in our genes.

## Why Meat Is Healthy

Over the eons, animals adapt to the food they regularly eat. Just as you'd expect, then, there's lots of evidence that eating meat is healthy.

We'll start with the repeated observation that hunter-gatherers—who generally eat lots of meat—get little to no heart disease[860] and little to no obesity (or even overweight).[861]

They also appear to get less cancer.[862]

A common fallacy is that hunter-gatherers don't live long enough to get these diseases. While it's true that the average hunter-gatherer dies quite young (their average life expectancy is only about 21-37 years) this low average is almost entirely due to their extremely high infant and child mortality rates, which are 30 and 100 times higher than ours, respectively.[863]

If a hunter-gatherer makes it to age 45, they can expect to

live another 14 to 24 years, on average. Their most common age of death is 72 years old.[864] And when they die, the most common cause is infectious disease, not heart disease or cancer. Contrary to popular belief, the near complete immunity to obesity and heart disease in traditional populations isn't based on a bunch of 25-year-olds.

For instance, in that Kitavan population where heart disease was nonexistent, there were 138 people between 60 and 95 years of age.[865]

(And heart disease was nonexistent.)

## Healthy Meat-Eaters

Hunter-gatherers are one thing, but what about meat-eaters in the developed world?

As a whole, vegetarians tend to get less heart disease and cancer than meat-eaters.[866] Vegetarians like to attribute this to avoiding meat, but vegetarians also smoke less, drink less, exercise more, and eat more fruits and vegetables.[867,868,869]

To tease out variables like these, one study compared vegetarians to health-conscious meat-eaters. 11,000 subjects (including 4,627 vegetarians) were recruited from health-food stores, health-food societies, and health-food magazine subscriber lists.

They followed everyone for 17 years.

The result? There were no significant differences in total mortality, heart disease, stroke, or cancer between vegetarians and meat-eaters.[870]

(The one exception was that vegetarians got more breast cancer.)

In the context of a healthy lifestyle, then, eating meat appears to be just fine. Most of the world's longest-lived (Blue Zone) populations eat at least a little meat.[871]

And it's worth noting that not all the findings on vegetarian diets have been positive.[872] A 2014 study found that, compared to meat-eaters, vegetarians were more likely to have cancer, allergies, and mental health problems.[873]

## Vitamin B-12

With very few exceptions, vitamin B-12 is only found in animal food.[874,875] For practical purposes, vitamin B-12 does not exist in plants. Vitamin B-12 is important for the health of nerve cells and blood cells, and for DNA synthesis.[876] Adolescents deficient in vitamin B-12 have been shown to do worse on cognitive tests.[877]

(It's a vitamin, after all.)

Even vegetarians—who may eat dairy and eggs—are at serious risk of vitamin B-12 deficiency.[878] One study found B-12 deficiency in 68% of vegetarians, 83% of vegans, and 5% of meat-eaters.[879]

And since the jury is still out on whether vitamin pills and supplements work at all, it's probably unwise to rely on vitamin B-12 pills to replace millions of years of evolution.

Compared to diets without meat, diets with meat also tend to have more zinc,[880] vitamin A,[881] vitamin D,[882] and omega-3 fatty acids.[883]

## Meat Hate

A large part of the anti-meat argument stems from ethics and environmental concerns, highlighting the inhumane and unsustainable nature of industrial meat production.

Indeed, animals in our food system are often treated abhorrently, and meat takes far more energy to produce than plant food.[884] With the human population ballooning like it is, this seems like a non-sustainable business model.

But while these concerns are important, they have nothing to do with health science. Not eating meat may be more ethical and better for the planet, but it isn't necessarily healthier. There seems to be a requirement for animal food in the human diet. Vegetarian diets include animal food, and can be quite healthy. But given what we know about our evolutionary past and vitamin B-12, vegan diets are probably not ideal. Having to plan your diet around supplements to ensure you're not deficient in key nutrients is a good sign of a bad diet.

## Just Don't Overcook It

There are only two kinds of meat to avoid: processed meat, and meat that's been overcooked. When meat has been cooked for a long time at high temperatures (over 300 °F), carcinogens called *heterocyclic amines* are formed, which cause cancer in animals.[885] In humans, eating well-done meats has been linked to colon cancer, breast cancer, and pancreatic cancer.[886] (Heterocyclic amines are much higher in *well-done* meat than *medium-rare* meat.[887])

Another concern with overcooked meats is *polycyclic aromatic hydrocarbons*,[888,889,890] which can be carcinogenic.

Here are some tips for healthy meat-cooking:

- Try using gentler cooking methods (steaming, boiling, baking, etc.).
- If there are black char marks on grilled meat, cut them off before eating.
- If your meat is on a grill or stove, flip it regularly.[891]
- Marinate your meat. This drastically reduces the formation of certain heterocyclic amines.[892,893]
- Try not to grill all the time.

## Take-Home

We've been eating meat for our entire evolutionary past. Like any other whole food, there's evidence that meat is healthy.

This is important, because meat is high in protein and widely considered enjoyable to eat. As long as it's not processed or overcooked, meat is a healthy way to fill the hole left behind from cutting out processed food.

# 26

# IN DEFENSE OF RED MEAT

In the popular imagination, red meat is only a step above cigarettes in the health department. Studies have found that eating red meat is associated with increased heart disease, cancer, and death.[894]

But scientific studies are only as good as their design. In several studies where red meat was associated with negative health outcomes, foods like hot dogs and hamburgers were counted as "red meat." [895,896,897]

By definition, a hot dog or hamburger contains a bun or a roll. Hot-dog buns and hamburger rolls are made of white flour, high-fructose corn syrup, and refined vegetable oil.[898,899] (Three for three.)

And that's not even counting the sugar and salt in ketchup,[900] the fact that hot dogs are highly processed, or that people who eat lots of hot dogs and hamburgers are likely to be unhealthy in general.

In their classification of "red meat," several of these studies included *processed* meats like bacon, sausage, cold cuts, and even "meats in foods such as pizza." [901,902,903,904]

This is important, because processed meat is consistently associated with worse health outcomes than any other food.[905,906]

Further complicating things, even people who eat a lot of *un*-processed red meat tend to eat fewer fruits and vegetables, smoke more, and drink more[907]—the usual unhealthy behaviors of people who throw official diet advice to the wind. A study of 84,555 women found that eating red meat was associated with eating french fries.[908]

## Unprocessed Red Meat

A 2010 meta-analysis deliberately separated red meat from processed meat. It found that eating unprocessed red meat wasn't associated with heart disease or diabetes, while eating *processed* meat led to much higher risks of both.[909]

A 2013 study also deliberately separated red meat intake from processed meat intake—in 448,568 people, over 13 years. Red meat intake wasn't associated with dying of heart disease, cancer, or any other cause. Even people with "very high consumption of red meat" were not more likely to die.[910]

On the other hand, processed meat intake was significantly associated with dying from heart disease, cancer, and other causes.[911]

## Colon Cancer?

We're often told that red meat gives us colon cancer.[912] But a 2011 meta-analysis of 34 prospective cohort studies found that the association between red meat and colon cancer was "weak," "inconsistent," and subject to "the likely influence of confounding by other dietary and lifestyle factors."[913]

(We've talked about those.)

But let's ignore confounding. Let's take the link at face value.

A large European study of almost half a million people

found that people who ate the most red meat had a 35% increased risk of colon cancer.[914]

While 35% may seem like a lot, it amounted to a person's 10-year odds of getting colon cancer increasing from to 1.28% to 1.71%.[915] Even if we assume these percentages are totally free of confounding, is it really worth cutting out a food you enjoy to achieve such a marginal reduction in theoretical risk of colon cancer?

## Take-Home

Unprocessed red meat is not bad for you. As a 2002 study concluded, "in terms of weight loss, elimination of red meat from the diet is unnecessary."[916] But far from just *not* being fattening, red meat can be a huge help for losing weight.

Eating high-protein foods makes people feel fuller, which helps them eat fewer total calories. But the thought of forsaking processed junk food for boneless skinless chicken breasts is neither palatable nor sustainable for most people.

A food like steak, however, is a more acceptable compromise.

# 27

# IN DEFENSE OF MEAT FAT

The theory that fatty meat is fattening and unhealthy is based on the premises that fat is fattening, and that saturated fat is unhealthy.

Neither of these premises is true.

Admittedly, lean meat is great for weight loss. Lean meat is high in protein, and protein is the most filling macronutrient.[917] It's been shown that high-protein diets help people lose weight and keep it off.[918] Lean meat helps keep you full on fewer calories, so it's good to eat a lot of lean meat when you're trying to lose weight.

But that doesn't make fatty meat fattening.

Fatty meat is high in protein, too.

The thing is, you can't live on lean meat. Most of your calories *have* to come from somewhere else. Lean meat is basically all protein. And unlike fat or carbs, the human body has no way to store surplus protein, which must be oxidized or eliminated.[919] This is partly why high-protein diets increase metabolic rate.[920]

Our bodies have a limited ability to process protein. The upper limit of using protein for energy seems to be when protein makes up around 50% of total calories.[921] Someone who weighs 176 pounds can only process about 300 grams of protein per day.[922]

If you ate nothing but boneless skinless chicken breasts, eventually you'd suffer a fate similar to early American explorers who were forced to live on rabbit meat—which is low in fat and high in protein[923]—when no other food was available. This led to a condition known as "rabbit starvation."

According to an early American pioneer forced to live on lean meat during the winter of 1857-1858:

> *We consumed the enormous amount of from five to six pounds of this* [very lean] *meat per man daily, but continued to grow weak and thin, until, at the expiration of twelve days, we were able to perform but little labor, and were continually craving for fat meat.*[924]

Despite eating lots of lean meat at every meal, the explorers constantly felt hungry and restless. They developed severe diarrhea, and many died after several weeks.[925]

In *The Voyage of the Beagle*, Charles Darwin quotes a doctor who says:

> *When people have fed for a long time solely upon lean animal food, the desire for fat becomes so insatiable, that they can consume a large quantity of unmixed or even oily fat without nausea.*[926]

In short, we can't live on lean meat. Protein can't be our only source of calories.

And since fat isn't fattening and saturated fat isn't unhealthy, it's fine if a portion of those other calories come from animal fat. Previously cited studies showing that unprocessed meat (including unprocessed *red* meat) is harmless were *not* specific to lean meat.[927,928]

As long as it's not processed, fatty meat is a high-protein whole food.

## Fattier Than the Past?

Some people argue that the meat we eat today is fattier than the meat from our evolutionary past—and that we shouldn't eat this modern fatty meat.

They're right about one thing: today's factory-farmed, hormone-enhanced meat is probably fattier than its Stone Age correlate.

But it's not that simple. Today, we basically only eat "muscle meat"—meat from an animal's muscle. Muscle meat is what most people call "meat": steak, chicken breast, chicken thigh, etc. Almost all of the meat people eat today is muscle meat.

But early humans were much different. If modern hunter-gatherers are any indication at all,[929] early humans ate the entire animal—including the organs and fat tissue. Many organs are naturally quite high in fat, such as the brain,[930] pancreas,[931] stomach,[932] tongue,[933] and bone marrow.[934]

After a kill, it was common for certain Indian tribes to eat the organs and leave the muscle meat for the dogs.[935]

(The dogs were happy.)

Aside from organs, early humans would have sought energy-dense fat wherever they could find it—like the big chunks of pure fat found in an animal's stomach region (omentum, mesentery), and under its skin (subcutaneous tissue).

We generally don't eat these fat stores today, but early humans surely did. These chunks of fat would have been highly prized, and quite large in some animals—like the many large mammals we hunted to extinction.

So while modern muscle meat may be fattier than Stone Age muscle meat, all the fatty organ meat and pure fat that our distant Stone Age ancestors probably ate makes that an apples-and-oranges sort of comparison.

## Is "Grass-Fed" Worth It?

They say you are what you eat. The same logic would seem to hold for animals: they are what *they* eat. And their meat is probably healthier for us to eat if they were eating healthy food (food they're adapted to).

Cows, for instance, evolved eating grass. So cow meat is probably healthier if the cow was eating *grass* than, say, the grain slushies commonly fed to cattle near the end of their lives. These slushies are usually based on corn or soy, and sometimes include candy, cotton, rice, and other cheap scraps of food.[936]

Compared to grain-fed beef, grass-fed beef has a better vitamin profile and more omega-3s.[937] It's also higher in something called CLA (*conjugated linoleic acid*),[938] which is claimed to help with weight loss.

Grass-fed lamb has similar nutritional advantages.[939] Eggs from chickens raised on pasture are twice as high in Omega-3s and Vitamin E as eggs from grain-fed chickens.[940]

So should we all switch to *grass-fed* and *pasture-raised*?

Despite clear differences, the health benefits of grass-fed meat and pastured eggs are mostly speculative.

And they're likely exaggerated.

For example, while grass-fed beef has more omega-3s than grain-fed beef, it still doesn't have much. Regular old farmed salmon has over 28 times the omega-3s as grass-fed beef, with fewer omega-6s.[941,942]

So even if omega ratios are important, eating salmon once a week is a much bigger game-changer than switching to grass-fed beef.

And most of the alleged weight-loss benefits of CLA come from mouse studies. Based on *human* trials, a 2013 review found that the relatively small amounts of CLA in grass-fed dairy (which has more CLA than grass-fed beef [943,944]) is likely to have "little or no effect on body weight." [945]

(Even taking CLA supplements, according to a 2018 meta-analysis, produces weight-loss results that are "not clinically relevant." [946])

The earlier studies showing that red meat is harmless were not based on grass-fed beef. While grass-fed beef is probably healthier, that doesn't make grain-fed beef unhealthy. The evidence indicates that it's fine the way it is.

It's kind of like the difference between organic produce and regular produce. If money is no object, sure: eat grass-fed meat and pastured eggs. They're probably better. But they're also much more expensive. (And regular meat is expensive already.)

There's no sense in letting the perfect be the enemy of the good. For the average person, the science isn't compelling enough to justify the much higher cost of grass-fed meat and pastured eggs.

When it comes to meat and health, the difference between chicken nuggets and steak is far more important than the difference between steak and grass-fed steak.

Grain-fed meat and regular eggs are whole foods.

## Take-Home

We can't live on lean meat.
Unprocessed fatty meat is a high-protein whole food.
(Even if it's grain-fed.)

# 28

# IN DEFENSE OF DAIRY

The low-fat movement clearly didn't prevent the obesity epidemic. In fact, it may have sparked it.

The mistaken belief that animal fat and cholesterol are unhealthy is the main reason skim milk and "low-fat" dairy products exist. Skim milk was uncommon in 1970.[947] Now it's one of the most common types of milk in the United States. I grew up drinking skim milk.

But a 2013 systematic review of 16 studies on dairy fat's relationship to obesity found that low-fat and no-fat dairy products either weren't associated with weight loss, or were actually associated with weight *gain*. As the authors stated:

> *None of the 16 studies found that low-fat dairy consumption was inversely associated with obesity risk...observational studies do not support the hypothesis that dairy fat is obesogenic, nor do they support the hypothesis that low-fat dairy protects against obesity.*[948]

So much for skim milk being slimming.

On the other hand, eating more full-fat dairy (whole milk, butter, full-fat cheese, and cream) was *inversely* correlated with weight gain. 11 out of the 16 studies found that people who ate more full-fat dairy were leaner. None of the studies found that they were fatter.

More dairy fat meant less body fat.

It seems that low-fat and no-fat dairy products have exactly the opposite of their intended effect.

Similarly, in large part because of the campaigns against fat and saturated fat, American butter consumption declined 75% over the 20th century.[949] But far from benefiting our health, evicting butter from the kitchen helped pave the way for one of the most unhealthy foods of all time: high-trans-fat margarine.

In men in the Framingham Heart Study, eating margarine was independently associated with heart disease, while eating butter had no association with heart disease.[950]

## The Skinny on Dairy Fat

Why might full-fat dairy products be slimming? It all comes back to satiety. To many people, skim milk tastes watery and bland. This isn't how milk is supposed to taste. Whole milk—*natural* milk—is more creamy and filling, keeping us fuller for longer.

In the satiety study, full-fat cheddar cheese did quite well. Full-fat cheddar was rated far more filling than almost every processed food, and beat out whole foods like lentils, brown rice, peanuts, and bananas.[951]

On the other hand, while low-fat dairy is high in protein, it isn't very satisfying. When you take the fat out of dairy, it leaves a hole.

That hole is usually filled with sugar.

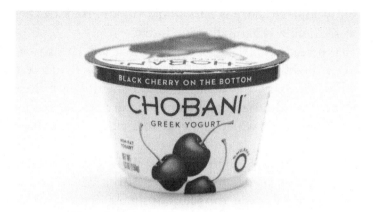

Photo Credit: Roman Tiraspolsky/ Shutterstock.com

**INGREDIENTS**: Nonfat yogurt (cultured pasteurized nonfat milk), **evaporated cane sugar**, black cherries, water, fruit pectin, **cherry juice concentrate**, locust bean gum, natural flavors, **lemon juice concentrate**.[952]

This petite serving of "non-fat" yogurt has 16 grams of sugar, most of which come from its three added sugars.

Yogurts like this are similar to low-fat and fat-free chocolate milk—you take a natural dairy product, suck the fat out, add a lot of sugar, and turn a whole food into a processed food.

## Full-Fat, Full Health Benefits

Every human being is designed to start life drinking full-fat milk—breast milk. Full-fat dairy products have been a staple in the diets of many human populations for thousands of years. For example, full-fat cheese and whole milk were staples in the traditional Sardinian diet, which produced some of the longest-lived people on Earth.[953]

*Full-fat* was the only kind of dairy available until quite

recently. Full-fat dairy is *natural* dairy. Skim milk has been processed; milk is naturally high in fat.

That preceding 2013 review found that full-fat dairy was associated with better metabolic health markers than low-fat and non-fat dairy, and wasn't associated with heart disease or diabetes.[954] "Low-fat" and "non-fat" dairy products usually have added sugar, which *is* associated with heart disease[955] and diabetes.[956]

Full-fat dairy is also nutritionally superior to non-fat dairy. Full-fat dairy products have vitamin A. But when you suck the fat out of dairy, you also suck out almost all the vitamin A (which is fat-soluble).[957,958] Artificial vitamin A is added back into skim milk, the same way that artificial vitamins are added back into white flour after they suck out the bran and germ.

But since vitamin A is *fat*-soluble, and fat-soluble vitamins require *fat* to be absorbed,[959,960,961] non-fat dairy products lack the necessary fat to absorb the artificial vitamin A that's added back into them.

Silly.

What else? Cheese and milk are two of the best sources of calcium out of any commonly eaten food,[962] and yogurt isn't far behind.[963]

Cheese, milk, and yogurt are high in vitamin B-12, riboflavin, and zinc, and milk and yogurt are high in potassium.[964,965,966,967,968]

And let's remind ourselves that butter is 20% less calorie-dense than vegetable oil. So if you're trying to lose weight, and you want to add some fat to your food, the smarter choice is butter, not vegetable oil.

Well done, dairy.

## Take-Home

Dairy fat appears to be *slimming*, not fattening.
If dairy agrees with you, eat full-fat dairy products to your heart's content. Just make sure there's no added sugar. *Read ingredients lists.*

# 29

# PROTEIN: THE X FACTOR

Part of the reason we went through so much trouble to show that unprocessed animal food is healthy is that unprocessed animal food is very high in protein. Protein is much more filling than fat or carbs,[969] and unprocessed animal food has more protein than any other food group. Certain plants have a decent amount of protein, but gram for gram, any plant pales in comparison to steak.[970]

In one trial, obese subjects ate diets made up of either 12% protein or 25% protein, with most of the protein coming from dairy and meat. After six months, the 12% protein group lost an average of 11 pounds. The 25% protein group lost an average of *20 pounds*, and had better triglyceride numbers.[971]

A 2012 meta-analysis of 24 controlled trials found that high-protein diets are superior to lower-protein diets for both weight loss and minimizing muscle loss *during* weight loss.[972]

In America, we tend to eat enough protein at lunch and dinner, but fall short at the breakfast table.[973] The main culprit is white flour in the form of bagels, muffins, breakfast bars, pancakes, waffles, and cereal. These processed foods have little protein compared to, say, eggs. Eating more protein at breakfast helps people eat fewer calories throughout the day, especially at night.[974]

## How Protein Causes Weight Loss

Food isn't just about taking calories *in*. In order to break food down, process it, and absorb it, your body also has to *expend* calories. And more than you might think.

The *thermic effect of food* is a measure of how many calories it takes to digest a certain food. This number of calories depends on the food. For carbs and fat, the thermic effect is relatively low. It's about 5-10% for carbs, and 0-3% for fat.[975] For every 100 calories of fat or carbs you eat, it takes anywhere from 0 to 10 of those calories just to digest the food.

But the thermic effect of protein is a whopping 20% to 30%.[976] For every 100 calories of protein you eat, it takes 20 to 30 of those calories just to break the protein down.

That's a big chunk.

A 2015 metabolic ward study split people into two groups. One group ate a high-protein diet, and the other group ate a low-protein diet. Both groups ate the same number of calories. On average, people in the high-protein group burned over 130 more calories per day.[977]

Eating more protein helps minimize the metabolic slowdown that accompanies weight loss,[978] and causes less preoccupation with food.[979] High-protein diets are easier to sustain than other diets,[980] and help people maintain weight loss.[981]

And you don't have to make drastic changes to reap rewards. Increasing protein from 15% to just 18% of total calories reduced the amount of weight people regained after weight loss by 50% in one randomized trial.[982]

Protein is so important to weight loss that some researchers are starting to think the success of low-carb diets has more to do with their being high in protein than low in carbs.[983] And it all comes back to satiety.

In the satiety study, the food with the most protein was ling fish. Out of 38 foods, it came in 2nd place. On average, the protein-rich food group was rated 66% more filling than white bread, and nearly twice as filling as bakery products.[984]

## Kidney Damage?

You may have heard that high-protein diets are bad for your kidneys. But that idea is completely based on people with pre-existing kidney disease—some of whom, admittedly, are probably better off avoiding high-protein diets.

But there is no convincing evidence whatsoever that high-protein diets cause *any* sort of kidney damage in people without preexisting kidney disease.[985]

It would be similar to arguing that, since exercise can be problematic for people with certain heart conditions, that exercise is bad for cardiovascular health in general.

Which is ridiculous, of course.

People who regularly eat high-protein diets have been found to have normal kidney function.[986] So have athletes and body-builders who regularly eat *very*-high-protein diets.[987]

But forget science. If eating lots of protein caused kidney disease, there would be countless stories of athletes and body-builders—many of whom eat staggering amounts of protein for years on end—suffering kidney disease later in life.

But this simply isn't the case. I've been around lots of athletes and bodybuilders and ex-athletes and ex-bodybuilders, and I've never even *heard* of a single case of kidney disease.

Even eating huge amounts of protein for years on end doesn't seem to cause kidney problems.

## Take-Home

High-protein diets are great for losing weight and keeping it off.

# 30

# THE BODY-FAT SET POINT

There's something deeper going on with food and fat. It's something beyond calories in and calories out, something that science doesn't yet fully grasp.

Apart from simply being more filling, there seems to be a deeper reason that whole foods can lead to a lifetime of leanness: *the body-fat set point.*

Although we don't know exactly how it works, it's obvious that the human body "defends" fat stores at certain levels, or "set points."

*Set points* are why weight tends to creep back on after weight loss.[988] On the other hand, set points are why, when someone goes on an uncharacteristic eating binge, they tend to lose the weight they gained.[989,990]

Most convincingly, set points are why many people manage to maintain nearly the exact same weight for years on end without any conscious thought or effort, somehow managing to eat exactly the same number of calories that they expend over very long stretches of time.[991]

Think about that.

Like a thermostat, despite fluctuating environments, the human body is capable of maintaining fat stores at very precise levels for very long periods.

Until quite recently, the vast majority of humans defended fat stores at relatively low levels. This is still the case for modern hunter-gatherers and people living in several traditional societies.[992,993,994]

Something in the modern environment has dramatically raised our body-fat set points.

Something has changed profoundly.

The most obvious culprit is diet.

Our body-fat set points are affected by the kind of foods we regularly eat. This has been demonstrated in animal models. When susceptible rats are fed highly palatable diets and allowed to eat freely, their body-fat set points increase dramatically: the rats gain lots of weight, and maintain this weight gain. (They don't just keep gaining weight forever.)

But when rats are switched back to less palatable diets and allowed to eat freely, their body-fat set points plummet: many rats lose lots of weight, and maintain this weight loss.[995,996]

(They don't just keep losing weight forever.)

Something similar happens to humans.

When processed food is freely available, humans spontaneously overeat and gain fat.[997,998,999] In other words, a diet of processed food causes the human body to store more fat.

But when humans start eating a *bland* diet and eat freely, trials show that they tend to lose weight quickly[1000]—*especially* when they're obese.[1001]

An interesting study from 1965 vividly illustrates how changing the *kinds* of foods you eat could dramatically lower your body-fat set point.

In a hospital setting, normal-weight and obese subjects were put on a bland liquid diet. The bland liquid contained 50%

carbs, 20% protein, 30% fat, and some vitamins and minerals. (It probably tasted like a watered-down Ensure.)

The subjects were allowed to drink as much of this liquid as they wanted, but could eat nothing else.

So what happened?

The leaner subjects drank enough of the bland liquid to maintain their weight over the study. The obese subjects, on the other hand, drank very small amounts of the bland liquid. They quickly started losing lots of weight.

In 12 days, one obese woman lost 23 pounds.

In 18 days, an obese man lost over 30 pounds. Despite consuming far fewer calories than his body needed to maintain his weight, the man never reported feeling hungry. Seeing the potential of this approach, he continued the diet at home, in a modified form, for 252 days after the study.

He lost 200 pounds.[1002]

His lack of hunger suggests that the bland liquid diet had somehow caused his body to start defending fat stores at a lower level. With nothing to eat except bland protein shakes, maybe his body decided it wasn't worth it storing all that fat.

Switching from a diet of processed foods to a diet of whole foods may accomplish something similar. While many whole foods are delicious, they do tend to be *blander* than hyper-palatable processed foods.

Indeed, the most common weight-loss strategy used by members of the National Weight Control Registry—a group of people who have lost a lot of weight and kept it off—is to modify their diet.[1003]

And the most common way that they modify their diet is by restricting certain foods.[1004] And dietary consistency is one of the best predictors of long-term success in the National Weight Control Registry.[1005]

In other words, people who successfully lose lots of weight and keep it off manage to lower their long-term body-fat set points by changing the foods they regularly eat—specifically, by restricting certain foods.

Sound familiar?

# 31

# PLANNING FOOD

If you fail to plan to eat healthy, you're planning to eat unhealthy. If you want to eat whole foods and lose weight, then there have to be satisfying whole foods around when you're hungry.

If there aren't, you'll probably eat processed food.

The key word here is *satisfying*.

Think of affordable whole foods that you actually *enjoy* eating. Make a list of them. This is your grocery list.

Go to the grocery store, and buy the items on the list.

Don't buy any processed food when you're there.

(Why would you *plan* to eat unhealthy?)

Buy enough whole foods to last you a while. Then put them in all the places where you usually eat—home, work, your car (nuts, apples, etc.) or wherever.

Then eat these whole foods when you're hungry.

And eat them until you're full.

If it won't get you in trouble with anyone, gather up all the processed food around you, put it in a big pile, and throw it away.

(Or donate it to charity.)

There is no reason to have processed food around if you're trying to lose weight and keep it off.

(Why would you *plan* to eat unhealthy?)

If processed food isn't around, it can't tempt you.

If you can't or won't throw out all the processed food, at least get it out of your sight. Hiding processed food in cabinets or drawers tends to decrease how much of it people eat.[1006,1007]

If you can't see it, it's not as tempting.

Make it harder for yourself to eat junk. One study found that secretaries ate far more Hershey's Kisses when the Kisses were on their desks rather than just *six feet* from their desks—which meant they had to stand up to get them.[1008]

Most importantly, surround yourself with tasty whole foods.

And just like humans have done since time immemorial, eat these whole foods when you're hungry.

And eat them until you're full.

# 32

# HOW TO EAT AT RESTAURANTS

If you want to lose weight and keep it off, restaurants generally belong in the "treat" category. You'll want to avoid them most days of the week.

The entire point of restaurants is to entice our taste buds enough to make us repeat customers, so that the restaurant can make money. This is almost never accomplished with whole foods. To woo our taste buds, restaurants slather most of their dishes with sugar and oil—even many "healthy" dishes at "healthy" restaurants.

It's not their fault. If restaurants don't do this, their competitors will. And they'll be out of business.

Eating out once or even twice a week can be fine. But if you're eating out three or more days of the week, even if you're trying to eat healthy when you're out to eat, you're fighting an uphill battle. And without an excellent strategy, you'll probably lose.

Say you're trying to eat healthy one day, minding your own business, and then you get dragged to a restaurant.

What should you order?

The best advice I can give the average person is to order steak (or some other whole-food meat) with a side of vegetables. And to not eat anything else.

Steak is high in protein, and will fill you up with far fewer calories than processed food. (This goes for any whole-food meat.) Even if the steak is coated in oily, sugary sauce, at least there's a lot of protein to balance things out.

Best of all, a steak doesn't feel like self-denial. Regularly ordering steak at restaurants is a sustainable habit that doesn't burn up loads of willpower. You'll need that willpower not to eat bread, appetizers, and dessert.

Steak tastes good—good enough to make your side-order of vegetables tolerable. The vegetables are there to provide fiber and nutrients, and to not be processed food. They're there because you're trying to eat healthy.

Remember, potatoes are vegetables. Feel free to order a baked potato without bacon or obscene amounts of butter. Steak, a baked potato, and greens is generally a more slimming option than salad, which tends to be swimming in vegetable oil (also known as "salad dressing"), not very filling, or both.

If you can stick to this meat-and-vegetables strategy—and not eat bread, appetizers, or dessert—you can probably eat at restaurants fairly often and lose a lot of weight.

## Vegetarian Options

If you're vegetarian or vegan, it pays to remember that added sugar, vegetable oil, and white flour are all vegan options.

Don't be afraid to ask how food is prepared.

Some of your best friends are baked potatoes, sweet potatoes, beans, brown rice, quinoa, peas, lentils, corn, and any other high-protein plant.

(Bread is not your friend.)

If you order salad, ask for a small side of olive oil to drizzle on yourself. Or you could even try the radical approach of not adding dressing at all.

## Damage Control

Sometimes we don't go to restaurants to eat healthy. Sometimes we go to treat ourselves. And sometimes we treat ourselves all the way.

But even if you've already decided you're not going to eat healthy, it's worth it to consider damage control. Damage control at restaurants is best accomplished by *portion control*.

With processed food, we can't count on our bodies to tell us when to stop eating. This is particularly important at restaurants, where typical portions are often cartoonishly large. If you rely on your body to tell you when to stop, you might eat thousands of calories.

The solution? Decide your portions *in advance*, and stop eating when you get there.

Where you decide to stop is arbitrary: two slices of bread, say, or one mini-plate of nachos.

But you have to stop somewhere.

For the main course, a good rule of thumb is to eat *half* the enormous portion that restaurants typically serve. It doesn't have to be exact. Just cut the food in half, pick a half, eat it, and don't eat the other.

Boom. You just cut the damage by 50%.

This is the point where most nutritionists would tell you to get a take-home box for the rest. But I don't recommend take-home boxes of processed food. Why would you *plan* on eating unhealthy in the future? You just had your cheat meal.

There's no reason to extend it. Give the food to a homeless person if you don't want it to go to waste.

One last point. When you *do* find yourself eating processed food at a restaurant (or anywhere else), try to slow down and really enjoy it. Savor the taste. Smell the roses. This can help you be satisfied with less of it.

## Take-Home

If you're trying to eat healthy at a restaurant, order meat with a side of vegetables. (Or some high-protein plants.)

If you're just there to enjoy yourself, you can still enforce practical stopping points: two slices of bread, half the main dish, etc.

# 33

# CHEAT DAYS

Experience has taught me to accept the *80-20 Rule*.

The 80-20 Rule states that as long as you're eating whole foods 80% of the time—and otherwise living a healthy lifestyle—you can get away with eating anything you want the other 20% of the time.

I have found this to be true.

In practice, the 80-20 Rule means the average person can probably stay lean despite eating just about anything one day a week.

Call it a "cheat day."

It's worked for me. For the past ten years, my regular diet has been strictly whole foods. But once or twice a week, I'd eat anything I wanted. And what I wanted was the Fat Four.

Despite these fairly regular junk-food excursions, I maintained significant weight loss the entire decade.

Many trainers and dietitians have similar experiences, both with themselves and their clients. Human metabolism seems to be regulated by the foods we *regularly* eat. It's what you do *most* of the time—your eating habits—that seems to have the biggest impact on your weight. If you're only eating whole foods most days, you can probably get away with a weekly cheat day.

But your mileage may vary. The 80-20 Rule assumes you're exercising regularly, sleeping well, and mostly eating great. It's not a free pass to indulge. And some people can get away with more than others.

Still, studies have found that, compared to people with rigid diet rules, so-called "flexible dieters" tend to lose more weight, have better weight-loss maintenance,[1009,1010] less depression and anxiety,[1011] and less frequent and severe binge-eating episodes.[1012]

In other words, understanding that you'll mess up sometimes and not being too hard on yourself—the essence of the 80-20 Rule—is associated with more weight loss.

You don't have to say goodbye to the Fat Four forever, or even for weeks at a time. You just have to say goodbye to the Fat Four *most days of the week*.

The way to think about junk food is "later," not "never."

This is a more sustainable, practical, and effective attitude.

Some gurus recommend designating a particular cheat day each week. Say, every Saturday. This can be effective for some people.

But for me, "life happens" at unpredictable times. I just try to avoid the Fat Four every day, with the understanding that I'll mess up sometimes.

Do whatever works for you.

## Take-Home

You don't have to be perfect. You *won't* be perfect.

If you eat whole foods about 80% of the time, you can probably eat whatever you want the other 20% of the time. This works out to one or two "cheat days" per week, on average.

It's fine to enjoy yourself sometimes.

## PART 2

# Exercise

# 34

# EXERCISE: INTRODUCTION

Exercise isn't something you do to lose weight. It's not a short-term fix. It's not a New Year's Resolution or a workout program.

It's much more than that.

For starters, regular exercise is an absolute requirement for anyone who wants to be healthy. The evidence for the health benefits of exercise is so overwhelmingly strong, and so well known, that if someone isn't in the habit of exercising regularly, it's safe to assume that they simply don't care about their health too much—like someone who smokes cigarettes.

These benefits include mental health. Humans are born to exercise. It's in our genes. Someone who never exercises is like a walrus that never swims, or a horse that never runs—completely out of sync with their bodies.

But "exercise" is a misnomer. When we hear that word, we think of going to the gym and sweating our brains out. We think of "working out," and of doing workouts that "kick our ass."

That's why so many people don't exercise.

(They think of hard work.)

But that's not what I mean by "exercise."

I just mean *physical activity*, in all its forms.

Physical activity includes standing, and it includes walking. Physical activity includes cleaning your room and mowing the lawn. It includes *anything* where you're up and moving.

I've changed. For years, I thought the only physical activity that mattered was the *intense* kind—the running, the lifting weights, etc. Anything else was child's play.

I couldn't have been more wrong. For health, weight loss, and everything else, science tells us that lots of light movement is probably *just* as important as the short and intense bouts we think of as "exercise." Maybe even more so.

For example, people dismiss walking. But walking is absolutely and unequivocally a form of cardiovascular exercise.

(It's physical movement that raises heart rate.)

In fact, walking is the most basic and essential exercise there is. People like to speculate about the running, sprinting, and lifting that may have characterized life in the Stone Age, but that's all it is: *speculation*. We can't see the past.

The only thing we can say for *certain* is that human beings evolved *walking*—a lot, every day.

Since time immemorial, walking was the only practical way to get around. Unless you have to get somewhere fast, walking is more efficient, thermodynamically, than running. And without question, walking was a daily activity of both hunter-gatherers and the early farmers they evolved into.

A lot of daily walking was mandatory for just about everyone who's ever lived—except those of us living today.

And that's a monster problem. Sure enough, when we look at the science, we don't find the greatest health benefits of exercise coming to gym rats who start doing P90X or CrossFit. Instead, the quickest, easiest, and most massive benefits—the lowest-hanging fruit—come to people who go from not exercising *at all* to simply *walking* for half an hour, three times per week.

For massive health benefits, that's all it takes.

And *that's* what I mean by caring about your health. Whether you want to do *intense* exercise on a regular basis is a personal choice—it's hard and draining. But if you're not *at least* walking, you're missing out on the mother of low-hanging fruit.

(Walking isn't torture, is it?)

All you *have* to do is walk.

If you want more, the next logical step is getting in the habit of resistance training, the *full-body* kind. Resistance training brings a panoply of unique health benefits that grow ever more important with age.

Nail these down—walking and resistance training—and you'll be so much better off than someone who does nothing that anything else is almost a moot point.

But if you have the ambition, vigorous cardio is the icing on the cake. It will take you to the loftiest peaks of physical wellness.

But all you *have* to do is walk.

(It's exercise.)


Exercise may not complete you, or make you a better person. But it *will* make you a better version of yourself. Start exercising regularly, and you'll feel better, you'll sleep better, and you'll think better.

You'll live better.

Oh, and science tells us that regular exercise is probably the one and only way the average human being can sustain significant, long-term weight loss.

So there's that.

But exercise is so much more than that.

# 35

# DIET, *THEN* EXERCISE

The phrase "diet and exercise" makes it sound like an equal partnership. *Diet and exercise*: two equally effective, equally necessary ingredients for weight loss.

*Diet and exercise*, like Bonnie and Clyde.

This is what we're led to believe.

But this isn't supported by science.

Think about it: exercise clearly isn't necessary for weight loss. You would be *much* lighter if you stayed in bed the next two months, only got up to use the bathroom, and only ate 500 calories per day. (This is true for any human.) This may sound ridiculous, but it's completely accurate.

You would lose a lot of weight.

You can't make a similar claim for exercise. Even doing *extreme* exercise—say, running six hours a day for two months—won't *guarantee* weight loss. Because it's *always* possible to eat back all the calories you burn. Michael Phelps was apparently eating 12,000 calories a day while training for the Olympics.[1013]

This isn't just theoretical, either. Hordes of football lineman and heavy weightlifters are walking, sweating proof that it's possible to regularly exercise at an elite level, and still look fat. Maybe they'd slim down if they lifted less and ran more?

## The Marathon's Effect on Weight

The marathon is a fitness paragon in our society, the Mount Olympus of cardio. It's enough of a feat, apparently, to warrant bumper stickers and tattoos. Of all the forms of exercise that might cause weight loss, you'd be hard-pressed to find something more extreme than working up to a 26.2-mile run. So how does training for a marathon affect runners' body weights? In a 1989 study, twenty-seven previously sedentary people were trained to run a marathon over the course of eighteen months.[1014]

What happened when, over that year and a half, those couch potatoes sprouted into marathoners? The men lost an average of five pounds of fat. *Five pounds.* In eighteen months.

But for the nine women in the study, "no change in body composition was observed." [1015]

The ladies didn't lose an ounce of fat. And remember, they were previously *sedentary.* Indeed, a lack of weight loss—and even weight *gain*—is a common story for aspiring marathoners (especially women[1016]).

Going for long runs—the iconic way to "sweat off the pounds"—is no guarantee you'll sweat off any pounds.

## The "Shape" of Exercise

I caught the exercise bug at eleven or twelve. Ever since, there's never been more than a week where I didn't exercise. Not even from the summer of 2007 to the spring of 2009, over which I gained forty pounds of fat.

That whole time, in fact, I was jogging and doing full-body weight training, twice or thrice a week.

And it didn't stop me from getting fat.

Ironically, the exercise was still "working"—I was in pretty good "shape." At my peak weight of a whopping 230 pounds, I ran on a treadmill at 8.0 mph for thirty minutes. That's fairly fast, for fairly long. Forty pounds lighter, I probably couldn't replicate that feat today (though I don't jog as much).

"Shape" is a slippery word. There's a fundamental difference between *being* in shape (whatever that means) and *looking* like you're in shape. I learned this the hard way, in eighth grade.

A skinny, three-sport athlete, I decided to run a grueling 10-mile road race called the Mountain Goat, in Syracuse, NY. On top of all my sports training, a month or two of dedicated jogging saw me in respectable "shape." And I was skinny.

I did well enough on race day. But something happened during that race that has stuck with me ever since. On mile 8, with the many long hills of the aptly named Mountain Goat exacting their toll, I was passed—rather casually—by a fellow runner who may have fallen in the "morbidly obese" range of the BMI scale. I'm not trying to be mean or insensitive; that's just how the person looked. But there they were, chugging right by skinny, "athletic," three-sport me.

And it didn't look like they were straining too hard.

Until then, I thought there was some essential connection between the shape of your body and the "shape" you're in.

There isn't.

## Exercise and Weight Loss

Like so much else in life, when it comes to exercise and weight loss, people are very different.[1017] For a minority of people, moderate exercise can actually lead to meaningful weight loss. But for most of us, the results of many exercise studies suggest that mere exercise (without dietary changes) leads to results ranging from "modest" to "useless."

What is "modest"? A 2011 meta-analysis of fourteen aerobic exercise trials found that, after *a year* of regular aerobic exercise, the mean weight loss was 3.74 pounds.[1018] That's less than one pound every three months.

Ouch. The authors concluded that "isolated aerobic exercise is not an effective weight loss therapy."[1019]

There's a fairly popular idea floating around that resistance training rules, and cardio drools. But the results of several long, randomized trials suggest that, like cardio, resistance training produces minimal weight loss on its own.[1020,1021,1022]

According to Dr. Eric Ravussin, an expert in obesity and diabetes and director of the Nutrition Obesity Research Center in Baton Rouge, Louisiana, "In general, exercise by itself is pretty useless for weight loss."[1023,1024]

I agree, Eric. (Can I call you Eric? Fine, *Dr. Ravussin.*)

## Diet, *THEN* Exercise

In 2007, a heavily cited meta-analysis of 59 studies found that exercise-only trials led to an average weight loss of 5 pounds over six months.

On the other hand, diet-only trials caused weight loss of between 11 and 39 pounds over six months, depending on the intervention.[1025] That's a lot of pounds.

Peering even deeper into the mists of time, a 1997 meta-analysis of the previous 25 years of research found that diet trials led to between three- and *five*-times as much of a change in body composition as exercise-only trials.[1026]

To be fair, the literature suggests that a *combined* diet-and-exercise program is the most effective approach.[1027,1028,1029,1030]

But the critical point remains.

**Diet is much more effective than exercise.**

# Basal Metabolism: Your 24-Hour Furnace

Don't you need to burn a lot of calories to lose weight?
You sure do. But all you have to do is sit there.
Your body will do the rest.

Your *basal metabolic rate* (BMR) is the number of calories
you burn per day by doing precisely *nothing*—no physical
activity whatsoever. Not even sitting up. (Not even *eating*.)
Human BMRs range from 1000 to 3000 calories per day. They
go up with weight, down with age, and are higher in men.[1031]

A woman who is 45 years old, 165 pounds, and 5-foot-6
will burn roughly 1400 calories per day by lying perfectly still
in a hospital bed. (Her BMR is ~1400 calories.)

In practice, though, even if this woman never exercises, she
will actually burn closer to 1700 calories per day,[1032] just by
virtue of not lying still all day. (You can quickly estimate your
BMR at www.bmrcalculator.org.)

Where do all those calories go? Well, when it comes to a
chemical system like your body, nothing is free. Even while you
sleep, your trillions of cells are constantly gobbling up energy
to do work—like pump ions, turn over proteins, fuel enzymes,
and maintain law and order amid nature's chaos.[1033,1034]

Going up a few levels, your *organs* are incessant calorie guz-
zlers. The brain alone makes up 19% of basal metabolic rate.
But it's the liver that's the real Hummer organ, accounting
for 27% of total BMR.[1035] The kidneys silently filter almost
800 liters of blood per day,[1036] making up 10% of BMR.[1037]

Then there's every heartbeat, every breath, every blink.
None of them are free. All of them cost energy.

These basic bodily processes slowly but surely devour tons
of calories. So many calories, in fact, that most of the calories the average Westerner burns in their lifetime will get
burned through basal metabolism, *not* physical activity and
exercise.[1038]

So the average person's body will burn more calories doing "nothing" than doing physical activity.

It takes a *lot* of exercise to out-burn your BMR. For example, an overweight woman who is forty, five-foot-six, and 195 pounds would have to jog nearly eight miles to burn more calories than her BMR.[1039,1040]

## Eating After Exercise

There's another problem with "sweating off the pounds." For many people (perhaps *half*,[1041,1042] and definitely me) exercise leads to *dietary compensation*: eating more than normal.

The more exercise that we "compensators" do, the more we eat.[1043] Indeed, strenuous workouts—*especially* cardio workouts—have always left me a ravenous bear.

The phrase *work up an appetite* didn't fall from the sky.

Worse yet, evidence indicates that right after exercising, compensators' food preferences change, and we explicitly crave junk food.[1044] And since difficult exercise burns willpower, we have less self-control than usual to restrain this junk-food impulse.

This is dangerous, because it's far easier to *eat* calories than to burn them. That 195-pound woman we met before has to jog over a mile to burn one Subway chocolate-chip cookie.[1045,1046] Combined with the rather narcissistic urge of many people to "treat themselves" after working out, and you start to see how exercising to lose weight can be an unmitigated disaster.

Nevertheless, many overweight people actually *do* eat the same amount—or *less*—after exercising. They are lucky. Predictably, they lose much more weight via exercising than we compensators do.[1047]

But even if that's you, your body will eventually find a way to compensate for exercise. Like reducing your BMR.[1048] If exercise never caused any energy compensation in a person, it would gradually burn through all their fat and muscle and whittle them down to a skeleton.

This doesn't happen, of course. For most people, calorie intake and calorie expenditure are matched to within a fraction of one percent over long periods of time.[1049]

One way or another, your body is programmed to replace the calories you burn.

## The Mindset

Why are you exercising? To improve your cardiovascular fitness? To get stronger? By all means, then: exercise away!

But if you're mostly exercising to lose weight, you need to get your priorities straight. It's diet, *then* exercise. Compared to diet, exercise is just a little bonus. It's the cherry on top, the sidekick.

Exercise is Robin. Diet is Batman.

If you're regularly eating processed food (food with more than one ingredient), then exercise is a waste of the limited willpower you're devoting to losing weight. If that's the case, you should leave the gym, head to the grocery store, buy acceptable foods made of one ingredient, go home, and start eating them. (And throw away your processed food.)

Only when you can honestly say that you don't eat processed food most days of the week should you even *toy* with the idea of exercising "to lose weight."

Diet comes first.

And remember: you don't need to go out of your way to "burn calories." Your body is a furnace that's always burning plenty of calories on its own.

Oh, and one more thing.

Don't treat yourself after working out.

You're not a dog.

# 36

# MIRACLE

We just came down hard on exercise. We established that it's no one-way ticket to Slim Town, and that diet comes first. But even though exercise is largely futile on its own, it turns out that regular exercise is one of the most important habits you can possibly develop for *long-term* weight loss. (The good kind.)

The strongest evidence of this probably comes from the National Weight Control Registry (NWCR).

## The National Weight Control Registry

The NWCR is a group of over 10,000 people (including me) who lost at least 30 pounds, kept the weight off at least a year, and are willing to share their story.[1050] The average weight loss is 66 pounds, kept off for 5.5 years.[1051] The goal is to figure out the common ground in this rare breed of weight losers—people who not only *lost* a lot of weight, but *kept* it off. (Most weight losers yo-yo.)

We regularly fill out questionnaires that assess what we did to lose weight, what we do now, and whether we're keeping the weight off. For many years, our habits have been synthesized, collated, and analyzed. And the results are in.

There is a lot of variation, but some approaches were nearly universal. 98% of us changed our diet in some way. (Big surprise.) **And 94% of us increased our level of physical activity.**[1052]

Isn't exercise useless for weight loss? By itself, usually. But as we saw last chapter, a *combined* diet and exercise program is the most effective weight-loss program.

And losing weight is only *half* the entrance requirement to the NWCR. The other half is *maintaining* weight loss.

And this is where exercise shines.

Many people go on diets and lose weight. In the next year, most of these people will regain one-third to two-thirds of the weight they lost. In the next five years, they will regain almost all of it.[1053] Those are pretty depressing stats.

Only a small fraction of dieters—perhaps 15%[1054]—succeed at long-term weight loss. And studies indicate that regular exercise is *crucial* for long-term weight loss (also known as *weight maintenance*).[1055,1056,1057,1058,1059,1060,1061]

In a 2004 review, eight scientists concluded that exercise is "perhaps the best predictor of weight maintenance."[1062]

The CDC's website sums up the critical consensus:

> *Most weight loss occurs because of decreased caloric intake. However, evidence shows the only way to maintain weight loss is to be engaged in regular physical activity.*[1063]

Translation: **If you're not willing to exercise regularly from now on, don't even bother trying to lose weight.**

Indeed, 90% of NWCR'ers continue to exercise regularly after they lose weight,[1064] for 40 to 60 minutes per day, on average.[1065,1066,1067]

But don't despair. I only work out two or three times a week, on average. You don't have to be a fitness fanatic to get massive benefits from exercise. It's good to emulate people who succeeded at what you're trying to succeed at. For someone trying to lose weight, there is probably no better approach than adopting habits that are nearly universal in people who succeed at long-term weight loss.

It's a no-brainer. You need to make changes to your diet. **And you need to exercise regularly.**

## What's Enough?

How much exercise is enough? Confusion sets in here. In studies, the link between physical activity and weight gain isn't terribly consistent,[1068] and it seems to take a lot of moderate exercise (around an hour a day)[1069,1070] to prevent weight gain.

But this is to be expected. After all, when it comes to body weight, diet is the Big Kahuna. And as we've seen, it's basically impossible to accurately capture someone's diet from a questionnaire. Diet quality is likely a big enough confounding variable in these studies to almost completely mask exercise's effects—so that only extreme exercisers seem to be able to keep weight off.

To illustrate, I gained 40 pounds of fat while doing vigorous workouts three days a week. But most days I was guzzling blue Powerade and eating processed foods, so the exercise didn't matter.

The point isn't that I might have avoided getting fat had I exercised for 75 minutes every day.

The point is that trying to fight a bad diet with exercise is bringing knives to a gun fight.

I don't work out any more or any less today than I did when I got fat. My exercise levels were constant; exercise wasn't the deciding factor in my getting fat. But it may have been a deciding factor in keeping the fat *off* once I lost it.

Evidence suggests that some people may need a lot of exercise to maintain their weight loss.[1071] Being obese for a long time often causes long-term metabolic changes that persist for at least a year after weight loss[1072] (and possibly much longer). To compensate for this, more exercise may be needed.

On the other hand, 25% of NWCR members maintain their weight loss with less than 30 minutes of moderate exercise per day, and 15% do less than 15 minutes of exercise per day.[1073] There is no cookie-cutter amount (or type) of exercise that works for everyone. Some people may simply need less exercise to maintain weight loss than others.[1074]

Only you can figure out the right amount (and type) of exercise for you.

But the evidence is clear: anyone who wants to keep weight off should exercise regularly. "Regularly" means multiple times per week. Twice a week is probably the bare minimum.

And if you're not planning on keeping the weight *off*, why bother?

## Exercise and Evolution

Why is exercise so crucial to lifelong fat loss? It's simple: we're built to move.

For almost the entire past of the *Homo* genus—over two million years—we were hunter-gatherers.[1075] Modern male hunter-gatherers seem to burn in the range of 600 to 1500 *more* calories per day from physical activity than the modern sedentary man.[1076] Since hunting and gathering have always required lots of movement, it's beyond question that we evolved doing lots of physical activity in those many millennia.

Evolution didn't stop after agriculture, and is still occurring today.[1077,1078]

Have we evolved to be more sedentary since our cavemen days? Contrary to popular belief, the average human may have become even *more* physically active after the dawn of agriculture.

Hunter-gatherers typically only spend two to three hours per day actively acquiring food[1079] (though that is not their only physical activity).

On the other hand, before modern technology, farming tended to be an all-day-long, wildly physically demanding job—and still can be.

Based on data from various population samples of hunter-gatherers and farmers, scientists have concluded that the physical activity levels of these two groups are similar—and, if anything, *farmers* are slightly more physically active than hunter-gatherers.[1080]

In 2004, a pedometer (step-counter) study was done on an Amish farming community. The Amish are a traditionalist Christian group who don't use electricity or gasoline, and lead simple lives.

10,000 steps per day is a popular goal of Fitbit users, and this amount of walking seems to have weight-management[1081] and health-promoting[1082] effects. How did the Amish stack up? The average Amish man took 18,425 steps per day, and the average Amish woman took 14,196 steps.[1083]

Even without the technological limitations of the Amish, it has been shown that modern Bolivian farmers burn more daily calories than Hadza hunter-gatherers.[1084]

The point is this: you are absolutely and unequivocally not adapted to a life of leisure.

## The Modern Sloth

The extent of sedentary living today is truly unprecedented. In evolutionary terms, farming remained the most common profession until extremely recently. In 1790, 90% of Americans were farmers. Here's how that number changed over time:

| Year | Americans who farmed |
|------|----------------------|
| 1790 | 90% |
| 1900 | 41% |
| 1970 | 4% |
| 2000 | **1.9%** |

Sources:[1085,1086]

Even after the masses stopped farming, until quite recently, most jobs still required a decent amount of physical activity. Factory jobs used to be about as common as desk jobs are today, and were far more physically demanding. Only since the rise of computers have so many people had the luxury of sitting all day and staring at screens.

But it hardly stops at your job. Well into the 20th century, most people were *forced* to be active in ways it's hard to fully appreciate today. Basic necessities like getting around, laundry, home care, dishes, shopping, and cooking required *far* more physical activity in days of yore—before cars, dishwashers, washing machines, ovens, and supermarkets made life easier.

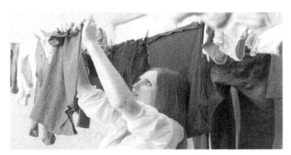

*People used clotheslines to dry clothes—after scrubbing them by hand.*
Photo Credit: Iakov Filiminov/Shutterstock.com

Once-routine chores like chopping wood and fetching water were completely eliminated in the West, and technology made other chores—like lawn mowing and snow removal—*far* easier than they once were.

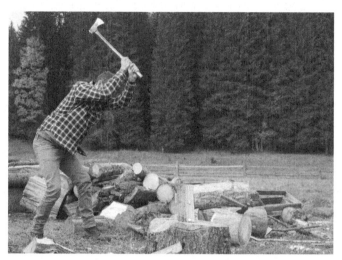

*Before thermostats, wood had to be chopped and carried.*
Photo Credit: rauloroca/Shutterstock.com

The plummeting of obligatory labor continued throughout the 20th century. In 1965, American women spent 25.7 hours per week on household activities (cooking, cleaning, laundry, etc.). By 2010, that number was 13.3 hours per week—a 48% decline.[1087] Over the same period, women spent 99% more time on "screen-based media."[1088]

Even buying food and supplies requires far less physical activity today. People used to walk to the local butcher, the baker, the candlestick maker.

Now they drive to the supermarket.

Soon, they may order all their groceries on Amazon.

Technology has slowly engineered nearly all the required

physical activity out of our lives, and will only continue to do so. But regular physical activity is our native state. Our bodies are built for it. They don't function properly without it.

You have to go out of your way to be active today.

**But unless you do, your body won't function properly.**

Going from sedentary to active isn't about "adding" something good to your life. It's about restoring yourself—physiologically, metabolically, mentally, and spiritually—to the state in which you were built to exist.

This comes with a smorgasbord of health benefits.

## Miracle

The Academy of Medical Royal Colleges issued a 2015 report that called exercise a "miracle cure" for the treatment and prevention of various diseases.[1089] Indeed, as a paper in the *Journal of Applied Physiology* in the year 2000 stated:

> *With the possible exception of diet modification, we know of no single intervention with greater promise than physical exercise to reduce the risk of virtually all chronic diseases simultaneously.*[1090]

Such superlatives are usually inappropriate in science.

In this case, however, they're wholly justified.

How does exercise make you healthier? Let me count the ways.

Exercise boosts immunity,[1091] reduces the risk of upper respiratory-tract infections,[1092] and reduces systemic inflammation[1093] (it lowers C-reactive protein, an inflammatory marker).

Exercise raises "good" HDL cholesterol,[1094] lowers "bad" LDL cholesterol, and lowers triglycerides.[1095]

Exercise reduces blood clotting,[1096,1097] significantly lowers blood pressure,[1098,1099] and reduces the risk of stroke.[1100]

One meta-analysis found that active people were almost

half as likely to die of heart disease.[1101] In general, there is a dose-response relationship (the more, the better) between exercise and reduction in heart-disease risk.[1102]

Active people are 30-40% less likely to get colon cancer, and active women are 20-30% less likely to get breast cancer.[1103] Physical activity probably reduces the risk of endometrial cancer, and may reduce the risk of prostate, stomach, and ovarian cancer.[1104]

Exercise prevents Type 2 diabetes,[1105] and improves glycemic control in Type 2 diabetics.[1106]

Exercise improves the functional capacity of people with multiple sclerosis,[1107] and is associated with a much lower chance of erectile dysfunction.[1108] (A fact which will inspire many men more than the dramatic effects on heart disease, cancer, and death.)

Exercise reduces lower back pain,[1109] reduces age-related loss of muscle mass[1110] and aerobic capacity,[1111] and reduces the risk of hip fractures,[1112] arthritis,[1113,1114] and osteoporosis.[1115]

Exercise improves memory[1116] and cognitive performance,[1117] and reduces the risk of Alzheimer's[1118] and Parkinson's Disease.[1119] Exercise improves depression treatment[1120] and has an "antidepressant effect."[1121]

Exercise improves sleep quality,[1122] enhances body image,[1123] reduces anxiety,[1124] and makes people happier.[1125,1126,1127,1128,1129,1130]

Exercise significantly reduces the risk of dying from any cause (all-cause mortality) in a dose-dependent fashion, with a 19% risk reduction for people exercising 2.5 hours per week.[1131]

Independent of any effect on weight loss, exercise reduces waist circumference and intra-abdominal ("visceral") fat.[1132] Since exercise can cut fat and build muscle at the same time,[1133] the bathroom scale isn't always a reliable measure of progress; exercise can improve body composition without weight loss.[1134]

A 2015 study assessed ten sets of identical male twins in

which one twin had exercised much more than the other twin over the previous three years. On average, the twin who exercised more had better insulin sensitivity, weighed less (despite having more lean body mass), had less body fat, and had more brain matter.[1135]

As noted in the textbook *Advanced Exercise Physiology*, "thousands of genes change expression during physical activity or inactivity,"[1136] and "exercise induces dramatic changes in the hormonal mileu."[1137]

This textbook goes on to state:

> *Physical activity is a natural cycle that is integrated into most other cycles in humans and animals. A disruption in the expected daily cycle of physical activity elicits disruptions in other cycles, leading to abnormal gene expression and systemic dysfunctions[1138] ... genes were optimized to support physical activity for survival. In the absence of historical physical activity levels, inherited genes "misfire" and function incorrectly.[1139]*

Regular exercise fixes that.

And it can help fix you.

# 37

# TAKE A STAND

Playing sports growing up, I used to think things like running and lifting weights were the only real forms of "exercise." If I'd run or lifted that day, I thought, it was okay to be a sloth for the other 23 hours.

After all, *I had already worked out.*

I was wrong. A 2013 meta-analysis showed that the more someone sits, the higher their risk of dying from any cause—and that exercise is only "partly protective."[1140] The study concluded that too much sitting causes 5.9% of all deaths, and that the risks "increase significantly" when you sit more than 7 hours per day (a span easily eclipsed by most people with desk jobs).

A 2015 meta-analysis concluded that lots of sitting caused a 24% higher chance of dying from any cause, and a *91%* higher risk of diabetes. This was *after* adjusting for physical activity.[1141]

A 2014 study of 16,586 Canadians found a 33% reduction in mortality (*death*) risk in people who stood "most of the day" compared to "almost none of the time," and that the biggest benefits of standing more come to otherwise inactive people.[1142]

## In Good Standing

In light of evolution, it's obvious why tons of sitting might be bad. Both common sense and various ethnographic reports of hunter-gatherers and traditional farming populations[1143,1144,1145,1146,1147,1148] indicate that for all of our relevant evolutionary past, the *Homo* lineage were on our feet at least a few hours per day.

Standing may not seem like "work," but it's much different than sitting. As a group of scientists wrote in the *International Journal of Cardiology* in 2014, "standing upright is a fundamental stressor that requires rapid and effective circulatory and neurological compensation to maintain blood pressure, cerebral blood flow, and associated consciousness."[1149] Simply standing in place requires several different muscle groups to contract, and we burn around 33% more calories standing than sitting.[1150]

But while sitting all day is surely bad, standing all day may cause problems of its own. Excessive standing at work has been associated with varicose veins[1151] and other circulatory problems,[1152] and a balanced amount of sitting and standing seems optimal. Extremes aren't ideal.

Rather than stand in place like a statue, experts urge us to regularly move around a bit while standing.[1153] This sort of non-statue lifestyle is more in line with our evolutionary past, and seems to have metabolic advantages over standing still.[1154]

## Exercise to the Rescue?

Some studies have found that more sitting time is associated with overweight and obesity—*independent of other physical*

*activity*.[1155,1156,1157] A 2014 follow-up study of bariatric surgery patients found that the people who sat more had worse
weight-loss outcomes, *independent of exercise*.[1158]

A 2015 study measured physical activity with an acceler-
ometer (a rather accurate measurement) in people at risk for
diabetes. More sitting time was heavily associated with more
heart fat, liver fat, and visceral (abdominal) fat.[1159]

(These are *not* "good fats.")

A 2015 study found that more standing was associated with
less obesity, and found a dose-response relationship between
more standing time and less obesity risk—*in people who already
met the Physical Activity Guidelines*.[1160]

Results like these seem to indicate that not only is exercise
ineffective at counteracting the effects of sitting all day, but
that exercise may actually be less important than total standing
time in keeping weight off.

Experts say to get up and move at least once every half hour
that you're sitting down,[1161] and they implore desk-jobbers
to spend at least two hours per day standing or doing some
sort of light movement while at work.[1162]

Breaking up long sits with very short bouts of very light
activity (walking to the bathroom, etc.) improves blood-sugar
responses[1163] and reverses the nasty effects of chronic sitting
on certain genes.[1164] Taking more breaks from sitting has been
associated with reduced BMIs, smaller waist circumferences,
and lower triglycerides.[1165]

It doesn't take much.

## Take-Home

A great deal of evidence indicates that it's optimal to stand at least a few hours per day. Whether it's getting a standing desk at work, standing and moving around while you're watching TV or taking a call, cooking instead of ordering out, or shopping in person instead of online, more time on your feet leads to more health—and less fat.

The amount of time you're on your feet seems to be just as important for weight loss as what most people call "exercise."

## 38

# WALK THE EARTH

For many, the word *exercise* is fraught with peril. It connotes unpleasantries like hard work, sweat, and soreness. We associate exercise with fitness boot camps, CrossFit, marathons, and the awful expression, "no pain, no gain."

Exercise is something that "kicks your ass," leaves you gasping for breath, and wipes you out.

But it needn't be so.

It's not that vigorous exercise doesn't have serious benefits. It's that the evidence indicates you can get *most* of the benefits of exercise just by doing moderate exercise—like walking.

No pain required.

In 2008, the US Department of Health and Human Services released its *Physical Activity Guidelines for Americans*. This illustrious report was done by thirteen experts in exercise and public health who extensively reviewed the relevant science since 1996. The report included a graph relating the amount of exercise someone did with their risk of dying from any cause. (A smaller chance you'll die from any cause is a great proxy for "health benefits.") Here's the graph:

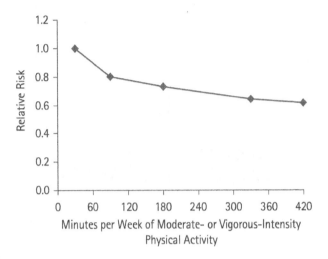

Source: US Department of Health and Human Services[1166]

As you can see, the steepest reduction in death risk comes at the very beginning—when people go from couch potatoes to doing the bare minimum of regular exercise.

The health benefits level off after that.

The report states:

> *It is not necessary to do high amounts of activity or vigorous-intensity activity to reduce the risk of premature death. Studies show substantially lower risk when people do 150 minutes of at least moderate-intensity aerobic physical activity a week.*[1167]

150 minutes. That's three *somewhat* brisk 50-minute walks per week (or five 30-minute walks, etc.). That's it. And 150 minutes is arbitrary. According to their own graph, there was major risk reduction well before that.

Doing more—and more intense—exercise will reap additional benefits, but *with diminishing returns*.

A 2009 meta-analysis of twelve studies found that walking

significantly reduces the risk of heart disease, and in a dose-dependent fashion.[1168] And for our noble purposes, a 2007 meta-analysis of twenty-four randomized controlled trials found that walking programs lead to statistically significant drops in body weight, body fat, and BMI.[1169]

Last—but certainly not least—walking is the most common form of physical activity of members of the National Weight Control Registry.[1170]

What does that tell you?

## A Walk Down Memory Lane

Walking is the most basic movement pattern of our species. It's the default way that humans go from point A to point B. If modern hunter-gatherers are any indication, we've been prolific walkers for quite some time. Hunter-gatherers cover a land range comparable to wild dogs and hyenas, with an average range larger than the city limits of Washington, D.C. (and an average of seven relocations per year in warm climates).[1171]

That's a lot of walking.

The Hadza, for example, walk an average of four to seven miles per day,[1172] which seems fairly typical for hunter-gatherers.[1173] Hadza women often spend hours walking in search of edible plants, while Hadza men hunt. Hunting includes running, but walking at moderate speeds seems to be the primary hunting activity.[1174]

As we've seen, physical activity levels didn't change much after agriculture, and traditional farmers may have walked even more than hunter-gatherers (remember how many steps the Amish took?).

Humans are adapted to a lifetime of walking.

And we're adapted to walk outside. Sunlight is the main way people get vitamin D, and vitamin D deficiency is linked to many serious chronic diseases.[1175] Vitamin D is rare in food, and exposure to sunlight is more effective at raising levels of vitamin D than taking 1000 IU of vitamin D3.[1176]

This is a likely reason why, compared to indoor exercise, outdoor exercise is associated with reduced anger, tension, and depression, increased energy, and "greater feelings of revitalization and positive engagement."[1177]

## Walk It Off

Despite the impression you get from watching *The Biggest Loser*, vigorous exercise is unnecessary to lose a lot of weight. As we've seen, exercise isn't terribly effective for weight loss to begin with. The key is making a habit of doing *some* form of exercise—for health and weight maintenance.

And you'd be *far* better off getting in the habit of walking than doing two months of vigorous exercise and then reverting back to nothing. Because if you're not going to sustain it, it doesn't matter what kind of exercise you do. It won't work.

According to a recent exercise physiology textbook:

> *For the sedentary, overweight person, moderate-intensity exercise is the proper choice because it can be done for longer periods of time in each exercise session and can be done each day.*[1178]

Right they are. And there are other reasons walking rules. First off, the heavier you are, the more calories you'll burn by walking. Exercise intensity is relative to the person. Given the same activity, obese people burn more calories.[1179] Walking at three miles per hour can fall in the "vigorous" category for a sedentary person with a low aerobic capacity.[1180]

In other words, walking can genuinely be a "great workout" for many people. The heavier you are, the more intense walking will be.

Walking is an excellent choice for anyone, but if you're sedentary or obese, there is no need to look any further. Walking doesn't require expensive equipment, new shoes, having to overcome the fear of doing something new in a public place (*a la* the popular fantasy that other gym-goers give you serious thought), or the need to psyche yourself up, pay for a personal trainer, or almost any of the litany of excuses people make not to exercise.

And walking is highly sustainable. For most people, vigorous exercise simply isn't sustainable—especially as they become elderly. The most important part of any exercise program is *adherence*. The ease and convenience of walking make it much more likely you'll stick with it in the long term—the only term that counts.

We shouldn't consider walking a "beginner" activity, or as something to graduate from. Walking is the most fundamental human movement, and the simple habit of walking several times a week will confer *most* of the immense benefits of exercise, including preventing weight gain.[1181]

It doesn't get more practical than that.

Whether you want to strain yourself any further is a personal choice.

# 39

# THE PATH OF MOST RESISTANCE

While walking is infinitely better than nothing, to even remotely approach exercise's *full* potential benefits, you need to strain those muscles. The American Heart Association and American Diabetic Association both recommend at least biweekly strength training.[1182,1183] The American College of Sports Medicine urges us to resistance train "a minimum of two days each week" with exercises that "target all major muscle groups."[1184]

## The Evolution of Strength

The physical activity of our past wasn't just a bunch of aerobics. As cavemen, we constantly used our muscles to do things like dig for tubers and roots, chop, carry meat and plants back to camp, make tools, and build shelters.[1185]

The !Kung are hunter-gatherers living in southern Africa. !Kung women routinely carry foraged plants weighing 15 to 22 pounds all the way back to camp.[1186] A typical !Kung woman will also carry her small child around 4,800 miles in its first four years of life.[1187]

Then there's hunting, which requires dragging heavy carcasses long distances—an activity women hunter-gatherers are known to help with.[1188]

Mandatory muscle-flexing continued unabated through our agricultural years. Old-school farming included clearing, plowing, digging, tilling, cutting, picking, carrying, grain-grinding, gathering wood, cutting wood, building, making repairs, animal care, and carrying water.[1189] In fact, it's thought that pre-modern farmers did more muscular work than hunter-gatherers.[1190]

In short, we've been using our muscles against resistance every step of the way. This is probably why a good deal of evidence suggests that combining cardio *and* resistance training is significantly better—for fat loss and general health—than either alone.

## Strong Muscles, Strong Health

Resistance training has a slew of health benefits, and it activates different cell-signaling pathways than cardio[1191]—which suggests unique benefits. Resistance training reduces blood pressure[1192] and blood clotting,[1193] improves blood-sugar control,[1194] and raises bone mineral density.[1195]

Contrary to popular belief, resistance training *improves* flexibility. A 2011 study found that resistance training was as effective as traditional stretching at improving flexibility.[1196]

Resistance training improves physical functioning in breast cancer survivors,[1197] and improves brain function[1198] and psychological well-being[1199] in the elderly.

Everyone can benefit from stronger bones and muscles, but they're especially vital for older people. Resistance training improves muscle strength[1200,1201] and bone mineral density[1202,1203] in elderly people, which helps limit and even *reverse* age-related loss of bone and muscle mass—and the associated risks of falls, fractures, osteoporosis, and arthritis. This is critical. About 50% of women over 65 who break a hip will never walk again.[1204]

It's *never* too late to start resistance training. Even people in their nineties have been clinically shown to make "significant gains in muscle strength, size, and functional mobility"[1205] from resistance training. In one study, after an eight-week resistance program, a group of nine participants—aged *86 to 96*—increased their average leg strength by 174%.[1206]

According to a recent exercise physiology textbook,

> *It is important to note that regular bouts of resistance exercise remains one of the most useful and practical means to delay age-related muscle loss.*[1207]

But perhaps the best measure of resistance training's effect on human health comes from a 2015 review of all-cause mortality and muscular strength. As we've seen, *reduced all-cause mortality* is a good proxy for "total health benefits." And this review of 23 studies found that muscular strength was independently and inversely associated with all-cause mortality.[1208]

In other words, *stronger people were less likely to die.*

Remarkably, this association was independent of cardiovascular fitness, which suggests a unique, life-supporting role of strength.

Think about it. Resistance training makes you stronger.[1209] Stronger people are less likely to die. It would seem to follow that resistance training makes you less likely to die.

As an added bonus, strength gains from resistance training

also tend to be more durable—and less vulnerable to quick detraining—than improvements in cardiovascular fitness.[1210]

Muscle is the main "sink" for all the fat and carbs we eat[1211,1212]—once fat and carbs are in your bloodstream after a meal, muscle is the main place they go. This makes muscle a crucial regulator of blood sugar and overall metabolism.

Indeed, the main defect of Type 2 diabetes is insulin resistance *in skeletal muscle.*[1213] Older men diagnosed with diabetes are significantly more likely to have weaker muscles, and there's even an association between muscle weakness and higher blood sugar in men *without* diabetes or impaired glucose tolerance.[1214] This suggests a graded continuum of muscle weakness and abnormal blood sugar.

Diabetes is hardly the only reason to fear blood-sugar problems; insulin resistance significantly increases heart-disease risk.[1215]

It's also worth noting that when a person starves to death, the ultimate cause of death is depleted muscle mass.[1216] Muscle acts as a sort of health insurance. During times of severe stress (major infections, serious injuries, advanced cancer, etc.) the body's need for protein increases considerably—sometimes beyond what you could reasonably eat.[1217] To make up the difference, your body breaks down skeletal muscle into protein.

So muscle plays a key role in recovery from illness and trauma—unless you don't have enough. Survival from severe burns is lowest in people with the lowest muscle mass,[1218] and lost muscle mass is a major factor in the high mortality rates of cancer[1219] and heart failure.[1220]

The upshot is that if you're already weak and frail, a serious health problem is more likely to be your last.

So muscle up.

## Resistance Training and Fat Loss

Compared to just cardio, a 2006 meta-analysis of exercise trials for diabetics found that a combined cardio and resistance-training program led to more weight loss, as well as better blood sugar, blood pressure, and cholesterol.[1221]

A 2011 meta-analysis of exercise trials in people with coronary heart disease found that a combined cardio-and-resistance program decreased body-fat percentage by a full 2.3 percentage points more than a cardio-only program (a rather large difference), and led to better heart function.[1222]

In a 2012 trial, 97 overweight/obese people were randomized into 12-week programs of cardio, resistance training, both, or nothing (the control group). After twelve weeks, the hapless control group *gained* body fat. The resistance-only and cardio-only groups both lost the same amount of fat, while the *combined* cardio-and-resistance group lost *twice* that amount of fat—including far more visceral fat (the uber unhealthy kind of fat).[1223]

So combining cardio and resistance training seems best.

Resistance training may be more effective than cardio. A 2015 study followed 10,500 men for twelve years and found that weight training was more predictive of smaller waistlines than was cardio.[1224] And several studies have found that resistance training causes fat loss, independent of calorie restriction.[1225,1226,1227,1228,1229]

Build muscle, lose fat.

## The Mechanism

Science tells us that a pound of muscle burns around *six* calories per day at rest[1230] (not 50 calories, as some have claimed). Six calories per day isn't much. But over time, little differences add up. If you put on five pounds of muscle, you'd burn an extra 109,500 calories over the next decade. Most of those calories would come from fat, as fat is the preferred fuel source of resting muscle.[1231]

More importantly, regular resistance training regularly burns a lot of calories. And the more muscle you have, the more calories you can burn. Resistance training has been shown to spike metabolism for up to two full days afterward,[1232] concomitant with increased protein synthesis.[1233]

In a 2002 study, young men's metabolic rates increased by an average of 20% (they burned almost 400 more calories a day) following strenuous bench presses, power cleans, and squats.[1234]

But keep in mind that intensity plays a major role in this post-workout metabolic spike.[1235] If the workout felt easy, fat won't start magically melting off.

## The Ideal Weight-Loss Exercise?

When people lose weight, anywhere from 25% to 40% of the weight they lose is actually "fat-free mass"—which is mostly muscle.[1236,1237] This isn't good. Muscle loss contributes to the metabolic slowdown that accompanies significant weight loss, which makes it harder to lose *more* weight.[1238]

But how much muscle you lose is up to you. Critically, resistance training preserves both lean mass[1239] and resting metabolic rate[1240] during weight loss. A 1999 study put ten women on a twelve-week program of severe dietary restriction and resistance training. After twelve weeks, an average of 32 pounds lighter, the women's resting metabolic rates slightly *increased*.[1241] Thanks, resistance training!

By maintaining metabolic rate during weight loss, resistance training helps bust stalls and plateaus, making it more likely you'll continue losing weight—and more likely you'll end up looking "toned" instead of just "skinny."

To be fair, studies indicate that aerobic exercise also helps preserve lean body mass[1242] and resting metabolic rate[1243] during weight loss. But resistance training seems to be more effective at both.[1244,1245,1246]

## The Secret Weapon of Being Big

Carrying lots of extra weight makes it harder to move around. Obese people have a much lower aerobic capacity than normal-weight people.[1247] But heavy people also have a secret weapon: stronger muscles. Contrary to popular belief, when people gain weight, it's not all fat. A significant portion of weight gained is actually lean mass[1248] (even *without* exercise).

That's just how the body works. On average, obese people have significantly more muscle than normal-weight people.[1249] And more muscle usually means more strength. A 2005 study compared the strength levels of obese and normal-weight people. Assessed by the leg press, obese people had between 23% and 32% more leg strength.[1250]

Lifting heavier weights means burning more calories. For most very heavy people, doing exercises like the leg press—a natural strength—makes more sense than trying to jog on a treadmill (a natural weakness).

Heavy people should capitalize on their strength.

## Compound Movements Are King

By "resistance training," I don't mean this:

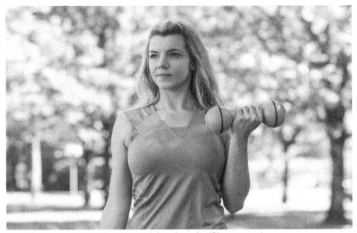

Photo Credit: wavebreakmedia/Shutterstock.com

Instead, I mean something more like this:

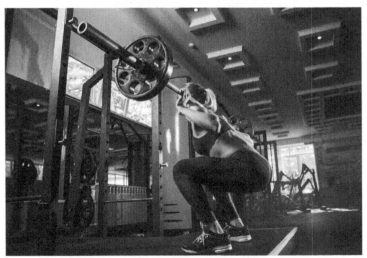

Photo Credit: Oleksandr Zamuruiev/Shutterstock.com

Our muscles are built to move in coordinated units, and that's how we should train them. "Isolation" exercises (curls, leg extensions, dumbbell flyes, etc.) tend to only work one muscle group at a time. These aren't nearly as effective metabolic stimuli as "compound" exercises—like squats, leg presses, pushups, seated rows, lunges, bench presses, deadlifts, lat pulldowns, chin-ups, overhead presses, and lots of other moves that work multiple muscle groups together.

Free-weights are generally better than machines because they promote balance and natural, functional movement patterns. Squats and deadlifts, for instance, are fantastic. These primal movements work over 200 muscles at a time.[1251] A 2007 study found that squats and deadlifts were more effective than hormone-replacement therapy at halting the loss of bone mineral density in the spines of postmenopausal women.[1252]

Are heavy squats and deadlifts safe? Powerlifting—which involves squatting, deadlifting, and bench pressing with huge weights for single repetitions—has a relatively low rate of injuries.[1253] Per 1000 hours of powerlifting, the injury rate is anywhere from half[1254] to *ten times less*[1255] than that of recreational running,[1256] for example.

According to the American College of Sports Medicine:

> *If appropriate guidelines are followed, the squat is a safe exercise for individuals without a previous history of injuries. The squat is a large-muscle-mass exercise and has excellent potential for adding lean muscle mass.*[1257]

In general, resistance training increases the strength of ligaments, tendons, and joints.[1258] The ACSM reports that former competitive weightlifters have *reduced* rates of lower back pain compared to the general population.[1259] Anecdotally, the only time I ever experience back or knee pain is when I *haven't* squatted in a while. However, you should assess your personal status and seek guidance from qualified trainers and medical experts.

Try to keep resistance training *progressive*, always trying to use more weight or do more repetitions—with excellent form—than before. It's this *overload* that forces muscles to adapt and get stronger.[1260] (Note to people without photographic memories: workout journals and tracking apps are great for keeping records.)

And to counter a potential self-limiting belief: although helpful, you don't need a gym or any equipment to start resistance training. Bodyweight squats, lunges, pushups from your knees, and regular pushups are just four of hundreds of bodyweight exercises you can Google how to do at home—and then do at home, for free.

Barring crippling disability, there is really no good reason not to resistance train. Remember: you don't need *any* baseline of fitness or skill to begin. The less fitness or strength you think you have, the *more* you need to start resistance training immediately. Guidance from a qualified trainer can be helpful.

## Note to Ladies

Many women worry that serious resistance training will make them "too muscular." They'd rather just be "toned."

They needn't worry. Men all over the world make Herculean efforts to put on muscle…and still don't look like Hercules. This is highly relevant for women, who have an average of *ten times* less circulating testosterone than men.[1261]

Testosterone plays a large role in muscle size.[1262,1263]

Think about it, ladies: if so many men can put in months of dedicated lifting and eating and *still* not look terribly muscular, what do you have to be concerned about?

Even in the wildly unlikely scenario that you lifted weights and became "too muscular," you could just stop. You'd lose most of the muscle you gained. Gains aren't permanent.

There is nothing to be scared of. The vast majority of people who look "too muscular" got that way via enormous dedication *and* steroids. It really doesn't happen by mistake.

Most women will simply *never* look "too muscular."

Even if they tried to.

# 40

# BREAK A SWEAT

## Running Through the Past

Sometimes you hear evolutionary arguments for jogging. Some modern hunter-gatherer men run and sprint during hunts,[1264] and some anthropologists speculate that *persistence hunting*—jogging after a faster animal for hours until it eventually collapses from heat exhaustion, the poor thing—may have played a crucial role in human evolution.[1265]

The implication is that we should jog today, too.

But this evo-running hypothesis is controversial among scientists,[1266,1267] and persistence hunting is uncommon among hunter-gatherers.[1268] The hunting methods of modern hunter-gatherers are highly variable, and some of their major weapons (the bow and arrow, etc.) may not have existed through much of our formative past.[1269] We don't know what ancient hunting looked like.

And there's another issue. However it happens, a great deal of ethnographic evidence indicates that hunting big game is overwhelmingly a *male* activity.[1270] This pattern is so pervasive that it seems safe to project it into the past. Indeed, the fossil record implies large differences in physical activity between ancient hunter-gatherer men and women.[1271]

This means men may be more adapted to the running-and sprinting-type movements of hunting than women—which could explain why female college athletes are about six times more likely to sustain ACL injuries than male college athletes.[1272]

The extent to which humans ever "ran from predators"—an ostensibly co-ed activity—is completely speculative, and probably illusory. Running away isn't a great strategy when you're a slow biped trying to flee a much faster quadruped predator.

In any case, after the spread of agriculture, the need to run and sprint for subsistence disappeared in many populations. We see this in human remains. In farmer bones, there's less of a difference between males and females ("sexual dimorphism") than there is in hunter-gatherer bones. This tells us that agriculture meant less running, and more equal physical activity patterns between the sexes.[1273,1274]

But some populations clung to their hunter-gatherer ways for far longer than others, which may explain why some ethnic populations are disproportionally dominant at competitive running.[1275]

The upshot is that, in the same way that different people are clearly adapted to different foods (wildly variable rates of lactose intolerance, etc.), different people may be adapted to different forms of exercise.

There's probably no one, "right" way to exercise.

Do what feels right for you.

## Vigorous Cardio

What counts as "vigorous" cardio? This is one of mankind's eternal questions. A nice rule of thumb is that moderate cardio is hard enough that you can't sing, while vigorous cardio is hard enough that you can't talk.[1276] For most people, walking at 3.0 miles per hour (fairly brisk) falls on the low end of the "moderate" range, while jogging at 5.0 miles per hour is "vigorous."[1277] However, "vigorous" is relative to the person.

Vigorous cardio can include biking, rowing, swimming, elliptical training, brisk walking, hiking, circuit training, cross-country skiing, various sports, and many other activities that make you sweat.

One benefit of vigorous cardio is that it's quicker. The American Heart Association and the ACSM both recommend at least 150 minutes of moderate activity, or at least 75 minutes of vigorous activity per week.[1278,1279] If you care about such guidelines, saving 75 minutes is nice.

And it turns out that sweating is very good for you.

## Health Benefits for Days

While walking will net you most of exercise's health benefits, more intense cardio brings more intense benefits.

Vigorous cardio increases *cardiovascular fitness* (a.k.a. *maximum aerobic capacity*, $VO_2$ *max*, *peak oxygen uptake*, etc.) to a much greater extent than moderate cardio—even *after* adjusting for the number of calories burned. In other words, short, intense workouts are better at making your heart work better than long, moderate ones.[1280]

Cardiovascular fitness isn't just good for jogging and sports. A 2009 meta-analysis found that, compared to people with low cardiovascular fitness, people with high cardiovascular fitness were **70% less likely to die**.[1281]

That's something to write home about.

Epidemiological studies have consistently found that, compared to moderate cardio, vigorous cardio is associated with a smaller risk of heart disease.[1282] Clinical trials show that vigorous cardio also trumps moderate cardio at improving blood pressure and blood-sugar control.[1283] In diabetics, exercise *intensity* is more important than exercise *volume* in improving blood-sugar control.[1284]

Crunching data from the massive Nurses' Health Study, researchers segregated the health outcomes of regular walkers based on their normal walking speed. Compared to women who usually walked at an "easy, casual pace," women who walked at a "normal, average pace" were 28% less likely to get diabetes. Women who walked at a "brisk" or "striding" pace were 59% less likely to get diabetes.[1285]

There's power in power walking.

Only vigorous exercise seems capable of reducing the risk of colon cancer,[1286] and in a study that analyzed three large Dutch data sets, vigorous exercisers took significantly less sick leave from work than moderate exercisers[1287] (though more days of work isn't universally cherished).

Poring over the self-reported habits and health outcomes of 13,485 men from the Harvard Alumni Health Study, researchers determined that "light activities" were not associated with mortality rates, that "moderate activities showed a trend toward lower mortality rates," and that "greater energy expended in vigorous activities clearly predicted lower mortality rates."[1288]

More intense exercise is better.

Finally, a 2014 cohort study of 8,960 people compared moderate to vigorous activity, controlling for the total volume of physical activity (which is rare in these studies[1289]). Vigorous activity was independently associated with lower mortality.[1290]

The harder you exercise, the longer you seem to live.

## Weight Loss?

Now that we've dispensed with general health, we come to the main event: weight loss. Unfortunately, there isn't clear evidence that vigorous cardio is innately better than moderate cardio for weight loss.[1291,1292]

The truth hurts.

In a 2003 randomized trial, 201 overweight women did either moderate or vigorous cardio—and dieted—for a year. The scientists made it so both groups burned roughly the same number of calories via exercise. Both groups lost weight, but there was no significant difference in how much they lost.[1293]

Similarly, a 2005 trial randomized 64 men to six months of either moderate- or high-intensity workouts on an exercise bike, with both groups burning 400 calories per workout. After six months, there was no significant difference in weight loss. In fact, the *moderate*-intensity group lost slightly more weight.[1294]

Finally, a 2002 randomized trial found that, over eight months, the equivalent of jogging twelve miles per week did not lead to significantly more weight loss than the equivalent of *walking* twelve miles per week—in fact, it caused slightly *less* weight loss.[1295]

Of course, given the same *duration* of exercise, some studies have found that vigorous cardio induces more fat loss than moderate cardio.[1296] But that's what you'd expect, since vigorous cardio burns far more calories per minute.

The above studies suggest that the main thing for weight loss is the *number* of calories you burn—not the *rate* at which you burn them. Do you like your workouts long and easy, or short and hard? It's up to you.

For weight loss, one doesn't seem inherently "better."

And remember: diet trumps all.

## Alternatives to Jogging

Jogging holds a hallowed place in our culture. But according to a recent exercise physiology textbook:

> *Jogging is not for everyone, and for those who are obese, or have ankle, knee, or hip problems, it might*

*be a good activity to avoid. Two activities that*
*reduce such stress are cycling (stationary or outdoor)*
*and swimming.*[1297]

Jogging is but one of many potentially productive forms of vigorous cardio. A 2015 study found that swimming lowered body fat and increased lean muscle mass in middle-aged women after three months.[1298] Swimming may be especially ideal for bigger people, as people with more fat are more buoyant in the water, and need less energy to swim at any given speed.[1299]

Rowing on an erg machine and cross-country skiing are both excellent, low-impact, full-body workouts. Rowing was a staple of my routine when I lost a boatload of weight.

Another gem is walking on a treadmill at a steep incline—"treadmill hiking," as I call it. The slope of the treadmill necessitates walking, which eliminates most of the impact forces of jogging, but provides a similar aerobic workout.

Many people hold on to the sides of the treadmill and lean back when they go treadmill hiking or use a StairMaster, which makes the exercise far easier—utterly defeating the purpose of the incline. A 2014 study found that walking at a 5% incline—unsupported—burned more calories than holding the rails and leaning back at a 10% incline.[1300]

Don't hold the rails.

## Take-Home

Vigorous cardio has greater health benefits, and lets you burn calories faster. But calorie for calorie, the science doesn't say it's better for weight loss. Whether you want to burn calories fast or slow is a personal choice. And vigorous cardio is much harder, which means it takes more willpower—with no obvious weight-loss payoff.

You should definitely do vigorous cardio if you enjoy it, but unless you make it a regular habit, it won't be productive in the long term. Compared to moderate exercise, adherence to intense exercise tends to be lower.[1301]

You'd be better off doing regular long walks for the rest of your life than sporadic jogs.

41

# GO ALL OUT

## High-Intensity Interval Training

*High-intensity interval training.* It even sounds hard.

The origins of HIIT can be traced through a 1996 paper by Japanese researcher Izumi Tabata. The aptly named "Tabata Protocol" featured seven sets of 20-second, all-out sprints on a stationary bike, with 10 seconds of rest between sets.[1302] This improved both the aerobic (with oxygen) and anaerobic (sans oxygen) capacities of the participants.

Since then, "HIIT" has been used to describe various protocols with various sets of various lengths.[1303,1304] According to the American College of Sports Medicine, HIIT can be done "on all exercise modes," with hard intervals (80% to 95% of max heart rate; "hard to very hard") lasting anywhere from five seconds to eight minutes, and easy intervals (40% to 50% of max heart rate; "very comfortable") lasting anywhere from one to *nine* times as long as the hard intervals.[1305]

How's that for specific? In practice, HIIT just means "light exercise with regular bursts of much harder exercise."

And the science indicates that this is very effective.

## A HIIT of Health

HIIT causes large improvements in insulin sensitivity (an excellent marker of health).[1306] A 2011 trial found that HIIT can "rapidly improve glucose control" in Type 2 diabetics.[1307] In a 2008 trial, interval training improved insulin sensitivity and blood-vessel function more than traditional, steady-state cardio in people with metabolic syndrome.[1308]

The list goes on. HIIT raises good cholesterol,[1309] and a meta-analysis of exercise in people with chronic disease found that HIIT increased cardiovascular fitness (another excellent health marker) *twice* as much as moderate cardio.[1310]

HIIT significantly improves anaerobic capacity,[1311] making it a rare bridge between the aerobic (breathing fuels it) and anaerobic (breathing doesn't fuel it) systems. HIIT causes a rapid increase in heart rate, followed by a much different hormonal response than moderate, steady-state cardio—one that may be particularly good for burning fat. Several studies have found that HIIT significantly reduces visceral fat, and modestly reduces weight.[1312]

So HIIT is great for your health.

And this is where the facts end, and the hype begins.

## HIIT: Overrated?

Some fitness gurus dogmatically proclaim that HIIT is far superior to traditional cardio for fat loss. The science, though, is much less convincing.

Studies directly comparing the fat-loss effects of HIIT and traditional cardio have had mixed results. Some found HIIT to cause more fat loss,[1313,1314] some found traditional cardio to cause more fat loss,[1315,1316] and some found that both were about the same.[1317,1318]

HIIT seldom causes significant weight loss, even in overweight subjects.[1319,1320] Critics will say that muscle weighs more than fat, but if HIIT were some kind of Shiva the Fat-Destroyer, you'd think overweight HIIT-ers might lose a few pounds.

A 2015 meta-analysis of 50 studies found no significant weight-loss difference between HIIT and traditional cardio.[1321] A year later, a 2016 meta-analysis of ten studies of exercise in people with coronary artery disease concluded that moderate cardio actually caused more weight loss than HIIT.[1322]

One of the studies most frequently used to tout the fat-burning prowess of HIIT took place in 1994 (Angelo Tremblay, et al.). It found that subjects doing HIIT lost far more subcutaneous fat than subjects doing steady-state cardio.[1323]

This study is often presented like a smoking gun.

But neither of the exercise groups in the study—which lasted *fifteen weeks*, by the way—lost any significant weight (the cardio group lost 1.1 pounds, on average, while the HIIT group lost 0.2 lbs).[1324] And all the subjects had previously been completely sedentary.

Critics will say the HIIT group gained muscle and lost fat, but if you go through the results of the study with a fine-tooth comb, you'll see that, while the HIIT group *did* lose more fat overall, there was no significant difference in abdominal fat loss (arguably the most important kind) between the two groups.[1325]

It's hard to claim the HIIT group got uniquely shredded when they didn't even lose more abdominal fat. Oh, and the study used the relatively inaccurate "skinfold" method to measure fat.

But I digress.

## Sprint Interval Training (SIT)

A similar but slightly different way to exercise is *sprint interval training*, or SIT (not to be confused with *sitting*). SIT doesn't even pretend to be cardio. It's just short, all-out sprints (30 seconds or less) with long periods of passive rest (around four minutes, possibly sitting) in between.

Even though SIT is completely anaerobic (breathing doesn't fuel it), it improves aerobic capacity[1326] (*cardiovascular fitness*, $VO_2$ *max*, etc.), which is wildly healthy. In fact, a 2014 meta-analysis found that SIT was just as effective as moderate-to-vigorous cardio at improving aerobic capacity.[1327]

SIT also improves insulin sensitivity and drops LDL (bad) cholesterol,[1328] and it improves blood-vessel function just as much as traditional cardio.[1329]

Bless SIT's heart.

A 2012 trial compared a short SIT session (two minutes of total sprinting) to thirty minutes of traditional cardio (70% $VO_2$ max). By measuring the amount of oxygen people breathed, they found that traditional cardio burned more calories *during* exercise, but SIT caused more calories to be burned *after* exercise (known as *excess post-exercise oxygen consumption*). By 24 hours, both groups had burned around the same number of calories.[1330]

Very short SIT workouts, then, can burn just as many calories as long cardio workouts.

(Note: This doesn't make SIT "better" or cardio "worse.")

A trial in 2014 put fifteen women through six weeks of SIT. Afterward, the women had lower body fat, smaller waists, and increased lean mass.[1331]

Another 2014 trial found that fifteen-second sprints caused the same increases in aerobic and anaerobic power as thirty-second sprints,[1332] implying that short sprints can be as effective as long ones.

If you want to exercise for as short as humanly possible, SIT is your best friend.

## HIIT and SIT: Final Thoughts

HIIT and SIT are very healthy. They seem to improve body composition and deliver lots of bang for your buck, time-wise. But keep them in perspective. Like any form of exercise, HIIT and SIT are not fat-loss panaceas. You can't outrun a bad diet.

And despite the hype, there's little evidence that HIIT and SIT are actually better for fat loss than traditional cardio.

And exercising very hard is…*very hard*. How likely are you to make SIT or HIIT a habit? To my shame, I haven't. And I exercise more than most, with a penchant for self-torture—have you seen all the citations in this book?

From a bird's-eye view of your lifetime fat stores, a two-month HIIT fad isn't going to make a big difference. And in a country where less than half of adults met the 2008 Physical Activity Guidelines[1333]—and 32% don't exercise at all[1334]—how practical is it to tell the average Joe or Jane to sprint three times a week?

Still, research tells us there are big benefits to moving as fast as you can. Maybe you're a better exerciser than I, and you start to HIIT and SIT on the regular. It's also possible to incorporate this sort of exercise—and its immense benefits—in a more sustainable way: maybe you pedal really hard for a minute during every other bike ride, or do a sprint every other time you go for a walk.

When it's not a crushing chore, sprinting can be fun.

And every sprint counts.

# 42

# EXERCISE: CONCLUSION

The most important thing about exercise and weight loss is that *diet comes first*.

Diet is more important than exercise.

Never forget that.

But you're built to move. Going from not exercising regularly to exercising regularly is one of the most profoundly healthy lifestyle changes a person can ever make. Exercise is the best medicine. There is no copay, no negative side effects or allergies, refills are free, and it can be taken anytime. Exercise reduces the risk of most major diseases simultaneously, and while it may not be the most effective way to *lose* weight, it's especially powerful in helping you *keep weight off* once you've lost it. Don't underestimate that one.

At the absolute minimum, the thing to do is walk—at a pace you feel comfortable with. Walking is cardio. It's convenient and easy, and regular walks will actually give you most of the health benefits of exercise (*most;* I didn't say *all*). If you never do anything but regular long walks, that's so much better than nothing that it's almost silly to criticize you.

But if you don't *at least* walk or do some other form of regular exercise, you simply don't care about your health too much.

It's that simple.

Once you're at least walking, the next logical step is resistance training. Resistance training has independent and broad health benefits, it helps with weight loss, and it becomes more and more important as you age. Combining cardio and resistance training brings greater health and weight-loss benefits than either alone. Try to focus on compound resistance movements.

If you still have gas in the tank after getting in the habit of resistance training, get in the habit of doing vigorous cardio and/or intervals. These will take you to the blessed heights of where exercise can bring the human body.

But whatever you do, at least walk.

And try to be on your feet a few hours per day.

**Habit 3: Exercise regularly. (At least walk regularly.)**

# PART 3

# Sleep

# 43

# SLEEP OFF THE POUNDS

As someone who struggled with sleeping problems for years, I can tell you that sleep touches everything. And the science tells us that getting enough sleep is one of the select few things with an impact on weight loss worth writing home about.

Why is this?

Let's play devil's advocate.

Let's assume you didn't sleep well last night.

## You Won't Feel Full

The hormone that makes you feel full is called *leptin*. Feeling "full" is, more or less, feeling leptin. If your body is in good working order, the more leptin in your blood, the fuller you will feel.

Inadequate sleep causes your body to produce *less* leptin.[1335,1336] And with less leptin, you'll feel less full.

Or in other words, *more hungry*.

## You'll Be *Extra* Hungry

The opposite of leptin is *ghrelin*, the "hunger" hormone.[1337] Ghrelin makes you feel hungry. The more ghrelin in your blood, the hungrier you will feel. Ghrelin is the yin to leptin's yang. Hungry and full. Full and hungry. Leptin and ghrelin.

Inadequate sleep causes your body to make *more* ghrelin.[1338]

And more ghrelin means...*more hunger*.

So inadequate sleep means you'll have less leptin to make you feel full, and more ghrelin to make you feel hungry. On average, this nasty one-two punch (less leptin, more ghrelin) will cause you to eat more food—*and gain more fat*.

A 2010 study found that, compared to eight hours of sleep, young men on just four hours of sleep ate an average of *559 more calories* per day.[1339]

That's an extra Big Mac.

A 2013 study found that just five days of sleep restriction led to nearly two pounds of weight gain.[1340]

And it gets worse.

## You WILL Crave Junk Food

Not only is Tired You hungrier and less full, but according to a 2013 study in *Nature*, you'll have a special craving for "weight-gain promoting high-calorie foods."[1341] In this study, they found that lack of sleep not only makes people crave more food in general, but specifically makes them crave junk food.

A well-controlled 2016 study may shed light here. It found that sleep-deprived people have more endocannabinoids in their blood.[1342] If you noticed the first seven letters of "cannabis" lurking in that word, you're on the right track: endocannabinoids bind to the same brain receptors as the THC of marijuana.[1343]

On a chemical level, being sleep deprived may be similar to having the munchies.

## You WILL Have Less Willpower

Willpower can be scientifically measured, and a broad range of studies have found that when people don't sleep enough, they have less willpower the next day.[1344,1345,1346,1347]

If this is true, can you really blame your tired self for gaining weight? It was practically inevitable. On top of feeling less full and more hungry, Tired You really craves junk food—and has less willpower to resist it.

Can you imagine a more fattening scenario?

This is why a 2008 meta-analysis of the sleep habits of 634,511 people found a "consistent increased risk of obesity amongst short sleepers [less than five hours per night]"[1348] and why a 2014 meta-analysis concluded that "short sleep duration was significantly associated with incidence of obesity."[1349]

It's why the twin who sleeps less is significantly more likely to be overweight,[1350] and why a 2009 study of 537 Canadians found that sleeping under six hours a night was *the single greatest risk factor for being overweight.*[1351] (Even more than dietary factors.)

Did lack of sleep make America fat? If sleep played a major role in the recent obesity epidemic, then Americans would be sleeping less today than they slept in the recent past.

Sure enough, between the 1960s and 2000—when obesity rates took off like the Apollo 11 space shuttle—average US sleep time dropped from about 8.5 hours to just 7 hours per night.[1352]

That's nearly 20% less sleep. And polls suggest that since the year 2000, we've been sleeping even less.[1353,1354]

And since then, we've gotten even fatter.[1355]

## How to Sleep More

The evidence is overwhelming. You need to get enough sleep.

But what's *enough*? We're all different, and there's no golden number. Experts generally recommend between seven and nine hours of sleep a night.[1356]

The important thing is to get enough sleep to feel rested most days. If you *don't* feel rested most days, then getting more sleep is probably one of the best things you can possibly do for weight loss.

So how do you get more sleep?

It depends. If you fall asleep easily, the answer is also easy: just go to bed earlier. Get some rough idea of how much sleep you need to feel rested, subtract that from the time you plan to wake up, and add 30 minutes for good measure.

Problem solved.

On the other hand, if your problem is falling asleep or staying asleep, my condolences. Here are some helpful, science-based tips:

- **Go to bed and wake up at consistent times.** Our circadian rhythms adapt to the time we're typically asleep,[1357] so try to give your body what it's expecting. Aim to sleep and wake at regular times.
- **Reduce artificial light at night.** Staring at bright screens tricks your body into thinking it's daytime; circadian rhythms are regulated in the eyes.[1358] Make it a rule not to look at bright screens (cell phones, laptops, TVs, etc.) in the hour before bed. If this is too much, at least download free software called f.lux. At night, this software reduces the *blue light* your screen emits. Blue light is the spectra of light with the worst impact on our circadian rhythms.[1359]

- **Move around during the day.** Physical activity improves sleep quality,[1360] among other things. We're not evolved to sit all day.
- **Get sunlight.** Morning sunlight can help reset your biological clock.[1361] We didn't evolve indoors. Vitamin D deficiency is caused by lack of sunlight, and it's a serious health problem.[1362] Get outside.
- **Avoid caffeine after noon.** Caffeine keeps you awake, and lingers in your system. The half-life of caffeine (how long it takes to clear *half* the caffeine you ingest) is almost six hours.[1363]
- **Avoid nicotine, big meals, and intense exercise within two hours of bedtime.** All of these can interfere with your sleep.[1364]
- **Make a to-do list for the next day.** Thinking about upcoming duties can keep you up, and writing them down can help relax your mind.[1365] If your mind is still racing after a bit, get out of bed and do something else.
- **Use relaxation techniques to fall asleep faster.** Deep breathing,[1366] listening to relaxing soundtracks,[1367] and progressive muscle relaxation[1368] can help people fall asleep faster. (That last one means tensing and then relaxing all the muscles in your body, starting at the head or toes and working down or up, respectively.)
- **Do cognitive behavioral therapy (CBT).** CBT effectively treats many mental disorders,[1369] including insomnia.[1370] Learn about CBT.

## Take-Home

If you sleep better, you'll *feel* better. You'll feel more full, less hungry, and less tempted by junk food.

And you'll have the willpower to make your dreams come true.

**Habit 4: Get enough sleep to feel rested most days.**

# PART 4

# Checks & Balances

## 44

# WEIGHT AND WAIST

If you don't drink sugar, generally avoid processed food, exercise regularly, and get enough sleep, you've eliminated the root causes of being overweight. You're doing a lot better than most people. (In fact, why don't you come up here and say a few words?)

But this may not be enough. Maybe you were heavy for years, and your metabolism stays altered long after you've lost weight[1371] (or even permanently) in a way that predisposes you to gain the weight back.[1372] Or, despite your best intentions, maybe processed food slithers into your life (as it slithers into mine).

Maybe you like to stuff yourself long past satiety. Maybe you binge eat for emotional reasons (which is possible even with whole foods). Maybe you have an unhealthy obsession with eating. Or maybe you have a naturally bigger body type, and it's harder for you to get skinny than it is for most people.

Rather than try to diagnose and cure every possible reason people struggle to lose weight, it's better to instill an objective system that lets you know how you're doing—and when you need to adjust.

That system starts with the bathroom scale.

People are great at self-deception. When I was 40 pounds overweight, I'd stand tall, retract my bulging gut, look in the mirror, and assure myself I looked lean. All that extra weight? Muscle. I'd been lifting. "It weighs more than fat."

Aside from lying to ourselves, we can also simply be wrong. Our judgment isn't perfect. In short, we can't be trusted to give ourselves honest, accurate assessments about the amount of fat on our bodies. We need something else to do that for us.

## The Scale of the Problem

It's important to get into the habit of weighing yourself most mornings. This will give you regular, objective feedback about how you're doing, and when you need to adjust.

Let's get it out of the way: scales aren't perfect. We're mainly interested in *fat*, not *weight*. Scales only give us weight. They don't differentiate between fat and muscle, between fat and food, between fat and glycogen stores, or between fat and water. All of these fluctuate, affecting your weight.

In a perfect world, there would be a device that would cheaply and accurately measure your *body fat*. You'd turn it on, hook it up to your body, and quickly get a readout that your body was, say, *18.3% fat*.

This device would be much better than a scale.

Unfortunately, it doesn't exist. Even gold-standard methods of measuring body fat like DEXA scans, which use x-rays and cost $59 to $359 per scan,[1373] and hydrostatic weighing, which involves going to a lab and getting weighed underwater, are based on *estimates*, and are surprisingly inaccurate on an individual basis.[1374]

(Not to mention inconvenient.)

The sort of consumer devices that shoot electricity through your body and use "bioelectrical impedance" to measure body fat—the kind you grab or stand on—are far more convenient than the gold-standard methods, but far more inaccurate.[1375,1376]

And if feedback isn't accurate, it isn't useful.

What else is there? The well-known *skinfold test* involves a qualified person pinching several different sites on your body with calipers (not fingers), and recording how much fat is there. Accurate results depend on the same qualified pincher repeating their pinchings in the future. Even then, the results aren't as accurate for very heavy people,[1377] and the entire method rests on equations that have been found to underestimate body fat.[1378]

That brings us to the tape measure.

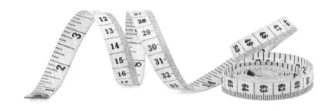

Photo Credit: Tetiana Rostopira/Shutterstock.com

Buy one of these. It will cost about five dollars on Amazon, and it can change your life.

You're going to use it to measure your waist.

Measuring your waist with a tape measure is extremely useful, for several reasons. Storing excess fat in the abdominal region is an especially strong predictor of diabetes,[1379] heart disease,[1380] and death.[1381] For all three of these, waist circumference seems to be a better predictor of risk than body mass index (BMI).[1382]

In other words, the tape is mightier than the scale.

Even in normal-weight people, excess fat in the midsection

is strongly associated with diabetes,[1383] heart disease,[1384] and death.[1385] Since these people are *normal* weight, the scale does not alert them to health risks.

But measuring their waist with a tape measure does.

According to major health institutions, you should aim for under a 40-inch waist if you're a man, and under a 35-inch waist if you're a woman.[1386,1387]

These numbers are very conservative. If your waist is bigger, then you have a problem. Losing weight should be a top priority in your life.

In reality, the risks exist on a continuum. The World Health Organization deems men at increased health risk if their waist measures over 37 inches, and women at increased risk if their waist measures over 31.5 inches.[1388]

And the risks probably start before that.

Every morning, standing relaxed, measure your waist.

Your waist is the midway point between the bottom of your ribs and the top of your hipbone. For most people, this will be somewhere around the belly button. The most important thing is to measure in the same place every time.

Breathe out, and wrap the tape measure around your waist. The tape measure should be parallel to the floor and fit a little snugly, without digging into your skin. Your waist measurement is the number where the zero end meets the slack end of the tape.

Why is abdominal fat so unhealthy? It seems to have to do with *visceral fat*, a metabolically active fat surrounding the liver and other abdominal organs.

Excess visceral fat is associated with insulin resistance and a general inflammatory state.[1389] Regularly measuring your waist will let you know if you have too much visceral fat.

But alerting you to major health risks that a scale can miss is only the beginning. Whenever you're trying to accomplish a goal, it's important to have regular, objective feedback.

Weighing yourself is one piece of objective feedback. Waist measurements are another.

With just the scale, weight loss can get discouraging. You might be excited to step on the scale after a day of dieting, only to see that you've gained a pound. Weight fluctuates in weird ways, which can make the whole thing seem hopeless.

But if you're in the habit of measuring your waist after you step on the scale, you may find that your waist is slightly smaller than yesterday. This can give you hope.

Similarly, if you start a new exercise routine, you might gain some muscle and lose some fat. But the fat loss and muscle gain may cancel each other out—even though your body composition has improved, you might not *weigh* any less.

This is where the tape measure shines. If you gain muscle and lose fat, the tape will find it. In general, the tape measure is much better at measuring body fat than a scale. After all, the tape literally measures the fat around your waist.

The scale measures *weight* loss.

The tape measures *fat* loss.

The tape is also far more universal than the scale. It doesn't matter whether you're short or tall, whether you have a big frame or a small frame, or how muscular you are: if you're a man with over a 40-inch waist, or a woman with over a 35-inch waist, you have a problem. If you're a man with over a 37-inch waist or a woman with over a 31.5-inch waist, you have elevated health risks.

There's no way to do that with weight; it's too variable.

Similarly, I have no idea how much you'd have to weigh to get a flat-looking stomach or a six-pack. But I *can* tell you that, if you're a man, you'll need to get down to a 34-inch waist (or less) for a flat-looking stomach, and a 32-inch waist (or less) for a six-pack.

This is probably true for 95% of guys.

Our *weight* is a personal number, but our *waist* gives us universal standards to shoot for. (And another personal number.)

In short, waist measurements are another easy, powerful, highly relevant data point to measure on our weight-loss journey.

When you wake up in the morning, weigh yourself on the scale, then measure your waist. Then record the numbers.

I made a Google Sheet called *Date, Weight, Waist.*

I try to update it every morning.

I suggest you do the same. It's a game-changer.

## Butt, Hips, or Thighs?

For some women, taking *butt, hip,* or *thigh* measurements may be better than taking waist measurements. Just ask yourself the following question: *When I gain weight, where does most of it go?*

Got it? That's where you should measure.

That's where your extra fat gets stored.

For me, that place is my gut. It bulges like a balloon when I get fat. Other hard-hit areas include my love handles, back, upper arms, and upper neck. But my *midsection* always takes the brunt of the trauma.

This goes for most men and many women. Hence the *waist* focus. But for many other women, extra fat mostly goes to their butt, hips, and/or thighs. And *that's* where they should measure. (Not their waist.)

Wherever your extra fat goes, measure that place the same way every morning, and track your progress. Measuring the same way every morning and tracking progress is more important than fussing over whether you're using "perfect" measuring technique.

## A Golden Habit

The scale is powerful by itself. But combine it with waist measurements (or butt, thigh, or hip measurements), and you have an extremely effective feedback system to keep you on track. Just keep in mind that these measurements will fluctuate a bit from day to day, for reasons that have nothing to do with fat (hydration levels, glycogen levels, etc.).

Don't think of these numbers as *tests* that make or break you. Instead, think of them as steady whispering *guideposts* that tell you how you're doing, and whether you need to adjust.

Scales and tapes are necessary, because people don't get fat overnight. Weight creeps up in imperceptible degrees. *You* might not feel the five pounds you gained over Thanksgiving, but the scale will.

Scales and tapes are necessary, because we need regular, accurate, objective feedback.

That brings us to the final Golden Weight-Loss Habit:

## Habit 5: Every morning, measure your weight and waist.

Regular self-weighing is one of the most common habits in the National Weight Control Registry (the gold standard of weight-loss power). 75% of NWCR members weigh themselves at least once a week,[1390] and 44% weigh themselves at least once a day.[1391] And remember, these people *already* lost a lot of weight, and kept it off at least a year.

I still weigh myself almost every day.

Despite the popular belief that regularly weighing yourself leads to some kind of unhealthy neurotic obsession, a 2015 review of 17 studies found that:

> *Regular self-weighing has been associated with weight loss and not with negative psychological outcomes.*[1392]

Less frequent weigh-ins—say, once a week—might be

better for someone prone to eating disorders or weight obsession. But when you're only getting feedback once a week, it can be hard to pinpoint what's causing your weight to change.

And there are fewer opportunities to adjust.

Infrequent feedback can make a higher-than-expected weight all the more discouraging. With daily weigh-ins, on the other hand, you'll care less about any *one* weight, and you'll have enough feedback to spot links between what you do and how much you weigh. Indeed, studies suggest that daily weighing causes more weight loss than weekly weighing.[1393,1394,1395]

So weigh and measure yourself every day.

And don't worry if you miss a day, a week, or even a month. "Every morning" is a goal, *not* a requirement.

The key is to keep getting back on the horse.

What else? Let's see. Notice how your clothes fit. Grab the parts of your body where you want less fat, and feel how much fat is there. Periodically look at your naked body in the mirror from several angles. (Don't suck in your gut. On the contrary, see how far you can push your gut *out*.)

Along with measuring your weight and waist, these quick-and-dirty metrics will give you a very accurate picture of how your body fat is changing.

## Take-Home

We need objective, regular feedback to stay on track.
The scale measures *weight* loss.
The tape measures *fat* loss.
Use both.

**Habit 5: Every morning, measure your weight and waist.**

# 45

# SHORT-TERM PROGRAMS

Say you weigh and measure yourself, and the numbers are higher than you want. What do you do? If you haven't already, let this motivate you to build The Five Golden Weight-Loss Habits. Cut out sugary drinks, only eat whole foods most days, exercise regularly, get enough sleep, and keep weighing and measuring yourself.

These habits are the main drivers of lifelong weight loss. They're the only way that most people can ever successfully lose weight—because they act in the *long term*.

Build these habits. Stick to them.

They're the most important thing.

But what if they're already established? Or what if you're working on building them, but you feel like you need something more—a radical change to kick things off? Maybe you want to do a short-term weight-loss strategy: a diet, program, etc.

This is fine. It may even be necessary for many people.

After great consideration, I decided that short-term strategies are mostly outside the scope of this book.

(It's long enough already.)

But quickly, some effective short-term strategies are fasting, intermittent fasting, calorie counting, and restricting yourself to certain foods (low-carb, low-fat, Whole30, etc.).

All of these approaches can work. The main idea is to take in fewer calories than you burn.

Despite some silly things you'll hear, at the end of the day, your body is a chemical system. Like all chemical systems, it obeys chemical laws.

The number of calories you burn each day is known as your *total daily energy expenditure* (TDEE). Your TDEE is the sum of your basal metabolic rate, the cost of digesting food, and all your physical activity.[1396]

When you eat more calories than you burn (your calorie intake is greater than your TDEE), you will gain weight.

When you eat as many calories as you burn (your calorie intake equals your TDEE), your weight will be stable.

When you eat fewer calories than you burn (your calorie intake is less than your TDEE), you will lose weight.

It's that simple.

For several reasons, it's hard to predict exactly how much weight you'll gain or lose. But these basic principles (eating less than you burn equals weight loss, and eating more than you burn equals weight gain) are very well-established in the scientific literature.[1397,1398,1399,1400,1401,1402,1403]

These principles follow directly from the laws of thermodynamics, and are basically indisputable. How do they fit with The Five Golden Weight-Loss Habits? By cutting out sugary drinks and processed food most days, you'll naturally feel fuller on fewer calories, eat below your TDEE, and gradually lose weight.

Sufficient sleep and regular exercise will help everything, and regularly measuring your weight and waist will keep you on track and help you avoid eating unnecessary calories.

If you decide to do a short-term strategy, be sure to eat

fewer calories than you burn. That's the only real requirement. If your program fails, it's because you didn't eat fewer calories than you burned. If it succeeds, you ate fewer calories than you burned. Period.

Here are three more guidelines that apply to all short-term weight-loss strategies:

## Short-Term Weight-Loss Guidelines

- **The less you eat, the more of your calories should come from protein.** Not only will more protein help you feel fuller on fewer calories (protein's campaign slogan: *"fuller on fewer"*), but it will minimize muscle loss.[1404] Sadly, in typical weight loss, a sizable portion of the lost weight is actually *muscle*. But you can minimize this by eating more protein. *More* protein is as important as *less* fat or carbs.

- **Drink lots of water.** Drinking more water will help you feel fuller and eat less.[1405] Drinking more water helps replace some of the oral fixation of eating, and actually causes you to burn significantly more calories. Your body has to process and filter all that water. This isn't free—one study found that drinking two extra liters of water (about half a gallon) caused people to burn almost 100 more calories per day.[1406]

- **Continue to follow The Five Golden Weight-Loss Habits.** When you're not eating as much, it's even more critical that what you *do* eat be whole foods (for both health and satiety). Regular exercise will speed up weight loss and preserve muscle. Getting enough sleep will maximize the willpower at your disposal to stick to the diet or program. Weighing and measuring yourself will keep you on track. Stick to the habits.

## Take-Home

Weight loss comes down to calories in versus calories out. If you follow a short-term program, be sure to eat fewer calories than you burn, drink a lot of water, try to eat a high-protein diet, and continue to follow The Five Golden Weight-Loss Habits.

# 46

# THE RAPID WEIGHT-LOSS OPTION

Most people don't realize this, but you have the option to lose weight quickly. You can accomplish this by eating a lot less.

Normal-weight people can survive around 60 days without a single calorie before starving to death.[1407] *60 days*. Heavy people can last far longer than that.[1408] Fat is just stored energy, after all. Remember that the next time you worry about missing a meal.

The higher your total daily energy expenditure (TDEE) soars over your calorie intake, the faster you'll lose weight. Taken to its logical extreme, the quickest short-term weight-loss strategy is to significantly cut your food intake, and exercise a lot more. Summon the willpower to do this, and you *will* lose weight quickly.

## Health Risks?

In general, the health risks of eating a lot less are greatly exaggerated. Even water fasting (consuming nothing but water) for long periods of time does not usually lead to any health complications. According to one scientific review,

> *Prolonged fasting is generally well tolerated with few and relatively minor complications.*[1409]

For example, in a 1968 study of 46 obese people who water-fasted for two weeks, no serious medical complications occurred.[1410]

46 people. Two weeks. No food.

No medical complications.

I've talked to many people who have fasted for long periods, and have never heard of any serious complications. (Though pregnant women should probably avoid fasting, and diabetics should be cautious.[1411])

In my experience, fasting feels *healthy*, not unhealthy.

## Lose Muscle?

In general, the risk of losing muscle from eating a lot less is greatly exaggerated. After three to four days of total starvation, it's estimated that a man will lose a gram of muscle for every 2.4 grams of fat he loses.[1412] But the vast majority (over 70%) of the weight he loses is still fat.

As the fast progresses, his muscle loss will shrink even further. Eventually, he'll lose a gram of muscle for every *nine* grams of fat he loses.[1413]

In any case, the average muscle loss from all-out fasting isn't much worse than traditional weight-loss diets. In the average successful diet, around 20% to 27% of total weight loss is muscle.[1414]

Muscle loss may be a concern if you're already very lean, but think about it: fat is just stored energy, right? When the body needs energy during a fast, why would it preferentially break down *muscle* if it's still got plenty of fat?

That wouldn't make sense.

And that's not what your body does. According to a biochemistry textbook:

> *Proteins are not stored, so any breakdown will necessitate a loss of function. Thus, the second priority of metabolism in starvation is to preserve protein, which is accomplished by shifting the fuel being used from glucose to fatty acids and ketone bodies.*[1415]

Fat—not protein—is the primary energy source your body uses during major calorie deficits.

If you've got visible fat to lose, you have little reason to worry that your body will cannibalize all your muscle.

## Starvation Mode?

In general, the risk of entering "starvation mode" from eating a lot less is greatly exaggerated. Contrary to popular belief, when you stop ingesting calories (water fasting), your metabolism doesn't slow down for quite some time.

After 21 days of water-fasting every other day, the 16 subjects of a 2005 study did not experience any slowdown in basal metabolism.[1416]

In a 1994 study, the metabolic rates of 29 subjects did not decrease between 12 hours and 36 hours of fasting (in fact, they slightly *increased*, though not significantly).[1417]

In a 2000 study, after four days of water fasting, the resting metabolic rates of the 11 subjects were *increased* by 10%, 13%, and 12% after two, three, and four days of fasting, respectively.[1418] Small increases in metabolic rate after a 48-hour fast were also shown in a 1990 study.[1419]

If anything, then, short-term fasting speeds up your metabolism. The idea of "starvation mode" came from studies of prolonged, intense calorie restriction—20 days of water fasting,[1420] for example, or three to six months of severe dieting.[1421]

These studies showed significant metabolic slowdown, but they're not relevant for the average person eating a lot less for a week.

## Gain It All Back? Unhealthy?

Finally, in general, whether a person "gains all the weight back" is determined by their habits. (Although people who have lost a lot of weight have slightly slower metabolisms than weight-matched people who haven't.[1422])

Gaining all the weight back is in no way inevitable. Eating a lot less is what worked for me, for example. I summoned oceans of willpower, ate a lot less, and exercised a lot more. I even started to perceive hunger as a tool of transformation, rather than a nagging pain. Hunger went from being a signal to eat, to a signal that my body was eating *fat*—and that I was accomplishing my goal. I learned to relish hunger.

This short-term, extreme mindset was extremely effective. I lost over 30 pounds in under a month. (And another 20 pounds the next month.) Aside from some relatively minor fluctuations, I've kept them off ever since.

(I stopped drinking sugary drinks.)

Was losing weight that quickly "unhealthy"? It certainly didn't feel that way. More than anything, it felt spiritual.

And in hindsight, having kept the weight off for a decade, that short period of rapid weight loss seems to be one of the healthiest things I've ever done.

Despite the popular belief that losing weight quickly is

"unhealthy," it's really only losing weight quickly in the context of yo-yo dieting—quickly losing and gaining and losing and gaining lots of weight—that is considered unhealthy.

But a 2014 review of 20 studies concluded that there was "no evidence" that a yo-yoing weight was any worse for your health than staying overweight or obese.[1423]

It's not like it's any healthier to be consistently fat.

And despite the popular belief that losing weight quickly is tied to yo-yo dieting, a 2016 study found that rapid weight loss did *not* lead to more weight regain than the slow and steady weight loss people preach.[1424]

Maybe you'd like to lose weight quickly. We are a world of very heavy people, and the thought of losing 50 pounds by losing a pound a week for a full year—the glacial pace recommended by most authority figures—may seem unbearably slow.

I don't recommend rapid weight loss for everyone. But everyone should at least understand that the option to lose weight quickly exists, and is generally well-tolerated. If you're highly motivated to change your life, you shouldn't let the "pound a week" dogma bore you into staying overweight.

There's nothing wrong with solving a problem fast.

## Take-Home

You'll lose weight quickly if you eat a lot less. The concerns people have about eating a lot less—potential health complications, losing muscle, and entering "starvation mode"—are greatly exaggerated.

# PART 5

# Stairway to Heaven

47

# THE ANATOMY
# OF WILLPOWER

Willpower is real. It may sound fluffy, but *willpower* is not a word like *karma*—there's convincing scientific evidence that willpower exists.

It wears many hats. *Self-discipline, self-control, self-regulation, self-denial, determination, grit,* etc. Willpower is the force that you use to pay attention to a boring talk, quit smoking, hold back fury, do laundry, or spend the long weekend with your in-laws. Willpower is what you use to swim against the current of the Lazy River. It's how you make yourself do things you don't want to do.

For the sake of style, it'll just be *willpower* from now on.

Willpower is partly innate. Differences in willpower at a very young age seem to persist for life.

One study monitored a thousand people from birth to age 32. From the tender ages of 3 to 11, they were subjected to regular willpower tests. The kids with more willpower turned into adults with more willpower—adults who made more money and were healthier, less addicted to drugs, and less likely to end up in jail.[1425]

Scientists are still fleshing out the details, but we know a front-brain structure called the anterior cingulate cortex plays a critical role in willpower.[1426]

And we know willpower is tightly linked to blood sugar. When blood sugar is high, willpower is generally high. And when blood sugar is low, willpower generally suffers.[1427]

This makes sense. The brain uses a whopping 19% of the body's total energy supply.[1428] Since blood sugar is the brain's main fuel, it's logical that when blood sugar is low, parts of the brain that aren't essential to survival on a minute-to-minute basis (like the anterior cingulate cortex) would get less blood sugar, and slow down.

(Willpower is important, but it's not *breathing*.)

And there are some uncanny links between willpower and blood sugar.

## Willpower and Blood Sugar

- Blood sugar is used most efficiently in the morning— right when willpower is the highest.[1429]
- Alcohol reduces self-control (willpower), and it reduces blood-sugar metabolism in the anterior cingulate cortex (the willpower hub).[1430]
- Diabetics, who struggle to use blood sugar efficiently, do poorly on tests of willpower.[1431]
- It's hard to focus (a form of willpower) when you're sleep deprived. Sleep deprivation decreases blood-sugar metabolism in brain regions associated with attention control.[1432]
- Criminal behavior is associated with both poor impulse control (a form of willpower) and poor blood-sugar control.[1433]

- "Hangry" people are less able to control their emotions. Being hangry (hungry + angry) is caused by low blood sugar.

**When you have low blood sugar, you have low willpower.**

## How Willpower Burns

Scientists study willpower with several different tests, like seeing how long someone works on an impossible geometry puzzle before they give up, or how long it takes them to yank their hand out of a bucket of ice water after plunging it in. The logic is that people burn willpower when they force themselves to do hard things.

And burning willpower leaves people with less willpower for *other* hard things. In one experiment, 67 college students skipped a meal and sat at a table with a stack of cookies and a bowl of radishes.[1434] To maximize temptation, the cookies were baked in the testing room. The researchers let one group of students eat the cookies, but forbade the other group from eating the cookies, only allowing them to eat the radishes (poor souls).

Right after, both groups were given an impossible geometry puzzle to solve. There was also a control group who simply skipped a meal and went straight to the impossible geometry puzzle.

On average, here's how long the different groups worked on the puzzle before quitting:

control group  21 minutes
cookie group  19 minutes
**radish group    8 minutes**

The radish group folded like a house of cards. According to the researchers, they caved so quickly because they'd already burned a blob of willpower resisting the cookies, so they had less willpower available for the geometry puzzle.

Burning willpower on one hard task (resisting cookies) left less willpower for a totally different hard task (the puzzle). In other words, willpower is *general-purpose*. We use it for many different things.

Kind of like money.

The question is, what will you spend your willpower on?

It's not just obvious things, like resisting cookies, that burn willpower. For instance, making decisions burns willpower.[1435] One study showed that judges were far more likely to grant parole in their first three decisions of a court session—before "decision fatigue" set in—than in their last three decisions.[1436]

You don't want a hangry judge.

The following things have all been found to deplete willpower: managing the impression you're making on someone, suppressing prejudices and stereotypes, coping with thoughts of death, controlling spending, restraining aggression, and controlling intake of food and alcohol.[1437]

A 2010 meta-analysis of 83 willpower studies concluded that there is "a significant effect of ego depletion on self-control task performance."[1438] In other words, this summary of 83 studies concluded that willpower is limited, that it's depleted by hard activities, and that after it's depleted, we do worse at other hard activities.

## The Flux of "You"

It's critical to realize that willpower is limited, and in constant flux. People fundamentally underestimate how different their future mental states will be from their present one. Psychologists call this the "hot-cold empathy gap." It refers to the poor ability of people in a calm, collected state to predict how they'll behave in the future—which may have churning emotions, low blood sugar (and willpower), and wicked temptations.

Studies show that this hot-cold empathy gap operates in areas as diverse as economics,[1439] eating,[1440] and sex.[1441]

It's easy to set goals when you're lounging on the couch watching holiday specials, your blood full of Christmas sugar, and your mind motivated to greet the New Year with a New You.

It's hard sticking to these goals on February 18th, after a poor night's sleep and a stressful day at work, with looming drudgeries and no major holidays (or even the weekend) anywhere in sight.

We usually set goals when we're feeling strong, and our tank of willpower is full. We project this strength into the future. That's why goals are often unrealistic: they don't account for our seesawing willpower—or our delusions. Studies have found that people tend to picture their future self as a sort of idealized saint.[1442]

Throughout my life, I've always pictured my future self as a paragon of human excellence, virtuous in all the ways that I am flawed. Alas, this person still hasn't shown up.

(But I'm expecting him any day now.)

When you're setting goals, remember that goals take willpower, and willpower fluctuates. Don't overestimate your future self when you're feeling strong, or underestimate your future self when you're feeling weak.

The point is, you are not a static entity. Your mind isn't bedrock. It's more like shifting sand, a 360° neuro-hormonal seesaw that's always tilting up and down and all around. To make successful changes in life, it helps to realize that you *are* change.

## Powering up Willpower

Willpower isn't a simple function of genetics and blood sugar. Other factors affect willpower, too. As if we needed another reason to exercise, it's been shown that regular exercise significantly improves willpower.[1443]

So does getting enough sleep.[1444,1445,1446,1447]

So does meditation.[1448]

Putting people in a positive mood increases their willpower.[1449] So does having them think more abstractly, rationally, and globally.[1450] Research indicates that motivation, beliefs, and incentives also affect willpower.[1451,1452]

In fact, believing your willpower is unlimited (and not a limited resource) has been shown to block willpower depletion in the lab, leading some researchers to speculate that willpower is "all in your head."[1453] Other studies have supported the idea that a belief in unlimited willpower makes people happier, and more likely to reach their goals.[1454]

But *other* research has shown that, while beliefs about willpower do make a difference when willpower depletion is mild, when willpower is severely depleted, beliefs don't matter.[1455] You can believe whatever you want, but willpower is still a limited resource.

Everyone needs to relax sometimes.

Even David Blaine, an endurance artist who did a medically documented water fast (consuming nothing but water) for 44 days.[1456] Blaine also held his breath underwater for 17 minutes on an episode of Oprah.[1457]

It's hard to imagine more incredible feats of self-control.

And yet, according to Blaine:

> *As soon as I'm done with that* [a stunt] *I go to the opposite extreme, where I have no self-control...After a stunt I'll go from 180 pounds to 230 pounds in three months...I'll eat perfectly for five days and then eat horrifically for ten days...I have self-discipline in work, but I have none in my life sometimes.*[1458]

David Blaine's epic willpower only seems to work in short bursts, after which it's severely depleted.

If he doesn't have unlimited willpower, neither do we.

Some studies have found that overestimating your willpower can lead to exposing yourself to more temptations than you can handle.[1459] Believing in unlimited willpower may work for some goals, but the last thing you need is to believe your willpower is unlimited, get disillusioned when you eat a cookie, and then quit.

Still, recent developments in the field suggest that beliefs and attitudes play a much larger role than previously thought, and that positive thinking has real, physical power.

Get motivated.

You can do this.

## Take-Home

Willpower is the rocket fuel we use to veer off the Lazy River and get what we want in life. It's the mental gasoline that powers us through hard tasks. It's our mighty agent of change.

But willpower is fickle. Like the blood sugar controlling it, willpower rises and falls, comes and goes, ebbs and flows.

And it's often in short supply.

When we burn willpower on *one* hard task, we have less willpower available for the next one. After enough consecutive hard tasks, our willpower tank is empty, and we're done with hard tasks.

Willpower is influenced by beliefs, motivation, and incentives. So believe in yourself.

(It's science.)

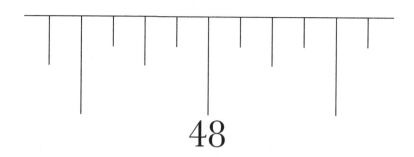

# 48

# THE PHYSIOLOGY OF HABITS

"We are what we repeatedly do.
Excellence, then, is not an act, but a habit."
-Aristotle

## Habits in Control

*We are what we repeatedly do.* What we repeatedly do are *habits.*

Despite feeling in control most of the time, research indicates that people spend around half their waking hours simply acting out of habit.[1460]

It's not just brushing your teeth and tying your shoes. Habits include the type of decisions you make, who you talk to, what you talk about, how you do things, and how you eat.

## Eating Habits

How many eating decisions do you make per day? In one experiment, 154 college students were asked to estimate how many eating decisions they made in a typical day.[1461]

Their average guess? 14.

Sounds reasonable.

To get a more accurate estimate, the students were given 15 questions about the specific components that went into their eating decisions: when, what, where, how much, and with whom to eat and drink every meal, snack, and beverage throughout an average day.

Using these more detailed guidelines, the students' average number of daily eating decisions was now 227.

This seemed high. So the researchers gave the students a digital counter to carry around. With the same guidelines as before, they were told to click their counter every time they made an eating decision. *Click.*

On average, the students clicked their counters 240 times per day. (This was slightly higher than their initial guess of 14.) It turned out that the students made 59 decisions a day simply deciding what to eat.

Why were they so far off in their initial estimates? Well, the students may have been decent estimators of their *conscious* eating decisions, but they didn't appreciate that most of their eating "decisions" weren't really *decisions*, at all—they were automatic reactions to their environments.

In other words, they were *habits.*

Changing these habits is the heart of weight loss.

## Habits in Your Brain

Changing your habits is supremely important, because willpower is limited—**and acting out of habit burns little, if any, willpower.**

When you act out of habit, whether the habit is good or bad, you burn far less willpower than when you act *against* habit.[1462] In fact, one definition of willpower is the force you use to *override* habits.[1463]

Acting out of habit is easy. Making decisions is hard.

Conscious decisions happen in an outer brain layer called the cerebral cortex.[1464,1465] This is where the tough choices go down, the ones that drain willpower.

But your brain is smart. If you keep making the same tough choices in the same situations, again and again, over and over, then new neural connections will form between your cortex and your basal ganglia,[1466] a structure near your brainstem that is heavily involved in habits.[1467]

Keep repeating these same choices, and the new neural connections will keep getting stronger until, eventually, the behavior becomes automatic: a *habit*. Instead of hemming and hawing over pros and cons, you'll just *react*—the way a frog's tongue darts out to catch a fly. These cortex-ganglia connections are the link between conscious thought and that part of our brain that only "thinks" to the extent that a frog thinks.

The point is, something that started as a *choice*—and cost willpower—got shunted to the basal ganglia, where it became an automatic habit.

**A choice repeated often enough becomes a habit.**

And whether that habit is good or bad, it will continue to make choices *for* you, for free. *Without* burning willpower.

(Your brain likes to save energy.)

The glorious upshot is that it takes willpower to *establish* a good habit, but once it's set, you're on cruise control, constantly doing good things *without* burning willpower.

You're in heaven.

For example, let's say you drink sugar. It can be tough the first few times you drink water instead of juice, soda, or some other liquid sugar. The water may taste dreadfully bland. You may have to almost gulp it down. It will take some willpower.

*But only the first few times.*

Stick it out, and pretty soon, drinking water will start to feel normal. You'll get used to it. It won't hurt anymore.

You'll just do it, automatically.

**And you won't burn willpower.**

And whenever you drink eight fluid ounces of water (just two-thirds of a can) instead of juice or soda, you'll save yourself about 100 of the world's most fattening calories.[1468,1469]

Every.

Single.

Time.

*Without effort.*

For some people, that's *hundreds* of calories per day.

That's the power of habit. Building a good habit is an initial investment that pays huge dividends in the long run.

Invest your precious willpower in building good habits.

## Cue, Routine, Reward

In practice, a habit kicks off when you perceive a *cue*, which is some relevant detail in your environment. A cue can be anything—hunger, your friend Pete, or the Netflix homepage.

A cue is something you respond to.

The first time you perceived a cue, you decided to act in a certain way—you did a *routine*. A routine is a response to a cue. A routine can be physical (you meet someone new, you shake their hand) or mental (Adele comes on the radio, you think of the one that got away).

Whatever the routine, it leads to a *reward* (or lack thereof) that helps determine if you'll repeat that routine in the future.[1470]

A reward is pleasure in your brain. Rewards are highly subjective. A reward could be the pleasure of eating chocolate cake, or the pleasure of pridefully *resisting* chocolate cake at a party.

Whatever you find rewarding, if a routine *doesn't* reward you, you'll be less likely to repeat it in the future. If a routine *does* reward you, you'll be more likely to repeat it. Keep repeating a rewarding routine in response to a cue—and keep getting rewarded—and the routine will eventually become a habit.

Cue.

Routine.

Reward.

*Repeat.*

There's a popular belief that it takes 21 days of repeating a certain routine for it to become a habit. This turns out to be a popular myth. Science indicates that how long it takes is actually extremely variable.[1471] It depends on the habit, the person, their level of motivation, and other factors. To be frank, "21 days" isn't even useful as a rough estimate.

However long it takes, though, science indicates that the more you repeat a routine, the more automatic it becomes—and that missing the odd day or occasion to do the routine has little to no impact on it becoming a habit.[1472] (That's a relief.)

Just keep trying.

## Suppression Is Futile

How do you change a bad habit? That discussion starts with how *not* to change a bad habit: trying to suppress it. Dozens of studies have shown that consciously trying to suppress bad thought patterns and behaviors is an awful strategy for changing bad thought patterns and behaviors.[1473]

These studies show that not only is suppression ineffective, it is downright counterproductive. Trying to suppress certain thoughts or behaviors tends to *increase* the frequency of those thoughts and behaviors.

In the classic suppression study, students were given a bell, and they were told *not* to think of a white bear. They were told to ring their bell whenever they thought of a white bear.

They rang their bells over once a minute, on average.[1474]

The profound implication? The students probably *never*

would have thought of a white bear if they hadn't consciously been trying *not* to.

This finding—that suppression is downright counterproductive, achieving the polar opposite of its goal—has been confirmed across a wide range of pathologies, including obsessive-compulsive disorder, depression, post-traumatic stress disorder, substance abuse, and eating disorders.[1475]

In each case, trying to suppress intrusive thoughts associated with the particular disorder caused reports of those nasty thoughts to *increase*, not decrease.

(Suppression may even *cause* certain mental disorders.)

It's a catch-22: you can't think of *not* doing something without thinking about it. And every time you think about it, the neural pathways in your brain that are associated with it are greased up and strengthened in a twisted Law of Attraction—so it will be even easier to think of it later.

It seems natural to try to suppress the parts of ourselves we want to change. But forget suppression. It doesn't work.

So how *should* you change a bad habit?

## Replace, Replace, Replace

Instead of trying to *suppress* a bad habit, research tells us that a much better strategy is *replacing* a bad habit with a good habit.[1476] (I can confirm this.)

In comes a cue. Your bad habit starts to fire. Instead of trying to beat it back down with a stick, make a conscious effort to do something else, something better. *Transfer* your reaction.

Before all this, you'll want to invest some willpower thinking about your bad habit—coldly, critically, like a scientist. Think about your bad habit's cues, about what sets it off. Then switch from science to zen, meditating on your bad habit, pondering its whys and hows, mindful of what it makes you feel and think and do.

Then invest willpower thinking of a good habit to replace it with. Like drinking water instead of juice or soda. Like eating your favorite whole foods instead of your favorite processed foods. Like going to the gym instead of feeling depressed. Like going to bed after an hour of Netflix instead of three hours of Netflix.

## Real-World Replacement

Let's say you have the bad habit of buying processed food at the grocery store (**processed food** *n* : *a food with an ingredients list longer than one item*). The cue? Maybe it's walking into the grocery store.

> **Highway to Hell**: *Don't buy processed food. Don't buy processed food. Don't buy processed food.*

This will just make you want processed food.

Instead, make a shopping list of strictly whole foods (**whole food** *n* : *a food composed of a single unprocessed ingredient*). Whole foods tend to snake the perimeter of grocery stores.

And instead, tell yourself something like this:

> **Stairway to Heaven**: *If I'm at the grocery store, then I'll only buy the whole foods on my shopping list. If I'm at the grocery store, then I'll only buy the whole foods on my shopping list.*

Then do it.

Then eat those whole foods when you're hungry.

Another example. Let's say you have a nasty habit of going to the break-room vending machine when you're bored at work around 3 p.m.

The cue? Being bored at work around 3 p.m.

**Highway to Hell**: *Don't go to the vending machine.*
*Don't go to the vending machine. Speaking of which,*
*did they restock the Reese's on the bottom row?*

Instead, think of something to *do* instead.
Maybe when you're bored around 3 p.m., you go for a walk.

**Stairway to Heaven**: *If I'm bored at work around*
*3 p.m., then I'll go for a walk. If I'm bored at work*
*around 3 p.m., then I'll go for a walk.*

## Program Your Brain for Success

I write software for a living. One of the foundations of software
is *if-then* statements. You tell the computer: *if* such-and-such
occurs, *then* do this action.

You tell the computer what to do in situation X.

Most of the magic comes from that.

It turns out that we can do the same thing with our brains:

**IF** (situation) **THEN** (action)

We've already seen this.

*If I'm at the grocery store, **then** I'll only*
*buy the whole foods on my shopping list.*

*If I'm bored at work at 3 p.m., **then** I'll*
*go for a walk.*

The scientific term for these statements is *implementation*
*intentions.* Many studies show that these implementation
intentions (*if-then statements*) increase your odds of success
at a number of things. They help people eat more fruits and

vegetables and exercise more. They help women give themselves regular breast exams, they help students get started on projects, and they help schizophrenics control their behavior.[1477,1478]

**And they help people lose weight.**[1479]

Implementation intentions are just specific plans for future situations.

For example:

> *If I'm at the grocery store,* **then** *I'll only buy the whole foods on my shopping list.*

When you think of something *new* to do in response to old cues, there are physical changes in your brain. When you think of being at the grocery store and only buying the whole foods on your shopping list, the neurons that register the grocery store will be primed and linked with the neurons associated with finding whole foods (which tend to snake the perimeter of grocery stores).

Repeat it to yourself a few times.

> *If I'm at the grocery store,* **then** *I'll only buy the whole foods on my shopping list.*

> *If I'm at the grocery store,* **then** *I'll only buy the whole foods on my shopping list.*

> *If I'm at the grocery store,* **then** *I'll only buy the whole foods on my shopping list.*

When you step foot in the grocery store, you'll know exactly what to do. You won't waste willpower hemming and hawing (and then buying junk food anyway).

You'll only buy the whole foods on your shopping list.

## Just Get Started

The main reason people haven't gotten started on their goals is that they haven't devoted willpower to making specific plans.

Let's say you want to learn Spanish.

**Highway to Hell**: *I want to learn Spanish.*

This won't help you learn Spanish.

Fuzzy, vague intentions like this are almost useless.

Instead, be specific:

**Stairway to Heaven**: *If I'm driving home from work, **then** I'm going to stop at OfficeMax, buy Rosetta Stone, go home, and spend 15 minutes setting it up.*

That will get you started. Precision is priceless.

When you don't make specific plans, things get left to chance. And when things get left to chance, habits take over. You may have the best intentions, but the future will be full of curveballs, fluctuating willpower, and constant distractions. A vague intention to do something is like a billboard on the side of the road when you're driving 100 miles per hour.

When people act according to specific plans, however, their reactions tend to be automatic, with little conscious effort.[1480]

In other words, *with little willpower.*

If you make specific plans with if-then statements, when important situations come up, your brain will automatically do what you programmed it to do.

To make your goals come true, then, make specific plans.

The key to long-term weight loss is to spend your willpower making specific plans to build effective habits.

Which habits? *These* habits:

# The Five Golden Weight-Loss Habits

1. Cut out all sugary drinks.
2. Only eat whole foods most days.
   **processed food** *n* : *a food with an ingredients list longer than one item*
3. Exercise regularly. (At least walk regularly.)
4. Get enough sleep to feel rested most days.
5. Every morning, measure your weight and waist.

It's best to focus on one habit at a time.

The Five Golden Weight-Loss Habits are ranked in order of importance, so start at the top.

Let me break down the thought process.

*If* you drink sugary drinks every day, *then* there's probably nothing more effective you can do for long-term weight loss than switching to water or other zero-calorie beverages. Nothing will give you more bang for your buck. There's really no sense in doing anything else until the habit of not drinking sugar is set in stone.

*If* you don't drink sugary drinks, but there's processed food in your regular diet (**processed food** *n* : *a food with an ingredients list longer than one item*), *then* there's probably nothing more effective you can do for long-term weight loss than getting in the habit of only eating whole foods most days of the week. Nothing will give you more bang for your buck. There's really no sense in doing anything else until the habit of only eating whole foods most days is set in stone.

(Repeat for Habits 3, 4, and 5.)

Build these habits, and you've eliminated the root causes of overweight and obesity, gotten much healthier, and set yourself up for lifelong success.

Only *then* should you think about diets or programs.

And even when you're on a diet or program, The Five Golden Weight-Loss Habits should *always* be working in the background.

## Take-Home

Habits are everything. Instead of trying to *suppress* bad habits, spend your willpower thinking of how you can *replace* bad habits with better habits.

Make specific plans for building The Five Golden Weight-Loss Habits.

Then follow your plans.

(*If-then.*)

# 49

# THE PLEASURE VACUUM

There's a critical concept in self-improvement that I've never really seen addressed. It is of great practical value, and fundamental to making most lasting changes.

Without further adieu, I give you: *the pleasure vacuum.*

A bit of groundwork. Barring a spiritual transformation like Saint Paul on the road to Damascus, you already work about as hard as you're going to work. You can sprinkle heroic efforts here and there, but your general, day-to-day work ethic and willpower will likely remain pretty stable over the next few years.

I hate to be the bearer of bad news, but Future You is no saint.

You only have so much blood, sweat, and tears in you. This is why most people are better off working *smarter*, not harder. *Smarter* means investing your willpower in the most effective places: *changing your habits.*

You already knew that.

But changing a habit means fighting the old-leather-couch comfort of established routine. Old habits tend to be relaxing and pleasurable. Changing an old habit—or building a new one—will temporarily cause discomfort and a *lack* of pleasure: a *pleasure vacuum*.

A "pleasure vacuum" is the mental hole left behind when you rip out a pleasant habit. Pleasure vacuums are why it's tough to quit smoking, drugs, and processed food.

Whichever way you lean politically, your brain is a staunch conservative. It likes things the way they are. To your stodgy old brain, your conscious intention to change a habit is an annoying young liberal, pushing radical reform and blasting loud music.

Your brain won't make things easy. In the trenches of habit change, you may find temporary pain and misery, torment and anguish, melancholy and despair—*the pleasure vacuum*.

**The pleasure vacuum is the price of positive change.**

It's what stops most people from *making* positive change.

There is no way around the pleasure vacuum. It's simply part of the process. You have to be motivated enough to overcome it.

But with the right approach, you can partially *fill* the pleasure vacuum, minimizing its depth and power, and maximizing your odds of success.

There are three main ways to do this.

## Make It Fun

If you're trying to replace a bad habit with a better habit, you're on the right track. (Suppression is an abysmal approach.)

But this isn't enough.

To be successful, your new habit has to be at least somewhat *palatable*—something that you don't mind doing, even when you're not drunk on motivation.

If you've been regularly eating processed food for a while, cutting it from your regular diet will leave a large pleasure vacuum in your brain.

And the problem with "eating healthy" is that it's often framed like this:

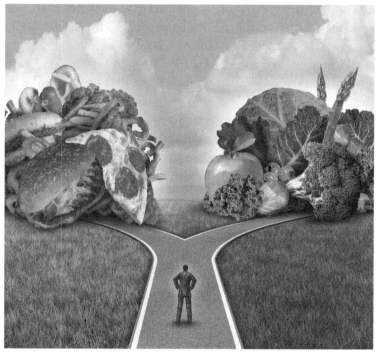

*Greasy delight... or green vegetables?*
Photo Credit: Lightspring/Shutterstock.com

According to popular nutrition, we basically have to choose between enthralling our taste buds with junk food or eating a plate of greens. For most people, choosing green plants instead of greasy pizza will leave such a massive pleasure vacuum in their brains that they won't stand a chance of sticking with it.

While most nutrition gurus have a more inclusive view of "healthy foods" than just green plants, the foods they tell us to eat are rarely exciting—which is precisely why we defended so many healthy whole foods before.

The very whole foods that popular nutrition has told us to *avoid*—eggs, fruit, red meat, potatoes, nuts, and cheese—are precisely the most *delicious* whole foods to the average person.

They are the very whole foods that give us the best chance of resisting the hedonic blitz of processed food, filling the pleasure vacuum, and sustaining a healthier diet.

Compared to processed junk food, *all* whole foods are slimming. Armed with the knowledge that cholesterol and saturated fat are harmless, that red meat is *not* the devil, that potatoes are filling and nutritious vegetables, that fruit is extremely healthy, and that nuts and full-fat dairy products are associated with weight loss, we can start to replace processed food with *satisfying* whole foods.

This is a much fairer fight:

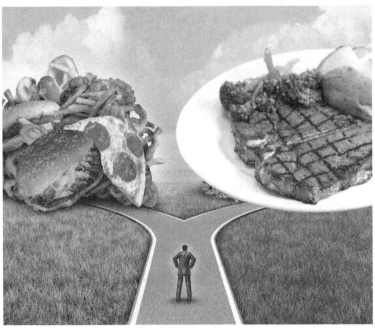

*Either one looks good.*
Photo Credit: Lightspring, farbled/Shutterstock.com

You may be tempted by pizza and french fries, but it doesn't take a hero to pick meat and potatoes (or full-fat cheese, full-fat yogurt, eggs, fruit, or whole grains). But choosing whole foods like these will make you much slimmer over time.

Basing your diet on whole foods you enjoy is the best way to fill the pleasure vacuum left behind from cutting out processed food. In fact, it's the only chance that most people have.

Similarly, in the last chapter, there was a reason we replaced our 3 p.m. vending-machine habit with *this*:

> **Stairway to Heaven**: *If I'm bored at work at 3 p.m., then I'll go for a walk.*

A walk may not be a bag of chips, but it's not miserable, either. It gives us a break from work, a change of scenery, and a chance to stretch our legs.

Maybe you chat with a colleague on the way.

Instead, though, imagine if we tried to replace the vending-machine habit with drudgery:

> **Highway to Hell**: *If I'm bored at work at 3 p.m., then I'll get a jump on next week's report.*

You may be able to pull this off once or twice. But as soon as your motivation flags for an instant (it will), you'll be face to face with Vending Machine vs. Unnecessary Work.

The giant discrepancy in fun between these two options will leave a massive pleasure vacuum in your skull. Your only chance will be to white-knuckle it, burning up loads of will-power—willpower that would have been better spent on selecting a more practical, sustainable replacement habit.

The same logic applies to letting yourself drink diet soda instead of just water (at least at first), starting off with easy workouts instead of brutal workouts, and letting yourself eat junk food once in awhile instead of trying to go cold turkey.

To fill the pleasure vacuum of habit change, make your replacement habits doable, palatable, and sustainable.

## Think Positive

No more negative self-talk. Life is too short. As we've seen, willpower is boosted by positive beliefs and motivation.

You're as good as your thoughts.

Tell yourself you're great for making an effort to change your life. (You *are*.)

Tell yourself you're strong. (You *are*.)

If you failed in the past, it's probably because you weren't using the right strategy. (You *weren't*; all short-term strategies are long-term failures.)

The Five Golden Weight-Loss Habits will change your life. (They *will*.)

Tell yourself you have a lot of willpower, and that you can lose weight and keep it off if you keep trying and stick it out. (You *can*.)

When you feel the pain of habit change, don't dwell on it.

Don't feel sorry for yourself. Self-pity is toxic, and almost never leads anywhere good. Instead, *transfer* your focus to feeling *good* about turning into someone *new*.

Focus on your better future self. Focus on feeling proud of yourself for having the guts to change. Focus on walking a higher path. Focus on feeling noble for trying.

Or come back down to earth, and dwell on how you're finally going to be better than someone you dislike.

Be petty and selfish if you have to.

Focus on something, *anything*, that brings you a nugget of joy.

The alternative is to focus on the pain, which can feed on itself, turning the pleasure vacuum into a hungry black hole that sucks you in, ripping your goals to shreds.

Think happy thoughts. Believe in yourself.

## Take It Easy

The third and final way to fill a pleasure vacuum has nothing to do with habits or attitudes.

It's about everything else in your life.

This is an important time for you. You're mustering your willpower to build great habits that will change your life, and going to war with the pleasure vacuum.

Don't fight a war on multiple fronts. When you're using willpower to build a Golden Weight-Loss Habit, it's best to be stingy with your willpower in other areas. During this pivotal time, you want to limit any unnecessary effort.

Unfortunately, you still have to spend willpower on the essentials, like going to work, doing your taxes, and putting up with certain people. But the buck stops here, with the *essentials*.

When you're trying to build a Golden Weight-Loss Habit, this is *not* the time to start a big home-improvement project, volunteer for a work assignment, or start spending 30 minutes a day learning Spanish.

Outside of building the Golden Habit, be stingy with your willpower. Avoid avoidable things that are hard, boring, and draining. Shirk the shirkable.

*Be stingy with your willpower in other areas.*

When you're trying to build a Golden Weight-Loss Habit, this is *just* the time for Netflix marathons, sleeping in, shopping sprees, and other guilty (non-food) pleasures.

The point is, when you're not explicitly focused on changing the habit—which is *hard*—you want to take life **nice and easy**.

Spend your willpower on building good habits, and replenish your willpower by taking it easy.

"No pain, no gain" was a misguided mantra for 1950s football coaches who thought that water breaks were for the weak.

Enduring maximal pain isn't noble or heroic.

It just makes you more likely to fail.

Habit change is inherently painful, so try to make it as painless as possible—by filling the pleasure vacuum as much as you can.

## Take-Home

Focus on one habit at a time, and fill the pleasure vacuum as much as you can. You can fill the pleasure vacuum by building *palatable* good habits, thinking positive (*if* you're feeling the pain of habit change, **then** think of something that makes you feel good) and taking it easy in other areas of life.

It will all be worth it.

Eventually, you'll have a Golden Weight-Loss Habit.

This habit will serve your best interests, for free.

Indefinitely.

Like winning a butler for life.

## 50

# TIME TO CHANGE

## Overweight and Healthy?

There is controversy over whether carrying a little extra weight is unhealthy or not. As 70% of US adults are overweight,[1481] this is not a trivial matter.

A rigorous 2013 meta-analysis got people talking when it found that people with an "overweight" body mass index (a BMI of 25-29.9) had a 6% *lower* risk of death than people with "normal weight" BMIs—and that these "normal weight" people were no less likely to die than people who were mildly obese (BMIs of 30-34.9).[1482]

Is it best to be a little overweight, then?

Should normal-weight people try to bulk up, and the mildly obese rest easy?

Don't get your hopes up.

These results were entirely based on body mass index (BMI).

*Ah*, BMI. We'll start with the famous caveat that BMI only takes height and weight into account. Height and weight. That's it. Nothing else. BMI doesn't take your body frame, body composition, or muscle into account at all. This is a serious limitation, of course. Champion bodybuilders, who have some of the lowest levels of body fat out of any athletes on Earth, are often "obese" according to the BMI scale (due to all their heavy muscle).

Then there are the cutoff points for "underweight," "normal weight," "overweight," and "obese" BMIs. These cutoff points are arbitrary, and in some ways, highly flawed.

Take "normal weight." This is defined as a BMI of 18.5-24.9. The upper part of this range is somewhat reasonable for most people, but that low end—18.5-19.9—is hardly "normal." Most people in this range are *extremely* thin, and would better be called "underweight."

This matters, because elderly people are the ones most likely to be death statistics, and underweight elderly people are even more likely to die than obese elderly people.[1483]

When you misclassify enough frail, sickly people as "normal weight," then "normal weight" stops appearing so healthy.

Take me. I'm 6-foot 2. My weight usually fluctuates between 180 and 190 pounds. But a few years ago, I cut down to 165 pounds. It wasn't easy. (Lots of counting calories, lots of weighing food.) This marked a rock-bottom weight for me—the least my adult body has ever weighed, by far.

I looked emaciated: very low body fat, fairly low muscle mass, an air of mild starvation. But at *that* point, I could have lost another *23 pounds* (weighed 142 pounds), and still had a "normal weight" BMI.

Let me tell you. At 142 pounds, I'd be a pencil. I wouldn't have a shred of muscle. As we saw, stronger people are much less likely to die.[1484] At 142 pounds, I wouldn't have the strength to fight a cold, let alone cancer.

There is nothing "normal" or "healthy" about me at 142 pounds.

I'd be much, *much* healthier at 192 pounds—a weight at

which, with my frame, most onlookers would call me "skinny," but the BMI scale rather impolitely labels me "overweight."

And there's the rub. Past age 50, many folks at the low end of "overweight" are actually quite healthy, while many at the low end of "normal weight" are frail, feeble, and sickly, possibly due to illnesses like cancer.

Are the results of that 2013 study starting to make sense?

Indeed, a 2010 study of 1.46 million adults found that the optimal BMI range was 22.5-24.9, with mortality increasing on either side.[1485] Compared to this sweet spot, people with BMIs of 18.5 to 19.9 (the low end of "normal weight") were 14% more likely to die in their 50s, and 32% more likely to die in their 70s and 80s.

BMIs that low generally aren't healthy.

You *can* be too skinny.

On the other side of that sweet spot, "overweight" women were 13% more likely to die, and "obese" women (BMIs of 30-34.9) were 44% more likely to die. Women with BMIs of 35.0-39.9 were **88% more likely to die**, and the poor women with BMIs over 40 were **251% more likely to die**.

Being a *little* overweight may be a bit of a grey area, but one thing is certain: past that point, the heavier you get, the worse it gets.

And it gets bad, *fast.*

(And it's a slippery slope.)

## Overweight *Is* Unhealthy

The *Harvard Medical School Guide to Healthy Eating* has this to say about weight and health:

> *Weight sits like a spider at the center of an intricate, tangled web of health and disease.*[1486]

When you look at most major diseases, you see a dose-response relationship with BMI. In other words, overweight people are more likely to get the disease, and obese people are even *more* likely to get it.

This is true for heart disease,[1487] which is the leading killer in the United States.[1488] It's also true for diabetes,[1489] depression,[1490] kidney disease,[1491] asthma,[1492] male infertility,[1493] arthritis,[1494] back pain,[1495] and a smattering of cancers: breast, endometrial, colon, esophageal, kidney, pancreatic, and gallbladder cancer.[1496,1497]

Lovely.

Obesity brings its own unique risk factors, too. Like significantly higher odds of dementia,[1498] sleep apnea,[1499] erectile dysfunction,[1500] female infertility and miscarriage risk,[1501] Crohn's disease,[1502] liver disease,[1503] and various skin diseases.[1504]

Contrary to popular belief, even so-called "metabolically healthy" obese people have increased risks of health problems[1505]—including heart disease[1506] and diabetes.[1507]

A word about diabetes. A 2010 meta-analysis found that **overweight people were 299% more likely to get diabetes, and obese people were 719% more likely to get diabetes**.[1508]

The evidence linking obesity and diabetes is so strong that some scientists simply call it "diabesity."[1509,1510]

Based on everything I've read, this seems like an accurate term to describe what's really going on in the body.

There is nothing good about diabetes. As one British doctor put it in 2014, "medically speaking, I'd rather have HIV than diabetes."[1511]

I can see his point. I have a friend that had to have his big toe amputated due to diabetic nerve damage. Big toes are crucial for balance, and my friend will have to walk with a cane for the rest of his life—assuming his diabetes doesn't put him in a wheelchair.

He's in his 30s.

## The Social Costs

Being too heavy is hardly just bad for your health. It takes a major toll in other areas, too. Like romance. Beauty may be in the eye of the beholder, but human attraction has some stark statistical realities. Obese people are not only generally judged to be less attractive,[1512] but actually elicit disgust.[1513]

Studies have found that obese people are judged less attractive than drug addicts, the mentally ill, people with STDs, people in wheelchairs, and people missing an arm.[1514,1515]

But it doesn't stop there. Obese people are discriminated against in their families, peer groups, schools, the healthcare system, and the workplace.[1516]

Studies have found that obese people are less likely to be hired, and are perceived as lazier, sloppier, less disciplined, and less competent than normal-weight people.[1517]

As a 2019 review put it, "people with obesity are blatantly dehumanized."[1518]

Obese people earn less money for doing the same jobs, and have worse job prospects.[1519] This makes it hard for them to afford the thousands of extra dollars in medical bills they pay each year[1520] due to all the foregoing health problems.

Given all this, is it any wonder that obese people have lower self-esteem,[1521] and are 55% more likely to be depressed?[1522]

None of this is fair. Obesity usually isn't a choice. But this is the way it is, unfortunately.

Being obese is no way to go through life.

If you're just overweight, keep in mind that there are still health risks, and that the path to obesity is a slow and steady and slippery slope that starts with being okay with being overweight.

This is your life, and it's ending one second at a time. It's time to change.

# The Five Golden Weight-Loss Habits

1. Cut out all sugary drinks.

2. Only eat whole foods most days.
   **processed food** *n : a food with an ingredients list longer than one item*

3. Exercise regularly. (At least walk regularly.)

4. Get enough sleep to feel rested most days.

5. Every morning, measure your weight and waist.

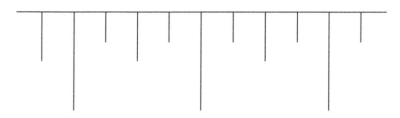

# REFERENCES

1.  "Obesity and Overweight." World Health Organization. https://www.who.int/en/news-room/fact-sheets/detail/obesity-and-overweight
2.  Ibid.
3.  Ibid.
4.  I'm a *citation*.
5.  I'm a *citation*.
6.  I'm a *citation*.
7.  "Appeal to Authority," *Your Logical Fallacy Is*. https://yourlogicalfallacyis.com/appeal-to-authority
8.  Korownyk et al., "Televised Medical Talk Shows—What They Recommend and the Evidence to Support Their Recommendations: A Prospective Observational Study," *BMJ* 349 (2014): g7346. doi: https://doi.org/10.1136/bmj.g7346
9.  James, William, "Talks to Teachers," Chapter 8: The Laws of Habit. https://www.uky.edu/~eushe2/Pajares/tt8.html
10. Wansink B and Sobel J, "Mindless Eating: The 200 Daily Food Decisions We Overlook," *Environment and Behavior* 39, no. 1 (2007): 106-23.
11. Hagger et al, "Ego Depletion and the Strength Model of Self-Control: A Meta-Analysis," *Psychological Bulletin* 136, no. 4 (2010): 495-525.
12. Baumeister et al., "Ego Depletion: Is the Active Self a Limited Resource?" *Journal of Personality and Social Psychology* 74, no. 5 (1998): 1252-65.
13. "Course Requirements in Years I and II," Harvard Medical School. https://hms.harvard.edu/departments/medical- education/md-programs/new-pathway-np/course-and-examination- requirements-md-degree
14. Adams et al., "Nutrition Education in U.S. Medical Schools: Latest Update of a National Survey," *Academic Medicine* 85, no. 9 (2010): 1537- 1542.
15. Ibid.
16. Ibid.
17. Mogre et al., "Nutrition in Medicine: Medical Students' Satisfaction, Perceived Relevance and Preparedness for Future Practice," *Health Professions Education* (2017): https://doi.org/10.1016/j.hpe.2017.02.003
18. Adams et al., "Nutrition Education in U.S. Medical Schools: Latest Update of a National Survey," *Academic Medicine* 85, no. 9 (2010): 1537- 1542.
19. Bruer et al., "Nutrition Counseling—Should Physicians Guide Their Patients?" *American Journal of Preventive Medicine* 10, no. 5 (1994): 308- 311.
20. Kuhn, Thomas. *The Structure of Scientific Revolutions*. Chicago: University of Chicago Press, 1970. Print.
21. Ibid.
22. Rohrmann et al., "Meat Consumption and Mortality—Results from the European Prospective Investigation into Cancer and Nutrition," *BMC Medicine* 11, no. 63 (2013): doi:10.1186/1741-7015-11-63
23. Hu et al, "Prospective Study of Major Dietary Patterns and Risk of Coronary Heart Disease in Men," *American Journal of Clinical Nutrition* 72, no. 4 (2000): 912-921.
24. Wallis, Claudia, "Hold the Eggs and Butter," Time Magazine. March 26, 1984. https://content.time.com/time/subscriber/article/0,33009,921647- 2,00.html
25. "Why Mouse Matters," National Human Genome Research Institute. National Institutes of Health. https://www.genome.gov/10001345
26. "New Genome Comparison Finds Chimps, Humans Very Similar at the DNA Level," NIH News. National Institutes of Health. August 31st, 2005.
27. Milton, K., "Nutritional Characteristics of Wild Primate Foods: Do the Diets of Our Closest Living Relatives Have Lessons for Us?" *Nutrition* 15, no. 6 (1999): 488-498.
28. Tweheyo et al., "Chimpanzee Diet and Habitat Selection in the Budongo Forest Reserve, Uganda," *Forest Ecology and Management* 188, no. 1-3 (2004): 267-78.
29. Chen, F., and Li, W., "Genomic Divergences between Humans and Other Hominoids and the Effective Population Size of the Common Ancestor of Humans and Chimpanzees," *American Journal of Human Genetics* 68, no. 2 (2001): 444-456.
30. Sauvageot et al., "Use of Food Frequency Questionnaire to Assess Relationships Between Dietary Habits and Cardiovascular Risk Factors in NESCAV Study: Validations and Biomarkers," *Nutrition Journal* 143, no.

12 (2013): DOI: 10.1186/1475-2891-12-143.

31. Woocher, Fredric, "Did Your Eyes Deceive You? Expert Psychological Testimony on the Unreliability of Eyewitness Identification," *Stanford Law Review* 29, no. 5 (1977): 969-1030.

32. Kristal et al., "Is it Time to Abandon the Food Frequency Questionnaire?" *Cancer Epidemiology, Biomarkers & Prevention* 14 (2005): 2826.

33. Archer et al., "The Inadmissibility of What We Eat in America and NHANES Dietary Data in Nutrition and Obesity Research and the Scientific Formulation of National Dietary Guidelines," *Mayo Clinic Proceedings* 90, no. 7 (2015): DOI: https://dx.doi.org/10.1016/j.mayocop.2015.04.009

34. Nurses' Health Study. 2014 Questionnaire (long version). https://www.nurseshealthstudy.org/participants/questionnaires

35. "The World's Biggest Industry," *Forbes*. https://www.forbes.com/2007/11/11/growth-agriculture-business-forbeslife- food07-cx_sm_1113bigfood.html

36. Lambert, Craig, "The Way We Eat Now: Ancient Bodies Collide with Modern Technology to Produce a Flabby, Disease-Ridden Populace," *Harvard Magazine*. May-June 2004. https://harvardmagazine.com/2004/05/the-way-we-eat- now.html

37. Kearns et al., "Sugar Industry and Coronary Heart Disease Research: A Historical Analysis of Internal Industry Documents," *JAMA Internal Medicine* 176, no. 11 (2016): 1680-1685.

38. Ibid.

39. "Fats 101," American Heart Association. Getting Healthy. https://www.heart.org/HEARTORG/Getting-Healthy/NutritionCenter/HealthyE Fats_UCM_301461_Article.jsp

40. "Health Cooking Oils," American Heart Association . https://www.heart.org/HEARTORG/HealthyLiving/HealthyEating/SimpleCoo Cooking-Oils_UCM_445179_Article.jsp - .V5buf5MrLox

41. "Foods Highest in Total Omega-6 Fatty Acids," Self Nutrition Data. https://nutritiondata.self.com/foods-000141000000000000000-w.html

42. Harris, et al., "Omega-6 Fatty Acids and Risk for Cardiovascular Disease," *Circulation* 119 (2009): 902-907.

43. "Who Owns Nature? Corporate Power and the Final Frontier in the Commodification of Life," ETC Group, 2008. https://www.etcgroup.org/files/publication/707/01/etc_won_report_final_color

44. "I Can't Believe It's Not Butter!, 79% Vegetable Oil Spread, Original," https://smartlabel.icantbelieveitsnot-butter.com/product/2746458/ingredients

45. Harris, et al., "Omega-6 Fatty Acids and Risk for Cardiovascular Disease," *Circulation* 119 (2009): 902-907.

46. Ibid.

47. Nestle, Marion, "Five More Industry-Sponsored Studies with Results Favorable to the Sponsor. The Score Since mid-March: 95:9," *Food Politics*. https://www.foodpolitics.com/2015/12/five-more-industry-spon-sored-studies- with-results- favorable-to-the-sponsor-the-score-since-mid-march-959/

48. Lesser et al., "Relationship Between Funding Source and Conclusion Among Nutrition-Related Scientific Articles," *PLOS Medicine* 4.1 (2007): e5. doi: 10.1371/journal.pmed.0040005.

49. Ibid.

50. Calder, P, "The American Heart Association Advisory on N-6 Fatty Acids: Evidence Based or Biased Evidence," *British Journal of Nutrition* 104, no. 11 (2010): 1575-15.

51. Ramsden et al., "N-6 Fatty Acid-Specific and Mixed Polyunsaturate Dietary Interventions Have Different Effects on CHD Risk: A Meta-Analysis of Randomised Controlled Trials," *British Journal of Nutrition* 104, no. 11 (2010): 1586-1600.

52. "About the US Department of Agriculture," USDA. https://www.usda.gov/wps/portal/usda/usdahome?navid=ABOUT_USDA

53. "Dietary Goals for the United States," Select Committee on Nutrition and Human Needs. 95th Congress, February 1977. https://zerodisease.com/archive/Dietary_Goals_For_The_United_States.pdf

54. Glueck, Charles, "Appraisal of Dietary Fat as a Causative Factor in Atherogenesis," *American Journal of Clinical Nutrition* (1979).

55. "Dietary Goals for the United States: Second Edition," Select Committee on Nutrition and Human Needs. 95th Congress. December 1977. https://thescienceofnutrition.files.wordpress.com/2014/03/dietary-goals-for- the-united-states.pdf

56. Minger, Denise, *Death by Food Pyramid*. Malibu: Primal Blueprint Publishing, 2013. Print. 40-47.

57. "Dietary Goals for the United States: Second Edition," Select Committee on Nutrition and Human Needs. 95th Congress. December 1977. https://thescienceofnutrition.files.wordpress.com/2014/03/dietary-goals-for-the-united-states.pdf

58. Oppenheimer et al., "McGovern's Senate Select Committee on Nutrition and Human Needs Versus the: Meat Industry on the Diet-Heart Question (1976-1977)," *American Journal of Public Health* 104, no. 1 (2014): 59-69.

59. Roache, Christina, "D. Mark Hegsted, National Force in Science of Huma Nutrition, Dies," *Harvard Gazette*. 06-20-2009. https://news.har vard.edu/gazette/story/2009/06/d-mark-hegsted-national-force-in-science-of-human-nutrition-dies/

60. Minger, Denise, *Death by Food Pyramid*. Malibu: Primal Blueprint Publishing, 2013. Print. 138-9.

61. Light, Luise, "A Fatally Flawed Food Guide," 2004. https://www.whale.to/a/light.html

62. Ibid.

63. Ibid.

64. Minger, *Death by Food Pyramid*. 138-9.

65. "Healthy Eating Pyramid," The Nutrition Source, Harvard School of Public Health. https://www.hsph.har-vard.edu/nutritionsource/pyramidtest/

66. "Table 50: U.S. Per Capita Caloric Sweeteners Estimated Deliveries for Domestic Food and Beverage Use, Per Calendar Year," Economic Research Service, USDA . https://www.ers.usda.gov/data-products/sug-ar-and- sweeteners-yearbook- tables.aspx#25512

67. *Dietary Guidelines for Americans, 1980 to 2000*. Center for Nutrition Policy and Promotion, USDA, May 30, 2000. https://health.gov/dietaryguidelines/1980_2000_chart.pdf

68. "Fiscal Year 2015 Annual Report," Academy of Nutrition and Dietetics Foundation. https://www.eatrightpro.org/-/media/eatrightpro-files/about-us/annual-reports/annualreport2015.pdf?la=en&hash=93BC65E570E5CD22711E030805FA23F251D1E34B

69. "Dietary Guidelines and MyPlate," Academy of Nutrition and Dietetics. https://www.eatright.org/resources/food/nutrition/dietary-guidelines-and-myplate

70. "Health Eating for Men," Academy of Nutrition and Dietetics. https://www.eatright.org/resource/health/

wellness/healthy-aging/healthy-eating-for-men

71. "Dietary Guidelines for Americans, 2015," Chapter 2. https://health.gov/dietaryguidelines/2015/guidelines/chapter-2/a- closer-look- at-current-intakes-and-recommended-shifts/#figure-2-5

72. "In Wake of New York Soda Ban Proposal, Academy of Nutrition and Dietetics Encourages Education, Moderation," Academy of Nutrition and Dietetics. 05/31/2012. https://www.eatright.org/Media/content.aspx?id=6442470211&terms=soda#.VMlW2Uvef8E

73. "Back to Basics for Healthy Weight Loss," Academy of Nutrition and Dietetics. 01/27/2014. https://www.eatright.org/resource/health/weight-loss/your-health-and-your-weight/back-to-basics-for-healthy-weight-loss

74. Brown et al., "Sugary Drinks in the Pathogenesis of Obesity and Cardiovascular Diseases," *International Journal of Obesity* 32 (2008): S28-S34.

75. Malik et al., "Intake of Sugar-Sweetened Beverages and Weight Gain: A Systematic Review," *American Journal of Clinical Nutrition* 84, no. 2 (2006): 274-288.

76. Smithers, Rebecca, "Food Standards Agency to Be Abolished by Health Secretary," *The Guardian*. 07/11/2010. https://www.theguardian.com/politics/2010/jul/11/food-standards-agency- abolished-health-secretary

77. Dobzhansky, Theodosius, "Nothing in Biology Makes Sense Except in the Light of Evolution," *The American Biology Teacher* 35 (1973): 125-129.

78. Jablonski, D., "Extinction: Past and Present," *Nature* 427 (2004): 589.

79. Hawking, Stephen, *A Brief History of Time*. New York: Random House, 2011. Print.

80. "Evolution," *Encyclopedia Britannica*. https://www.britannica.com/science/evolution-scientific-theory

81. Overbye, Dennis, "A Scientist Takes on Gravity," *The New York Times*. 07-12-2010.

82. Ley et al., "Ecological and Evolutionary Forces Shaping Microbial Diversity in the Human Intestine," *Cell* 124.4 (2006): 837-848.

83. Akcil et al. "Biological Treatment of Cyanide by Natural Isolated Bacteria (Pseudomonas sp. )," *Minerals Engineering* 16, no. 7 (2003): 643-649.

84. Frassetto et al., "Metabolic and Physiologic Improvements from Consuming a Paleolithic, Hunter-Gatherer Type Diet," *European Journal of Clinical Nutrition* 63, no. 8 (2009): 947-955.

85. Ryberg et al., "A Paleolithic-Type Diet Causes Strong Tissue-Specific Effects on Ectopic Fat Deposition in Obese Postmenopausal Women," *Journal of Internal Medicine* 274, no. 1 (2013):67-76.

86. Österdahl et al., "Effects of a Short-Term Intervention with a Paleolithic Diet in Healthy Volunteers," *European Journal of Clinical Nutrition* 62 (2008): 682-685.

87. Lindeberg et al., "A Paleolithic Diet Improves Glucose Tolerance More Than a Mediterranean-Like Diet in Individuals with Ischaemic Heart Disease," *Diabetologia* 50, no. 9 (2007): 1795-1807.

88. Jönsson et al., "Beneficial Effects of a Paleolithic Diet on Cardiovascular Risk Factors in Type 2 Diabetes: A Randomized Cross-Over Pilot Study," *Cardiovascular Diabetology* 8, no. 35 (2009): 1-14.

89. Jönsson et al., "Subjective Satiety and Other Experiences of a Paleolithic Diet Compared to a Diabetes Diet in Patients with Type 2 Diabetes," *Nutrition Journal* 12 (2013): 105.

90. Genoni et al., "Cardiovascular, Metabolic Effects and Dietary Composition of Ad Libitum Paleolithic vs. Australian Guide to Healthy Eating Diets: A 4-Week Randomised Trial," *Nutrients* 8, no. 5 (2016): 314.

91. Boers et al., "Favourable Effects of Consuming a Palaeolithic-Type Diet on Characteristics of the Metabolic Syndrome: A Randomized Controlled Pilot-Study," *Lipids in Health and Disease* 13, no. 1 (2014): 160.

92. Mellberg et al., "Long-Term Effects of a Paleolithic-Type Diet in Obese Postmenopausal Women: A Two-Year Randomized Trial," *European Journal of Clinical Nutrition* 68, no. 3 (2014): 350-357.

93. Cochran, Gregory and Harpending, Henry, *The 10,000 Year Explosion: How Civilization Accelerated Human Evolution*. New York: Basic Books, 2009. Kindle File, Page 2.

94. Ibid., 5.

95. Cochran, Gregory and Harpending, Henry, *The 10,000 Year Explosion: How Civilization Accelerated Human Evolution*. New York: Basic Books, 2009. Kindle File.

96. Orr, H., "The Population Genetics of Beneficial Mutations," *Philosophical Transactions of the Royal Society of London B: Biological Sciences* 365, no. 1544 (2010): 1195-1201.

97. Cochran, Gregory and Harpending, Henry, *The 10,000 Year Explosion: How Civilization Accelerated Human Evolution*. New York: Basic Books, 2009. Kindle File. Page 65.

98. Ibid.

99. Ibid., 91.

100. Ibid., 149.

101. Olalde et al., "Derived Immune and Ancestral Pigmentation Alleles in a 7000-Year-Old Mesolithic European," *Nature* 225 (2014): 225-228.

102. Cochran, Gregory and Harpending, Henry, *The 10,000 Year Explosion: How Civilization Accelerated Human Evolution*. New York: Basic Books, 2009. Kindle File. Page 94.

103. Ibid.

104. Ibid., 95.

105. Ibid., 88.

106. Ibid., 161.

107. Ibid., 181.

108. Ibid., 79.

109. Polley et al., "Evolution of the Rapidly Mutating Human Salivary Agglutinin Gene (DMBT1) and Population Subsistence Strategy," *Proceedings of the National Academy of Sciences* 112, no. 16 (2015): 5105- 5110.

110. Cochran, Gregory and Harpending, Henry, *The 10,000 Year Explosion: How Civilization Accelerated Human Evolution*. New York: Basic Books, 2009. Kindle File, Page 79.

111. Taylor, R. "Type 2 Diabetes: Etiology and Reversibility," *Diabetes Care* 36, no. 4 (2013): 1047-1055.

112. Cochran, Gregory and Harpending, Henry, The 10,000 Year Explosion: How Civilization Accelerated Human Evolution. New York: Basic Books, 2009. Kindle File, Page 80.

113. Ibid., 77.

114. "The Molecular Explanation," Lactose Intolerance. *Concepts in Genomics*. The NCMHD Center of Excellence for Nutritional Genomics. https://nutrigenomics.ucdavis.edu/?page=Information/Concepts_in_Nutrigenomics/Lactose_Intolerance

115. Perry et al., "Diet and the Evolution of Human Amylase Gene Copy Number Variation," *Nature Genetics* 39, no. 10 (2007): 1256-60.

116. Mandel et al., "High Endogenous Salivary Amylase Activity Is Associated with Improved Glycemic Homeostasis Following Starch Ingestion in Adults," *The Journal of Nutrition* 142, no. 5 (2012): 853-8.
117. Ibid.
118. Vesa et al., "Lactose Intolerance," *Journal of the American College of Nutrition* 19.2 (2000): 165S-175S.
119. "World Population Clock," *Worldometers*. https://www.worldometers.info/world-population/
120. "Milk, whole, 3.25% milkfat." Self Nutrition Data. https://nutritiondata.self.com/facts/dairy-and-egg-products/69/2
121. "Bread, whole-wheat, prepared from recipe," Self Nutrition Data. https://nutritiondata.self.com/facts/baked-products/4878/2
122. Tack et al., "The Spectrum of Celiac Disease: Epidemiology, Clinical Aspects, and Treatment," *Nature Reviews Gastroenterology and Hepatology* 7 (2010): 204-13.
123. "Sources of Gluten," Celiac Disease Foundation. https://celiac.org/live- gluten-free/glutenfreediet/sources-of-gluten/
124. Sicherer, S., and Sampson, H., "Food Allergy: Epidemiology, Pathogenesis, Diagnosis, and Treatment," *The Journal of Allergy and Clinical Immunology* 133, no. 2 (2014): 291-307.
125. Kurowski, Kurt, and Boxer, Robert, "Food Allergies: Detection and Management," *American Family Physician* 77, no. 12 (2008): 1678-1686.
126. Sicherer, S., and Sampson, H., "Food Allergy: Epidemiology, Pathogenesis, Diagnosis, and Treatment," *The Journal of Allergy and Clinical Immunology* 133, no. 2 (2014): 291-307.
127. Soller et al., "Overall Presence of Self-Reported Food Allergy in Canada," *The Journal of Allergy and Clinical Immunology* 130, no. 4 (2012): 986-988.
128. Kurowski, Kurt, and Boxer, Robert, "Food Allergies: Detection and Management," *American Family Physician* 77, no. 12 (2008): 1678-1686.
129. Ibid.
130. Wu et al., "Cruciferous Vegetable Intake and the Risk of Colorectal Cancer: A Meta-Analysis of Observational Studies," *Annals of Oncology* 24, no. 4 (2013): 1079-1087.
131. Joshipura et al., "The Effect of Fruit and Vegetable Intake on Risk for Coronary Heart Disease," *Annals of Internal Medicine* 134, no. 12 (2001): 1106-1114.
132. Zhang et al., "Cruciferous Vegetable Consumption Is Associated with a Reduced Risk of Total and Cardiovascular Disease Mortality," *American Journal of Clinical Nutrition* 94, no. 1 (2011): 240-246.
133. "Hypothyroidism (underactive thyroid)," Overview. Mayo Clinic. https://www.mayoclinic.org/diseases-conditions/hypothyroidism/home/ovc-20155291
134. Bajaj et al., "Various Possible Toxicants Involved in Thyroid Dysfunction: A Review," *Journal of Clinical Diagnosis and Research* 10, no. 1 (2016): FE01-FE03.
135. Cho, Y., and Kim, J., "Dietary Factors Affecting Thyroid Cancer Risk: A Meta-Analysis," *Nutrition and Cancer* 67, no. 5 (2015): 811-817.
136. "Hypothyroidism," University of Maryland Medical Center https://umm.edu/health/medical/altmed/condition/hypothyroidism.
137. Felker et al., "Concentrations of Thiocyanate and Goitrin in Human Plasma, Their Precursor Concentrations in Brassica Vegetables, and Associated Potential Risk for Hypothroidism," *Nutrition Reviews* (2016): 1-11.
138. Canaris et al., "The Colorado Thyroid Disease Prevalence Study," *JAMA* 160, no. 4 (2000): 526-534.
139. "What Is Hypothyroidism?" Understanding Hypothyroidism. *Synthroid*. https://www.synthroid.com/hypothyroidism/definition
140. Fatourechi, V., "Subclinical Hypothyroidism: An Update for Primary Care Physicians," *Mayo Clinic Proceedings* 84, no. 1 (2009): 65-71.
141. Unnikrishnan et al., "Prevalence of Hypothyroidism in Adults: An Epidemiological Study in Eight Cities in India," *Indian Journal of Endocrinology and Metabolism* 17, no. 4 (2013): 647-652.
142. Chambers et al., "Integration of Satiety Signals by the Central Nervous System," *Current Biology* 23, no. 9 (2013): R379-R388.
143. Guyenet, S., and Schwartz, M., "Regulation of Food Intake, Energy Balance, and Body Fat Mass: Implications for the Pathogenesis and Treatment of Obesity," *The Journal of Clinical Endocrinology and Metabolism* 97, no. 3 (2012): 745-755.
144. Holt et al., "A Satiety Index of Common Foods," *European Journal of Clinical Nutrition* 49, no. 9 (1996): 675-690.
145. Geliebter et al., "Effects of Oatmeal and Corn Flakes Cereal Breakfasts on Satiety, Gastric Emptying, Glucose, and Appetite-Related Hormones," *Annals of Nutrition & Metabolism* 66, no. 2-3 (2015): 93-103.
146. Soto et al., "The Form of Energy-Containing Food Alters Satiety and fMRI Brain Responses in Humans," *The Journal of the Federation of American Societies for Experimental Biology* 29, no. 1 (2015): Supplement 983.1
147. Bligh et al., "Plant-Rich Mixed Meals Based on Paleolithic Diet Principles Have a Dramatic Impact on Incretin, Peptide YY and Satiety Response, but Show Little Effect on Glucose and Insulin Homeostasis: An Acute Effects Randomised Study," *British Journal of Nutrition* 113, no. 4 (2015): 574-84.
148. Holt et al., "A Satiety Index of Common Foods," *European Journal of Clinical Nutrition* 49, no. 9 (1996): 675-690.
149. Duncan et al., "The Effects of High and Low Energy Density Diets on Satiety, Energy Intake, and Eating Time of Obese and Nonobese Subjects," *American Journal of Clinical Nutrition* 37, no. 5 (1983): 763-7.
150. Risling et al., "Food Intake Measured by an Automated Food-Selection System: Relationship to Energy Expenditure," *American Journal of Clinical Nutrition* 55, no. 2 (1992): 343-9.
151. Larson et al., "Ad Libitum Food Intake on a 'Cafeteria Diet' in Native American Women: Relations with Body Composition and 24-H Energy Expenditure," *American Journal of Clinical Nutrition* 62, no. 5 (1995): 911-7.
152. Larson et al., "Spontaneous Overfeeding with a 'Cafeteria Diet' in Men: Effects on 24-hour Energy Expenditure and Substrate Oxidation," *International Journal of Obesity and Related Metabolic Disorders* 19, no. 5 (1995): 331-7.
153. Poti et al., "Is the Degree of Food Processing and Convenience Linked with the Nutritional Quality of Foods Purchased by US Households?" *American Journal of Clinical Nutrition* (2015): doi: 10.3945/ajcn.114.100925
154. "Obesity and Overweight," Centers for Disease Control and Prevention. https://www.cdc.gov/nchs/fastats/obesity-overweight.htm
155. "Kashi® GOLEAN Crunch Cereal," Ingredients. *Kashi*. https://www.kashi.com/our-foods/cold-cereal/

kashi-golean-crunch-cereal
156. "Whole Grains: 100% Whole Wheat," *Oroweat*. https://www.oroweat.com/products/sliced-breads/whole-grains/100-whole-wheat?gclid=EAIaIQobChMI_dafuvyp3AIVAtRkCh2TyAHWEAAYASAAEgLScv
157. "Oats 'N Honey Granola Crunch," Ingredients. *Nature Valley*. https://www.naturevalley.com/product/granola-oats-n-honey-granola-crunch/
158. "Sugars, granulated [sucrose]." Self Nutrition Data. https://nutritiondata.self.com/facts/sweets/5592/2
159. "Oil, Soybean, Salad or Cooking," Self Nutrition Data https://nutritiondata.self.com/facts/fats-and-oils/507/2
160. "Nutrients in Wheat Flour: Whole, Refined and Enriched," Whole Grains Council. https://wholegrainscouncil.org/whole-grains-101/what-is-a-whole-grain
161. Cordain, Loren. "Implications of Plio-Pleistocene Hominin Diets for Modern Humans." In *Evolution of the Human Diet. The Known, the Unknown, and the Unknowable*, edited by P.S. Ungar, 363-83. Oxford, UK: Oxford University Press. 2007
162. Ibid.
163. Ibid.
164. "The History of Canola," Canola Council of Canada. https://www.canolacouncil.org/oil-and-meal/what-is-canola/the-history-of-canola/
165. Poti et al., "Is the Degree of Food Processing and Convenience Linked with the Nutritional Quality of Foods Purchased by US Households?" *American Journal of Clinical Nutrition* (2015): doi: 10.3945/ajcn.114.100925
166. Moss, Michael. *Salt Sugar Fat: How the Food Giants Hooked Us*. New York: Random House, 2014. Kindle File, Location 508.
167. Ibid., Location 804-815, 991.
168. Holt et al., "A Satiety Index of Common Foods," *European Journal of Clinical Nutrition* 49, no. 9 (1996): 675-690.
169. Leidy et al., "The Role of Protein in Weight Loss and Maintenance," *American Journal of Clinical Nutrition* 101, no. 6 (2015): 1320S-1329S.
170. Barr, S., and Wright, J., "Postprandial Energy Expenditure in Whole-Food and Processed-Food Meals: Implications for Daily Energy Expenditure," *Food & Nutrition Research* 54 (2010): doi: 10.3402/fnr.v54i0.5144.
171. Paddon-Jones et al., "Protein, Weight Management, and Satiety," *American Journal of Clinical Nutrition* 87, no.5 (2008): 1158S-1561S.
172. Oostindjer et al., "The Role of Red and Processed Meat in Colorectal Cancer Development: A Perspective," *Meat Science* 97, no. 4 (2014): 583-96.
173. Santarelli et al., "Processed Meat and Colorectal Cancer: A Review of Epidemiologic and Experimental Evidence," *Nutrition and Cancer* 60, no. 2 (2008): 131-44.
174. Larsson et al., "Processed Meat Consumption, Dietary Nitrosamines and Stomach Cancer Risk in a Cohort of Swedish Women," *International Journal of Cancer* 119, no. 4 (2006): 915-9.
175. Rohrmann et al., "Meat Consumption and Mortality—Results from the European Prospective Investigation into Cancer and Nutrition," *BMC Medicine* 11, no. 63 (2013): doi:10.1186/1741-7015-11-63
176. Schwingshackl et al., "Food Groups and Risk of All-Cause Mortality: A Systematic Review and Meta-Analysis of Prospective Studies," *The American Journal of Clinical Nutrition* (2017): ajcn153148.
177. Larsson, S., and Orsini, Nicola, "Red Meat and Processed Meat Consumption and All-Cause Mortality: A Meta-Analysis," *American Journal of Epidemiology* 179, no. 3 (2014): 282-89.
178. Micha et al., "Red and Processed Meat Consumption and Risk of Incident Coronary Heart Disease, Stroke, and Diabetes Mellitus: A Systematic Review and Meta-Analysis," *Circulation* 121, no. 21 (2010): 2271-2283.
179. Chan et al., "Red and Processed Meat and Colorectal Cancer Incidence: Meta-Analysis of Prospective Studies," *PLOS One* 6, no. 6 (2011): e20456.
180. Cohen, Rich, "Sugar Love: A Not So Sweet Story," *National Geographic*, August 2013. https://www.nationalgeographic.com/magazine/2013/08/sugar-love/
181. "Timeline of Sugar," *Sugar History*. http://www.sugarhistory.net/who-made-sugar/sugar-timeline/
182. "19th Century Sugar Boxes in Poland," Association of Small Collectors of Antique Silver (ASCAS). http://www.ascasonline.org/articoloDICEM89.html
183. Cordain, Loren. "Implications of Plio-Pleistocene Hominin Diets for Modern Humans." In *Evolution of the Human Diet. The Known, the Unknown, and the Unknowable*, edited by P.S. Ungar, 363-83. Oxford, UK: Oxford University Press. 2007.
184. Guyenet, Stephen, "By 2606, the US Diet Will Be 100% Sugar," *Whole Health Source*. 02-18-12. https://wholehealthsource.blogspot.com/2012/02/by-2606-us-diet-will-be-100-percent.html (updated version through 2016 provided via personal correspondence with Dr. Guyenet).
185. Johnson et al., "Potential Role of Sugar (Fructose) in the Epidemic of Hypertension, Obesity, and the Metabolic Syndrome, Diabetes, Kidney Disease, and Cardiovascular Disease," *American Journal of Clinical Nutrition* 86, no. 4 (2007): 899-906.
186. Ibid.
187. Ibid.
188. Morenga et al., "Dietary Sugars and Body Weight: Systematic Review and Meta-Analyses of Randomised Controlled Trials and Cohort Studies," *BMJ* (2013): 346, e7452. doi: https://doi.org/10.1136/bmj.e7492
189. Yang et al., "Added Sugar Intake and Cardiovascular Diseases Mortality Among U.S. Adults," *JAMA Internal Medicine* 174, no. 4 (2014): 516-524.
190. Katschinski et al., "Smoking and Sugar Intake Are Separate but Interactive Risk Factors in Crohn's Disease," *Gut* 29 (1988): 1202-1206.
191. Bostick et al., "Sugar, Meat, and Fat Intake, and Non-Dietary Risk Factors for Colon Cancer Incidence in Iowa Women (United States)," *Cancer Causes and Control* 5, no. 1 (1994): 38-52.
192. Seely, S., "Diet and Breast Cancer: The Possible Connection with Sugar Consumption," *Medical Hypotheses* 11, no. 3 (1983): 319-27.
193. Klein, Richard, *The Human Career: Human Biological and Cultural Origins*. Chicago: University of Chicago Press, 1999.
194. Alinia et al., "The Potential Association Between Fruit Intake and Body Weight—A Review," *Obesity Reviews* (2009): 10.1111/j.1467-789X.2009.00582.x
195. Slavin, J., and Green, H., "Dietary Fibre and Satiety," *Nutrition Bulletin* 32: 32-42.

196. Burton-Freeman, B., "Dietary Fiber and Energy Regulation," *The Journal of Nutrition* 130, no. 2 (2000): 2725-2755.
197. Marlowe et al. "Honey, Hadza, Hunter-Gatherers, and Human Evolution," *Journal of Human Evolution* 71 (2014): 119- 128.
198. Ibid.
199. Yang et al., "Added Sugar Intake and Cardiovascular Diseases Mortality Among U.S. Adults," *JAMA Internal Medicine* 174, no. 4 (2014): 516-524.
200. Alvarez-Suarez et al., "Contribution of Honey in Nutrition and Human Health: A Review," *Mediterranean Journal of Nutrition and Metabolism* 3, no. 1 (2010): 15-23.
201. Wyrick, J., "Honey Makes Up Nearly 20 Percent of Diet in Tanzanian Group," Scientific American. 9/3/2014. https://blogs.scientificamerican.com/food-matters/honey-makes-up-nearly- 20-percent-of-diet-in-tanzanian-group/
202. Ibid.
203. Marlowe, F.W., and Berbesque, J.C., "Tubers as Fallback Foods and their Impact on Hadza Hunter-Gatherers," *American Journal of Physical Anthropology* 4 (2009): 751-8.
204. Pontzer et al., "Hunter-Gatherer Energetics and Human Obesity," *PLOS One* 7 (2012): e40503. doi:10.1371/journal.pone.0040503
205. "BMR Calculator," *BMR Calculator*. https://www.bmrcalculator.org
206. Pontzer et al., "Hunter-Gatherer Energetics and Human Obesity," *PLOS One* 7 (2012): e40503. doi:10.1371/journal.pone.0040503
207. Westerterp, K.R., and Speakman, J.R., "Physical Activity Energy Expenditure has not Declined Since the 1980s and Matches Energy Expenditure in Wild Mammals," *International Journal of Obesity* 32 (2008): 1256-1263.
208. Johnson et al., "Potential Role of Sugar (Fructose) in the Epidemic of Hypertension, Obesity, and the Metabolic Syndrome, Diabetes, Kidney Disease, and Cardiovascular Disease," *American Journal of Clinical Nutrition* 86, no. 4 (2007): 899-906.
209. "Apple juice, canned or bottled, unsweetened, without ascorbic acid." Self Nutrition Data. https://nutritiondata.self.com/facts/fruits-and-fruit-juices/1822/2
210. "Is Agave Worse Than High Fructose Corn Syrup?" *Team Planet Green*. https://health.howstuffworks.com/wellness/food-nutrition/facts/agave-fructose-corn-syrup.htm
211. "Orange juice, canned, unsweetened," Self Nutrition Data. https://nutritiondata.self.com/facts/fruits-and-fruit-juices/1972/2
212. Stanhope et al., "Twenty-Four Hour Endocrine and Metabolic Profiles Following Consumption of High-Fructose Corn Syrup-, Sucrose, Fructose- and Glucose-Sweetened Beverages with Meals," *American Journal of Clinica Nutrition* 87, no. 5 (2008): 1194-1203.
213. Monsivais et al., "Sugar and Satiety: Does the Type of Sweetener Make a Difference," *American Journal of Clincial Nutrition* 86, no. 1 (2007): 116-123.
214. Rippe et al., "Sucrose, High-Fructose Corn Syrup, and Fructose, Their Metabolism and Potential Health Effects: What Do We Really Know?" *Advances in Nutrition: An International Review Journal* 4, no. 2 (2013): 236-245.
215. "How It's Made, Sugar," *YouTube*. https://www.youtube.com/watch? v=cWl141Bu7fc
216. "Crystallization," Sugar. *Encyclopedia Britannica*. https://www.britannica.com/EBchecked/topic/571880/sugar/50464/Crystallization
217. Schultz, David, "Evaporated Cane Juice: Sugar in Disguise?" The Salt, *NPR*. https://www.npr.org/blogs/thesalt/2012/10/18/163098211/evaporated-cane-juice-sugar-in-disguise
218. "DRAFT Guidance for Industry: Ingredients Declared as Evaporated Cane Juice; Draft Guidance," US Food and Drug Administration, October 2009. https://www.fda.gov/Food/GuidanceRegulation/GuidanceDocumentsRegulator
219. Holt et al., "A Satiety Index of Common Foods," *European Journal of Clinical Nutrition* 49, no. 9 (1996): 675-690.
220. Risling et al., "Food Intake Measured by an Automated Food-Selection System: Relationship to Energy Expenditure," *American Journal of Clinical Nutrition* 55, no. 2 (1992): 343-9.
221. Larson et al., "Ad Libitum Food Intake on a "Cafeteria Diet" in Native American Women: Relations with Body Composition and 24-H Energy Expenditure," *American Journal of Clinical Nutrition* 62, no. 5 (1995): 911-917.
222. Larson et al., "Spontaneous Overfeeding with a 'Cafeteria Diet' in Men: Effects on 24-Hour Energy Expenditure and Substrate Oxidation," *International Journal of Obesity and Related Metabolic Disorders* 19, no. 5 (1995): 331-337.
223. Moss, Michael. *Salt Sugar Fat: How the Food Giants Hooked Us*. New York: Random House, 2014. Kindle File, Location 699-710.
224. "Rice, white, long-grain, regular, raw, unenriched," Self Nutrition Data. https://nutritiondata.self.com/facts/cereal-grains-and-pasta/5812/2
225. "Sugars, granulated [sucrose]," Self Nutrition Data. https://nutritiondata.self.com/facts/sweets/5592/2
226. "Banana, raw," Self Nutrition Data. https://nutritiondata.self.com/facts/fruits-and-fruit-juices/1846/2
227. Sun, S., and Empie, E., "Fructose Metabolism in Humans – What Isotopic Tracer Studies Tell Us," *Nutrition & Metabolism* 9, no. 1 (2012): 89.
228. Tappy, L., and Le, K., "Metabolic Effects of Fructose and the Worldwide Increase in Obesity," *Physiological Reviews* 90, no. 1 (2010): 23-46.
229. Teff et al., "Dietary Fructose Reduces Circulating Insulin and Leptin, Attenuates Postprandial Suppression of Ghrelin, and Increases Triglycerides in Women," *Journal of Clinical Endocrinology and Metabolism* 89, no. 6 (2004): 2963-2972.
230. Kyriazis et al., "Sweet Receptor Signaling in Beta Cells Mediates Fructose-Induced Potentiation of Glucose-Stimulated Insulin Secretion," *PNAS* 109, no. 8 (2012): E524-E532.
231. Holt et al., "An Insulin Index of Foods: The Insulin Demand Generated by 1000-kj Portions of Common Foods," *American Journal of Clinical Nutrition* 66, no. 5 (1997): 1264-1276.
232. Pal, S., and Ellis, V., "The Acute Effects of Four Protein Meals on Insulin, Glucose, Appetite, and Energy Intake in Lean Men," *British Journal of Nutrition* 104, no. 8 (2010): 1241-8.
233. Hallschmid et al, "Postprandial Administration of Intranasal Insulin Intensifies Satiety and Reduces Intake of Palatable Snacks in Women," *Diabetes* 61, no. 4 (2012): 782-9.

234. Debons et al, "A Direct Action of Insulin on the Hypothalamic Satiety Center," *American Journal of Physiology* 219, no. 4 (1970).
235. Woods et al, "Chronic Intracerebroventricular Infusion of Insulin Reduces Food Intake and Body Weight of Baboons," *Nature* 282 (1979): 503-5.
236. Labouebe et al., "Insulin Induces Long-Term Depression of Ventral Tegmental Area Dopamine Neurons Via Endocannabinoids," *Nature Neuroscience* 16 (2013): 300-308.
237. Jauch-Chara et al., "Intranasal Insulin Suppresses Food Intake via Enhancement of Brain Energy Levels in Humans," *Diabetes* 61, no. 9 (2012): 2261-2268.
238. Boden et al., "Effects of Prolonged Hyperinsulinemia on Serum Leptin in Normal Human Subjects," *Journal of Clinical Investigation* 100 (1997): 1107-13.
239. Barr et al., "Insulin Stimulates Both Leptin Secretion and Production by Rat White Adipose Tissue," *Endocrinology* 138, no. 10 (1997): 4463-72.
240. Kolaczynski et al., "Acute and Chronic Effects of Insulin on Leptin Production in Humans," *Diabetes* 45 (1996): 699-701.
241. Wabitsch et al., "Insulin and Cortisol Promote Leptin Production in Cultured Human Fat Cells," *Diabetes* 45 (1996): 1435-1438.
242. Harris, R., "Leptin—Much More Than a Satiety Signal," *Annual Reviews of Nutrition* 20.1 (2000): 45-75.
243. Guyenet, S., and Schwartz, M.," Regulation of Food Intake, Energy Balance, and Body Fat Mass: Implications for the Pathogenesis and Treatment of Obesity," *The Journal of Clinical Endocrinology and Metabolism* 97, no. 3 (2012): 745-755.
244. Page et al., "Effects of Fructose vs Glucose on Regional Cerebral Blood Flow in Brain Regions Involved in Appetite and Reward Pathways," *Journal of the American Medical Association* 309, no. 1 (2013): 63-70.
245. Teff et al., "Dietary Fructose Reduces Circulating Insulin and Leptin, Attenuates Postprandial Suppression of Ghrelin, and Increases Triglycerides in Women," *The Journal of Clinical Endocrinology and Metabolism* 89, no. 6 (2004): https://dx.doi.org/10.1210/jc.2003-031855
246. Stanhope et al., "Consuming Fructose-Sweetened, Not Glucose-Sweetened, Beverages Increases Visceral Adiposity and Lipids and Decreases Insulin Sensitivity in Overweight/Obese Humans," *The Journal of Clinical Investigation* 119, no. 5 (2009): 1322-34.
247. Johnson et al., "Potential Role of Sugar (Fructose) in the Epidemic of Hypertension, Obesity, and the Metabolic Syndrome, Diabetes, Kidney Disease, and Cardiovascular Disease," *American Journal of Clinical Nutrition* 86, no. 4 (2007): 899-906.
248. Ibid.
249. Stanhope et al., "Consuming Fructose-Sweetened, Not Glucose-Sweetened, Beverages Increases Visceral Adiposity and Lipids and Decreases Insulin Sensitivity in Overweight/Obese Humans," *The Journal of Clinical Investigation* 119, no. 5 (2009): 1322-34.
250. Zhang et al., "Very High Fructose Intake Increases Serum LDL- Cholesterol and Total Cholesterol: A Meta-Analysis of Controlled Feeding Trials," *Journal of Nutrition* 143, no. 9 (2013): 1391-1398.
251. Ouyang et al., "Fructose Consumption as a Risk Factor for Non-Alcoholic Fatty Liver Disease," *Hepatology* 48, no. 6 (2008): 993-999.
252. Esmaillzadeh et al., "Fruit and Vegetable Intakes, C-Reactive Protein, and the Metabolic Syndrome," *American Journal of Clinical Nutrition* 84, no. 4 (2006): 1489-97.
253. "Honey," Self Nutrition Data. https://nutritiondata.self.com/facts/sweets/5568/2
254. Larson-Meyer et al., "Effect of Honey versus Sucrose on Appetite, Appetite-Regulating Hormones, and Postmeal Thermogenesis," *Journal of the American College of Nutrition* 29, no. 5 (2010): 482-493.
255. Bogdanov et al., "Honey for Nutrition and Health: A Review," *American Journal of the College of Nutrition* (2008): 677-689.
256. Avena et al., "Evidence for Sugar Addiction: Behavioral and Neurochemical Effects of Intermittent, Excessive Sugar Intake," *Neuroscience & Behavioral Reviews* 32, no. 1 (2007): 20-39.
257. Stice et al., "Relation Between Obesity and Blunted Striatal Response to Food is Moderated by TaqIA AI Allele," *Science* 322 (2008): 449-452.
258. Colantuoni et al., "Excessive Sugar Intake Alters Binding to Dopamine and Mu-Opioid Receptors in the Brain," *Neuroreport* 12 (2001): 3549-3552.
259. Drewnowski et al., "Taste Responses and Preferences for Sweet High-Fat Foods: Evidence for Opioid Involvement," *Physiology & Behavior* 51, no. 2 (1992): 371-379.
260. Bray et al., "Consumption of High-Fructose Corn Syrup in Beverages May Play a Role in the Epidemic of Obesity," *American Journal of Clinical Nutrition* 79, no. 4 (2004): 537-54.
261. Malik et al., "Intake of Sugar-Sweetened Beverages and Weight Gain: a Systematic Review," *American Journal of Clinical Nutrition* 84, no. 2 (2006): 274-288.
262. Ludwig et al., "Relation Between Consumption of Sugar-Sweetened Drinks and Childhood Obesity: A Prospective, Observational Analysis," *Lancet* 357 (2001): 505-508.
263. Zheng et al., "Sugar-Sweetened Beverage Consumption in Relation to Changes in Body Fatness over 6 and 12 Years among 9-Year-Old Children: The European Youth Heart Study," *European Journal of Clinical Nutrition* 68, no. 1 (2014): 77- 83.
264. Odegaard et al, "Soft Drink and Juice Consumption and Risk of Physician-Diagnosed Incident Type 2 Diabetes: The Singapore Chinese Health Study," *American Journal of Epidemiology* 171, no. 6 (2010): 701-8.
265. Faith et al., "Fruit Juice Intake Predicts Increased Adiposity Gain in Children from Low-Income Families: Weight Status-by-Environment Interaction," *Pediatrics* 118, no. 5 (2006): 2066-75.
266. Dennison et al., "Excess Fruit Juice Consumption by Pre-School Aged Children Is Associated with Short Stature and Obesity," *Pediatrics* 99, no. 1 (1997): 15-22.
267. Bes-Rastrollo et al., "Predictors of Weight Gain in a Mediterranean Cohort: The Seguimiento Universidad de Navarra Study," *American Journal of Clinical Nutrition* 83, no. 2 (2006): 362-370.
268. Hu, F., and Malik, V., "Sugar-Sweetened Beverages and Risk of Obesity and Type 2 Diabetes: Epidemiological Evidence," *Physiology & Behavior* 100, no. 1 (2010): 47-54.
269. Chen et al., "Reduction in Consumption of Sugar-Sweetened Beverages is Associated with Weight Loss: The PREMIER Trial," *American Journal of Clinical Nutrition* 89, no. 5 (2009): 1299-1306.
270. Vartanian et al., "Effects of Soft Drink Consumption on Nutrition and Health: A Systematic Review and Meta-Analysis," *American Journal of Public Health* 97, no. 4 (2007): 667-675.
271. Wojcicki, J., and Heyman, M., "Reducing Childhood Obesity by Eliminating 100% Fruit Juice," *American Journal of Public Health* 102, no. 9 (2012): 1630-1633.

272. Schulze et al., "Sugar-Sweetened Beverages, Weight Gain, and Incidence of Type 2 Diabetes in Young and Middle-Aged Women," *Journal of the American Medical Association* 8 (2004): 927-934.
273. Mozaffarian et al., "Changes in Diet and Lifestyle and Long-Term Weight Gain in Men and Women," *New England Journal of Medicine* 364, no. 25 (2011): 2392-2404.
274. Tanasescu et al., "Biobehavioral Factors are Associated with Obesity in Puerto Rican Children," *Journal of Nutrition* 130, no. 7 (2000): 1734-42.
275. Sangiorski et al., "Association of Key Foods and Beverages with Obesity in Australian Schoolchildren," *Public Health Nutrition* 10, no. 2 (2007): 152-157.
276. Kral et al., "Beverage Consumption Patterns of Children Born at Different Risk of Obesity," *Obesity* 16, no. 8 (2008): 1802-1808.
277. Carlson et al., "Dietary-Related and Physical-Activity Related Predictors of Obesity in Children: A 2-Year Prospective Study," *Childhood Obesity* 8, no. 2 (2012): 110-115.
278. James et al, "Preventing Childhood Obesity by Reducing Consumption of Carbonated Drinks: Cluster Randomised Controlled Trial," *British Medical Journal* 328 (2004): 1237. doi: https://dx.doi.org/10.1136/bmj.38077.458438.EE
279. Berkey et al., "Sugar-Added Beverages and Adolescent Weight Change," *Obesity Research & Clinical Practice* 12, no. 5 (2004): 778-788.
280. Liebman et al., "Dietary Intake, Eating Behavior, and Physical Activity-Related Determinants of High Body Mass Index in Rural Communities in Wyoming, Montana, and Idaho," *International Journal of Obesity and Related Metabolic Disorders* 27, no. 6 (2003): 684-692.
281. Troiano et al., "Energy and Fat Intakes of Children and Adolescents in the United States: Data from the National Health and Nutrition Examination Surveys," *American Journal of Clinical Nutrition* 72 (2000): 1343S-1353S.
282. Dhingra et al., "Soft Drink Consumption and Risk of Developing Cardiometabolic Risk Factors and the Metabolic Syndrome in Middle-Aged Adults in the Community," *Circulation* 116 (2007): 480-88.
283. Malik et al., "Sugar-Sweetened Beverages and BMI in Children and Adolescents: Reanalyses of a Meta-Analysis," *American Journal of Clinical Nutrition* 89, no. 1 (2009): 438-9.
284. Olsen N., and Heitmann, B., "Intake of Calorically Sweetened Beverages and Obesity," *Obesity Reviews* 10, no. 1 (2009):68-75.
285. Phillips et al., "Energy-Dense Snack Food Intake in Adolescence: Longitudinal Relationship to Weight and Fatness," *Obesity Research & Clinical Practice* 12, no. 3 (2004): 461-472.
286. Ebbeling et al., "Effects of Decreasing Sugar-Sweetened Beverage Consumption on Body Weight in Adolescents: A Randomized, Controlled Pilot Study," *Pediatrics* 117, no. 3 (2006): 673-680.
287. Dubois et al., "Regular Sugar-Sweetened Beverage Consumption Between Meals Increases Risk of Overweight Among Preschool-Aged Children," *Journal of the American Dietetic Association* 107, no. 6 (2007): 924-934.
288. Nissinen et al., "Sweets and Sugar-Sweetened Soft-Drink Intake in Childhood in Relation to Adult BMI and Overweight. The Cardiovascular Risk in Young Finns Study," *Public Health Nutrition* 12, no. 11 (2009): 2018-26.
289. Viner R., and Cole, T., "Who Changes Body Mass Between Adolescence and Adulthood? Factors Predicting Change in BMI Between 16 Year and 30 Years in the 1970 British Birth Cohort," *International Journal of Obesity* 30, no. 9 (2006): 1368-74.
290. Palmer et al., "Sugar-Sweetened Beverages and Incidence of Type 2 Diabetes Mellitus in African American Women," *Archives of Internal Medicine* 168, no. 14 (2008): 1487-92.
291. Giammattei et al., "Television Watching and Soft Drink Consumption: Associations with Obesity in 11- to 13-Year-Old School Children," *Archives of Pediatrics and Adolescent Medicine* 157, no. 9 (2003): 882-886.
292. Gillis L., and Bar-Or, O., "Food Away from Home, Sugar-Sweetened Drink Consumption and Juvenile Obesity," *Journal of the American College of Nutrition* 22, no. 6 (2003): 539-45.
293. Nicklas et al., "Eating Patterns and Obesity in Children: The Bogalusa Heart Study," *American Journal of Preventive Medicine* 25, no. 1 (2003): 9-16.
294. Welsh et al., "Overweight Among Low-Income Preschool Children Associated with the Consumption of Sweet Drinks: Missouri, 1999-2002," *Pediatrics* 115, no. 2 (2005): 223-229.
295. Lim et al., "Obesity and Sugar-Sweetened Beverages in African-American Preschool Children: A Longitudinal Study," *Obesity* 17, no. 6 (2009): 1262-8.
296. Malik et al., "Sugar-Sweetened Beverages and Weight Gain in Children and Adults: A Systematic Review and Meta-Analysis," *American Journal of Clinical Nutrition* 98, no. 4 (2013): 1084-1102.
297. Inoue et al., "Lifestyle, Weight Perception and Change in Body Mass Index of Japanese Workers: MY Health Up Study," *Public Health* 124, no. 9 (2010): 530-7.
298. Field et al., "Association of Sports Drinks with Weight Gain Among Adolescents and Young Adults," *Obesity* 22, no. 10 (2014): 2238-2243.
299. Hu, F., "Resolved: There is Sufficient Evidence That Decreasing Sugar-Sweetened Beverage Consumption Will Reduce the Prevalence of Obesity and Obesity-Related Diseases," *Obesity Reviews* 14, no. 8 (2013): 606-619.
300. DiMeglio, D.P., and Mattes, R.D., "Liquid Versus Solid Carbohydrate: Effects on Food Intake and Body Weight." *International Journal of Obesity* 24, no. 6 (2000): 794-800.
301. Mourao et al., "Effects of Food Form on Appetite and Energy Intake in Lean and Obese Adults," *International Journal of Obesity* 11 (2007): 1688-95.
302. Ogden et al., "NCHS Health E-Stat: Prevalence of Overweight, Obesity, and Extreme Obesity Among Adults: United States, Trends 1960-1962 through 2007-2008," Centers for Disease Control and Prevention. https://www.cdc.gov/nchs/data/hestat/obesity_adult_07_08/obesity_adult_07_0
303. Han E., and Powell, L., "Consumption Patterns of Sugar-Sweetened Beverages in the United States," *Journal of the Academy of Nutrition and Dietetics* 113, no. 1 (2013): 43-53.
304. "Milk, lowfat, fluid, 1% milkfat, with added Vitamin A," Self Nutrition Data. https://nutritiondata.self.com/facts/dairy-and-egg-products/74/2
305. Paddon-Jones et al., "Protein, Weight Management, and Satiety," *American Journal of Clinical Nutrition* 87, no.5 (2008): 1158S-1561S.
306. Cordain et al., "Plant-Animal Subsistence Ratios and Macronutrient Energy Estimations in Worldwide Hunter-Gatherer Diets," *American Journal of Clinical Nutrition* 71, no. 3 (2000): 682-692.
307. Taylor, W., "The Hunter-Gatherer Nomads of Northern Mexico: A Comparison of the Archival and

Archeological Records," *World Archaeology* 4, no. 2 (1972): 167-178.

308. Wolf et al., "A Short History of Beverages and How Our Body Treats Them," *Obesity Reviews* 9, no. 2 (2008): 151-164.

309. "Orange Juice - Full of Vitamin C," *Professor's House*. https://www.professorshouse.com/orange-juice/

310. Boucher, D., "Cocaine and the Coca Plant," *Bioscience* 41, no. 2 (1991): 72-76.

311. He et al., "Changes in Intake of Fruits and Vegetables in Relation to Risk of Obesity and Weight Gain Among Middle-Aged Women," *International Journal of Obesity* 28 (2004): 1569-1574.

312. Bazzano et al., "Intake of Fruit, Vegetables, and Fruit Juices and Risk of Diabetes in Women," *Diabetes Care* 31, no. 7 (2008): 1311-1317.

313. Faith et al., "Fruit Juice Intake Predicts Increased Adiposity Gain in Children From Low-Income Families: Weight Status-by-Environment Interaction," *Pediatrics* 118, no. 5 (2006): 2066-75.

314. Wojcicki, J., and Heyman, M., "Reducing Childhood Obesity by Eliminating 100% Fruit Juice," *American Journal of Public Health* 102, no. 9 (2012): 1630-1633.

315. Muraki et al., "Fruit Consumption and Risk of Type 2 Diabetes: Results from Three Prospective Longitudinal Cohort Studies," *British Medical Journal* 347 (2013): doi: https://dx.doi.org/10.1136/bmj.f5001

316. Faith et al., "Fruit Juice Intake Predicts Increased Adiposity Gain in Children From Low-Income Families: Weight Status-by-Environment Interaction," *Pediatrics* 118, no. 5 (2006): 2066-75.

317. Walker, A., "Ask an Academic: Orange Juice," *The New Yorker*. May 12, 2009. https://www.newyorker.com/books/page-turner/ask-an-academic-orange-juice

318. Klein, A., and Kiat, H., "Detox Diets for Toxin Elimination and Weight Management: A Critical Review of the Evidence," *Nutritional Sciences* 28, no. 6 (2015): 675-686.

319. Wannamethee S., and Shaper A., "Alcohol, Body Weight, and Weight Gain in Middle-Aged Men," *American Journal of Clinical Nutrition* 77, no. 5 (2003): 1312-1317.

320. Wannamethee et al., "Alcohol Intake and 8-Year Weight Gain in Women: A Prospective Study," *Obesity Reviews* 9 (2004): 1386-96.

321. Röjdmark et al., "Alcohol Ingestion Decreases Both Diurnal and Nocturnal Secretion of Leptin in Healthy Individuals," *Clinical Endocrinology* 55, no. 5 (2001): 639-647.

322. Wannamethee et al., "Alcohol Intake and 8-Year Weight Gain in Women: A Prospective Study," *Obesity Reviews* 9 (2004): 1386-96.

323. Lavalle, R., and Hsiao-ye Y., "Surveillance Report #92: Apparent Per Capita Alcohol Consumption: National, State, and Regional Trends, 1977- 2009," National Institute on Alcohol Abuse and Alcoholism: Division of Epidemiology and Prevention Research. Alcohol Epidemiologic Data System. https://pubs.niaaa.nih.gov/publications/Surveillance92/CONS09.pdf

324. Ogden et al., "NCHS Health E-Stat: Prevalence of Overweight, Obesity, and Extreme Obesity Among Adults: United States, Trends 1960-1962 through 2007-2008," Centers for Disease Control and Prevention: Publications and Information Products. https://www.cdc.gov/nchs/data/hestat/obesity_adult_07_08/obesity_adult_07_0

325. Wang et al., "Alcohol Consumption, Weight Gain, and Risk of Becoming Overweight in Middle-Aged and Older Women," *Archives of Internal Medicine* 170, no. 5 (2010): 453-461.

326. Liu et al., "A Prospective Study of Alcohol Intake and Change in Body Weight Among US Adults," *American Journal of Epidemiology* 140, no. 10 (1994): 912-20.

327. Catenacci et al., "Low/No Calorie Sweetened Beverage Consumption in the National Weight Control Registry," *Obesity* 22, no. 10 (2014): 2244- 2251.

328. Raben et al., "Sucrose Compared with Artificial Sweeteners: Different Effects on Ad Libitum Food Intake and Body Weight After 10 WK of Supplementation in Overweight Subjects," *American Journal of Clinical Nutrition* 76, no. 4 (2002): 721-9.

329. Tordoff, M., and Alleva, A., "Effect of Drinking Soda Sweetened with Aspartame or High-Fructose Corn Syrup on Food Intake and Body Weight," *American Journal of Clinical Nutrition* 51, no. 6 (1990): 963-969.

330. de Ruyter et al., "A Trial of Sugar-Free or Sugar-Sweetened Beverages and Body Weight in Children," *The New England Journal of Medicine* 367 (2012): 1397-1406.

331. Tate et al., "Replacing Caloric Beverages with Water or Diet Beverages for Weight Loss in Adults: Main Results of the Choose Healthy Options Consciously Everyday (CHOICE) Randomized Clinical Trial," *American Journal of Clinical Nutrition* 95, no. 3 (2012): 555-563.

332. Peters et al., "The Effects of Water and Non-Nutritive Sweetened Beverages on Weight Loss During a 12-Week Weight Loss Treatment Program," *Obesity* 22.6 (2014): 1415-1421.

333. Miller, P., and Perez, V., "Low-Calorie Sweeteners and Body Weight and Composition: A Meta-Analysis of Randomized Controlled Trials and Prospective Cohort Studies," *American Journal of Clinical Nutrition* (2014): doi: 10.3945/ajcn.113.082826

334. Rogers et al., "Does Low-Energy Sweetener Consumption Affect Energy Intake and Body Weight? A Systematic Review, Including Meta-Analyses, of the Evidence from Human and Animal Studies," *International Journal of Obesity* 40 (2015): 381-394.

335. Tey et al., "Effects of Aspartame-, Monk Fruit-, Stevia and Sucrose-Sweetened Beverages on Postprandial Glucose, Insulin and Energy Intake," *International Journal of Obesity* 41 (2017): 450-7.

336. Rogers et al., "Does Low-Energy Sweetener Consumption Affect Energy Intake and Body Weight? A Systematic Review, Including Meta-Analyses, of the Evidence from Human and Animal Studies," *International Journal of Obesity* 40 (2015): 381-394.

337. Fagherazzi et al., "Consumption of Artificially and Sugar-Sweetened Beverages and Incident Type 2 Diabetes in the Étude Epidémiologique Auprès des Femmes de la Mutuelle Générale de l'Education Nationale–European Prospective Investigation into Cancer and Nutrition Cohort," *American Journal of Clinical Nutrition* (2013): doi: 10.3945/ajcn.112.050997

338. Pereira M., and Odegaard A., "Artificially Sweetened Beverages—Do They Influence Cardiometabolic Risk," *Current Atherosclerosis Reports* 15, no. 12 (2013): 375. doi: 10.1007/s11883-013-0375-z.

339. Ma et al., "Sugar Sweetened Beverages but Not Diet Soda Consumption Is Positively Associated with Insulin Resistance and Prediabetes," *The Journal of Nutrition* 146, no. 12 (2016): 2544-2550.

340. Weihrauch, M.R., and Diehl, V., "Artificial Sweeteners—Do They Bear a Carcinogenic Risk?" *Annals of Oncology* 15, no. 10 (2004): 1460-1465.

341. Magnuson et al., "Aspartame: A Safety Evaluation Based on Current Use Levels, Regulations, and Toxicological and Epidemiological Studies," *Critical Reviews in Toxicology* 37, no. 8 (2007): 629-727.

342. Mallikarjun, S., and Sieburth, R., " Aspartame and Risk of Cancer: A Meta-Analytic Review," *Archives of*

*Environmental and Occupational Health* 3 (2015): 133-141.
343. "Artificial Sweeteners and Cancer," National Cancer Institute. Fact Sheets: Risk Factors and Possible Causes. https://www.cancer.gov/cancertopics/factsheet/Risk/artificial-sweeteners
344. "Aspartame," American Cancer Society. *Learn About Cancer*. https://www.cancer.org/cancer/cancercauses/othercarcinogens/athome/aspartame
345. "Coca Cola Nutrition," *The Coca-Cola Company*. https://productnutrition.thecoca-colacompany.com
346. "White Chocolate Mocha," Starbucks. https://www.starbucks.com/menu/drinks/espresso/white-chocolate-mocha-?foodZone=9999
347. "Coca Cola Nutrition," *The Coca-Cola Company*. https://productnutrition.thecoca-colacompany.com
348. "Original," Product Facts. *The Coca-Cola Company*. https://www.coca-colaproductfacts.com/en/products/coca-cola/original/12-oz/
349. "Basic Report: 09206, Orange Juice, Raw (Includes Foods for USDA's Food Distribution)," USDA. https://ndb.nal.usda.gov/ndb/foods/show/09206
350. Westerterp, K.R., and Speakman, J.R., "Physical Activity Energy Expenditure Has Not Declined Since the 1980s and Matches Energy Expenditure in Wild Mammals," *International Journal of Obesity* 32 (2008): 1256-1263.
351. Ibid.
352. "FAQs: Popular 20th Century American Foods," *Food Timeline*. https://www.foodtimeline.org/fooddecades.html#70snewproducts
353. "Timeline of Events in Food History, 1971-'75, 1976-1980," *FoodReference.*
354. White, J., "Straight Talk About High-Fructose Corn Syrup: What It Is and What It Ain't," *American Journal of Clinical Nutrition* 88, no. 6 (2008): 1716S-1712S.
355. "The History of Canola," Canola Council of Canada. https://www.canolacouncil.org/oil-and-meal/what-is-canola/
356. "FAQs: Popular 20th Century American Foods," *Food Timeline*. http://www.foodtimeline.org/fooddecades.html#70snewproducts
357. "Timeline of Events in Food History, 1971-'75, 1976-1980," *FoodReference.*
358. "Food Processing: A History," *Food Processing*. 10-05-2010. https://www.foodprocessing.com/articles/2010/anniversary/?show=all
359. Cutler et al., "Why Have Americans Become More Obese?" *Journal of Economic Perspectives* 17, no. 3 (2003): 93-118.
360. Guyenet, Stephan, "Calorie Intake and the US Obesity Epidemic," *Whole Health Source*. https://wholehealthsource.blogspot.com/search?q=obesity+in+the+us
361. Gerrior et al., "Nutrient Content of the US Food Supply, 1909-2000," *Home Economics Research Report*, no. 56, Center for Nutrition Policy and Promotion, USDA. 2004.
362. "Kellogg's Froot Loops Cereal," Ingredients. *Kellogg's*. https://www.kelloggs.com/en_US/kelloggs-froot-loops-cereal.html
363. "Learning to Like Foods: An Interview with Anthony Sclafani," *Observer*. Association for Psychological Science. https://www.psychologicalscience.org/index.php/publications/observer/2010/m 10/learning-to-like-foods.html
364. Ibid.
365. Martire et al., "Extended Exposure to a Palatable Cafeteria Diet Alters Gene Expression in Brain Regions Implicated in Reward, and Withdrawal from This Diet Alters Gene Expression in Brain Regions Associated with Stress," *Behavioral Brain Research* 265 (2014): 132-141.
366. Sampey et al., "Cafeteria Diet is a Robust Model of Human Metabolic Syndrome with Liver and Adipose Inflammation: Comparison to High-Fat Diet," *Obesity* 19, no. 6 (2012): 1109-17.
367. Guyenet, S., and Schwartz, M., " Regulation of Food Intake, Energy Balance, and Body Fat Mass: Implications for the Pathogenesis and Treatment of Obesity," *The Journal of Clinical Endocrinology and Metabolism* 97, no. 3 (2012): 745-755.
368. Risling et al., "Food Intake Measured by an Automated Food-Selection System: Relationship to Energy Expenditure," *American Journal of Clinical Nutrition* 55, no. 2 (1992): 343-9.
369. Ibid.
370. Larson et al., "Spontaneous Overfeeding with a 'Cafeteria Diet' in Men: Effects on 24-hour Energy Expenditure and Substrate Oxidation," *International Journal of Obesity and Related Metabolic Disorders* 19, no. 5 (1995): 331-337.
371. Larson et al., "Ad Libitum Food Intake on a 'Cafeteria Diet' in Native American Women: Relations with Body Composition and 24-H Energy Expenditure," *American Journal of Clinical Nutrition* 62, no. 5 (1995): 911-917.
372. Risling et al., "Food Intake Measured by an Automated Food-Selection System: Relationship to Energy Expenditure," *American Journal of Clinical Nutrition* 55, no. 2 (1992): 343-9.
373. Holt et al., "A Satiety Index of Common Foods," *European Journal of Clinical Nutrition* 49, no. 9 (1996): 675-690.
374. Marsh, P., "Dental Plaque as a Biofilm and a Microbial Community—Implications for Health and Disease," *BMC Oral Health* 2006 (Supplement 1): S14. doi:10.1186/1472-6831-6-S1-S14.
375. Yang et al., "Added Sugar Intake and Cardiovascular Diseases Mortality Among U.S. Adults," *JAMA Internal Medicine* 174, no. 4 (2014): 516-524.
376. Katschinski et al., "Smoking and Sugar Intake Are Separate but Interactive Risk Factors in Crohn's Disease," *Gut* 29 (1988): 1202-1206.
377. Bostick et al., "Sugar, Meat, and Fat Intake, and Non-Dietary Risk Factors for Colon Cancer Incidence in Iowa Women (United States)," *Cancer Causes and Control* 5, no. 1 (1994): 38-52.
378. Seely, S., "Diet and Breast Cancer: The Possible Connection with Sugar Consumption," *Medical Hypotheses* 11, no. (1983): 319-327.
379. Masterjohn, C., "The Scientific Approach of Weston Price, Part 1: Nature's Closest Thing to a RCT," *The Weston A. Price Foundation*. https://www.westonaprice.org/
380. Price, Weston, *Nutrition and Physical Degeneration*. Lemon Grove: Price Pottenger Nutrition, 2012. Print.
381. Ibid., Chapter 1, page 6.
382. Ibid., Chapter 9, page 120.
383. Ibid., Chapter 18, page 296.
384. Ibid., Chapter 3, page 23.

385. Ibid., Chapter 6, page 83.
386. Ibid., Chapter 6, page 71.
387. Ibid., Chapter 9, pages 119-120.
388. Ibid., Chapter 11, page 179.
389. Willett, Walter, "Diet, Nutrition, and Avoidable Cancer," *Environmental Health Perspectives* 103, Supplement 8 (1995): 165-170.
390. Burkitt, D.P., "Some Diseases Characteristic of Modern Western Civilization," *British Medical Journal* 1 (1973): 274-278.
391. Cleave, T.L. *The Saccharine Disease: Conditions Caused by the Takings of Refined Carbohydrates Such as Sugar and White Flour*. Bristol: John Wright & Sons Limited, 1974.
392. Slome et al., "Weight, Height, and Skinfold Thickness of Zulu Adults in Durban," *South African Medical Journal* 34 (1960): 505-509.
393. "whole food," *Merriam Webster's Collegiate Dictionary*, Eleventh Edition. 2012.
394. "whole," *Merriam Webster's Collegiate Dictionary* , Eleventh Edition. 2012.
395. Cordain, Loren. "Implications of Plio-Pleistocene Hominin Diets for Modern Humans." In *Evolution of the Human Diet. The Known, the Unknown, and the Unknowable*, edited by P.S. Ungar, 363-83. Oxford, UK: Oxford University Press. 2007.
396. Guyenet, S., and Schwartz, M., " Regulation of Food Intake, Energy Balance, and Body Fat Mass: Implications for the Pathogenesis and Treatment of Obesity," *The Journal of Clinical Endocrinology and Metabolism* 97, no. 3 (2012): 745-755.
397. "Ingredients," Stroehmann Dutch Country 100% Whole Grain Bread. *Stroehmann*. https://stroehmann. com/Products/Stroehmann-Dutch-Country-100-Whole-Wheat-(1-pack)/Default.aspx#
398. Moss, Michael. *Salt Sugar Fat: How the Food Giants Hooked Us*. New York: Random House, 2014. Kindle File, Location 557-572.
399. "Kashi GOLEAN Crunch Cereal," *Kashi*. https://www.kashi.com/our-foods/cold-cereal/ kashi-golean-crunch-cereal
400. Ibid.
401. "Product Nutrition," Lucky Charms Product List. *General Mills*. https://www.generalmills.com/en/Brands/ Cereals/lucky-charms/brand-product-list
402. "205.600: Evaluation Criteria for Allowed and Prohibited Substances, Methods, and Ingredients," The National List of Allowed and Prohibited Substances. USDA. https://www.ams.usda.gov/AMSv1.0/getfile? dDocName=STELPRDC5068682
403. Smith-Spangler et al., "Are Organic Foods Safer or Healthier Than Conventional Alternatives? A Systematic Review," *Annals of Internal Medicine* 157, no. 5 (2012): 348-366.
404. "Who Owns Organic," *The Cornucopia Institute*. https://www.cornucopia.org/who-owns-organic/
405. "Organic Industry Structure: Acquisitions & Alliances: Top 100 Food Processors in NorthAmerica," *Cornucopia*. https://www.cornucopia.org/wp-content/uploads/2014/02/Organic-chart-feb-2014.jpg
406. Ibid.
407. Pollan, Michael. *The Omnivore's Dilemma*. New York: Penguin, 2007. Page 159.
408. Smith-Spangler et al., "Are Organic Foods Safer or Healthier Than Conventional Alternatives? A Systematic Review," *Annals of Internal Medicine* 157, no. 5 (2012): 348-366.
409. Bradbury et al., "Organic Food Consumption and the Incidence of Cancer in a Large Prospective Study of Women in the United Kingdom," *British Journal of Cancer* 110 (2014): 2321-2326.
410. "U.S. Organic Industry Survey 2014," Market Analysis. *Organic Trade Association*. https://www.ota.com/ what-ota-does/market-analysis
411. "ClifBar: Chocolate Chip," Nutrition Facts. *ClifBar*. https://www.clifbar.com/products/clif-bar/clifbar/ chocolate-chip
412. Ibid.
413. "Kit Kat Milk Chocolate," Nutrition Information. *Hersheys*. https://www.hersheys.com/kitkat/products/kit-kat-milk-chocolate.aspx
414. Moss, Michael. *Salt Sugar Fat: How the Food Giants Hooked Us*. New York: Random House, 2014. Kindle File, Location 285 of 7325.
415. "2009-2013 Flavor and Fragrance Industry Leaders," *Leffingwell and Associates*. https://www.leffingwell.com/ top_10.htm
416. Moss, Michael. *Salt Sugar Fat: How the Food Giants Hooked Us*. New York: Random House, 2014. Kindle File, Location 805 of 7325.
417. Ibid., Location 1074 of 7325.
418. Cordain, Loren. "Implications of Plio-Pleistocene Hominin Diets for Modern Humans." In *Evolution of the Human Diet. The Known, the Unknown, and the Unknowable*, edited by P.S. Ungar, 363-83. Oxford, UK: Oxford University Press. 2007.
419. Lake A., Townsend T., "Obesogenic Environments: Exploring the Built and Food Environments," *The Journal of the Royal Society for the Promotion of Health* 126, no. 6 (2006): 262-267.
420. "The World's Biggest Industry," *Forbes*. 11-15-2007. https://www.forbes.com/2007/11/11/growth-agriculture-business-forbeslife-food07-cx_sm_1113bigfood.html
421. Moss, Michael. *Salt Sugar Fat: How the Food Giants Hooked Us*. New York: Random House, 2014. Kindle File, Location 3280 of 7325.
422. "Why Is It Important to Consume Oils?" *MyPlate*. United States Department of Agriculture. https://www. choosemyplate.gov/food-groups/oils-why.html
423. "Use Olive, Canola, Corn, or Safflower Oil as Your Main Kitchen Fats," American Heart Association. https://www.heart.org/HEARTORG/GettingHealthy/NutritionCenter/HealthyE Olive-Canola-Corn-or-Safflower-Oil-as-Your- Main-Kitchen-Fats_UCM_320268_Article.jsp
424. Confessore, N., "Corn: Vegetable, Fruit or Grain," *The New York Times*. 06-11-2007.
425. "Fruit," *Encyclopaedia Britannica*. https://www.britannica.com/EBchecked/topic/221056/fruit
426. Ibid.
427. "Question: Is Coconut a Fruit, Nut, or Seed," *Fun Science Facts from the Library of Congress*. The Library of Congress. https://www.loc.gov/rr/scitech/mysteries/coconut.html
428. "Oil Palm," Food and Agriculture Organization of the United Nations. https://www.fao.org/3/t0309e/ T0309E01.htm#ch1.2
429. "Twenty Facts About Cottonseed Oil," National Cottonseed Products Association. https://www.cottonseed.

com/publications/facts.asp
430. "Olive Oil Times Special: Extra Virgin Olive Oil," *Olive Oil Times*. https://www.oliveoiltimes.com/extra-virgin-olive-oil
431. Namdar et al., "Olive Oil Storage During the Fifth and Sixth Millennia BC at Ein Zippori, Northern Israel," *Israel Journal of Plant Sciences*. DOI: 10.1080/07929978.2014.960733
432. "The History of Canola," Canola Council of Canada. https://www.canolacouncil.org/oil-and-meal/what-is-canola/
433. "Global Consumption of Vegetable Oils from 1995/1996 to 2014/2015, by Oil Type, in Million Metric Tons," *Statista*. https://www.statista.com/statistics/263937/vegetable-oils-global-consumption/
434. "How It's Made—Canola Oil," YouTube. https://www.youtube.com/watch?v=Cfk2IXlZdbI
435. "Solvent Extraction," Edible Oil Processing. *The AOCS Lipid Library*. https://lipidlibrary.aocs.org/processing/solventextract/index.htm
436. Mag, Ted, "Canola Seed and Oil Processing," Oklahoma State. https://canola.okstate.edu/canolaoilmeal/oilprocessing.pdf
437. Holt et al., "A Satiety Index of Common Foods," *European Journal of Clinical Nutrition* 49, no. 9 (1996): 675-690.
438. Ibid.
439. Weaver, C., and Marr, E., "White Vegetables: A Forgotten Source of Nutrients: Purdue Roundtable Summary," *Advances in Nutrition* 4 (2013): 318S- 326S.
440. "Lay's Classic Potato Chips," *Frito-Lay*. https://www.fritolay.com/snacks/product-page/lays/lays-classic-potato-chips
441. "RUFFLES Original Potato Chips," *Frito-Lay*. https://www.fritolay.com/snacks/product-page/ruffles/ruffles-original-potato-chips
442. "Oil, Soybean, Salad or Cooking," Self Nutrition Data. https://nutritiondata.self.com/facts/fats-and-oils/507/2
443. "Carbohydrate, Proteins, and Fats," Merck Manual. https://www.merckmanuals.com/home/disorders-of-nutrition/overview-of-nutrition/carbohydrates,-proteins,-and-fats
444. "Water in Meat and Poultry," United States Department of Agriculture. https://www.fsis.usda.gov/wps/portal/fsis/topics/food-safety-education/get-answers/food-safety-fact-sheets/meat-preparation/water-in-meat-and-poultry/ct_index
445. Marciani et al., "Additive Effects of Gastric Volumes and Macronutrient Composition on the Sensation of Postprandial Fullness in Humans," *European Journal of Clinical Nutrition*. doi: 10.1038/ejcn.2014.194
446. Ibid.
447. Hellmig et al, "Gastric Emptying Time of Fluids and Solids in Healthy Subjects Determined by $^{13}$C Breath Tests: Influence of Age, Sex and Body Mass Index," *Journal of Gastroenterology and Hepatology* 21, no. 12 (2006): 1832-1838.
448. Holt et al., "A Satiety Index of Common Foods," *European Journal of Clinical Nutrition* 49, no. 9 (1996): 675-690.
449. Mendoza et al., "Dietary Energy Density is Associated with Obesity and the Metabolic Syndrome in U.S. Adults," *Diabetes Care* 30, no. 4 (2007): 974-979.
450. "Strawberries, Raw," Self Nutrition Data. https://nutritiondata.self.com/facts/fruits-and-fruit-juices/2064/2
451. "Kale, Raw," Self Nutrition Data. https://nutritiondata.self.com/facts/vegetables-and-vegetable-products/2461/2
452. "Potato, Flesh and Skin, Raw," Self Nutrition Data. https://nutritiondata.self.com/facts/vegetables-and-vegetable-products/2546/2
453. "Bananas, Raw," Self Nutrition Data. https://nutritiondata.self.com/facts/fruits-and-fruit-juices/1846/2
454. "Beef, Ground, 95% Lean Meat/ 5% Fat, Raw [Hamburger]," Self Nutrition Data. https://nutritiondata.self.com/facts/beef-products/6188/2
455. "Fish, Salmon, Atlantic, Wild, Raw," Self Nutrition Data. https://nutritiondata.self.com/facts/finfish-and-shellfish- products/4102/2
456. "Egg, Whole, Raw, Fresh," Self Nutrition Data. https://nutritiondata.self.com/facts/dairy-and-egg-products/111/2
457. "Beef, Ground, 70% Lean Meat / 30% Fat, Raw," Self Nutrition Data. https://nutritiondata.self.com/facts/beef-products/8004/2
458. "Cheese, Parmesan, Hard," Self Nutrition Data. https://nutritiondata.self.com/facts/dairy-and-egg-products/32/2
459. "Candies, Kit Kat Wafer Bar," Self Nutrition Data. https://nutritiondata.self.com/facts/sweets/5418/2
460. "Snacks, Potato Chips, Plain, Salted," Self Nutrition Data. https://nutritiondata.self.com/facts/snacks/5627/2
461. "Butter, Without Salt," Self Nutrition Data. https://nutritiondata.self.com/facts/dairy-and-egg-products/133/2
462. "Oil, Industrial, Canola with AntiFoaming Agent, Principal Uses Salads, Woks and Light Frying," Self Nutrition Data. https://nutritiondata.self.com/facts/fats-and-oils/7946/2
463. "Nuts, Almonds, [Includes USDA Commodity Food A256, A264]," Self Nutrition Data. https://nutritiondata.self.com/facts/nut-and-seed-products/3085/2
464. "Nuts, Cashew Nuts, Raw," Self Nutrition Data. https://nutritiondata.self.com/facts/nut-and-seed-products/3095/2
465. "Nuts, Walnuts, English [Includes USDA Commodity Food A259, A257], Self Nutrition Data. https://nutritiondata.self.com/facts/nut-and-seed- products/3138/2
466. "Oil, Soybean, Salad or Cooking," Self Nutrition Data. https://nutritiondata.self.com/facts/fats-and-oils/507/2
467. "Oil, Vegetable Safflower, Salad or Cooking, Linoleic, (Over 70%)," Self Nutrition Data. https://nutritiondata.self.com/facts/fats-and-oils/573/2
468. "Oil, Vegetable, Sunflower, High Oleic (70% and Over)," Self Nutrition Data. https://nutritiondata.self.com/facts/fats- and-oils/623/2
469. "Oil, Vegetable, Corn, Industrial and Retail, All Purpose Salad or Cooking," Self Nutrition Data. https://nutritiondata.self.com/facts/fats-and-oils/580/2
470. "Oil, Vegetable, Palm," Self Nutrition Data. https://nutritiondata.self.com/facts/fats-and-oils/510/2
471. "Oil, Peanut, Salad or Cooking," Self Nutrition Data. https://nutritiondata.self.com/facts/fats-and-oils/506/2
472. "Oil, Vegetable, Cottonseed, Salad or Cooking," Self Nutrition Data. https://nutritiondata.self.com/facts/

fats-and-oils/571/2

473. "Oil, Olive, Salad or Cooking," Self Nutrition Data. https://nutritiondata.self.com/facts/fats-and-oils/509/2

474. "Vegetable Oil, Coconut," Self Nutrition Data. https://nutritiondata.self.com/facts/fats-and-oils/508/2

475. Moss, Michael. *Salt Sugar Fat: How the Food Giants Hooked Us.* New York Random House, 2014. Kindle File, Location 2809 of 7325.

476. "The Original," Flavor Finder. *Pringles.* https://www.pringles.com/en_US/products/favorites/the-original. html#nutrition-modal

477. "Lay's Classic Potato Chips," *Frito-Lay.* https://www.fritolay.com/snacks/product-page/lays/lays-classic-potato-chips

478. "DORITOS Nacho Cheese Flavored Tortilla Chips," *Frito-Lay.* https://www.fritolay.com/snacks/product-page/doritos

479. "CHEETOS Crunchy Cheese Flavored Snacks," *Frito-Lay.* https://www.fritolay.com/snacks/product-page/cheetos

480. "FRITOS Original Corn Chips," *Frito-Lay.* https://www.fritolay.com/snacks/product-page/fritos

481. "KIT KAT Milk Chocolate," *The Hershey Company.* https://www.thehersheycompany.com/brands/kit-kat-wafer-bars/milk-chocolate.aspx?cat=cat

482. "Nestle Butterfinger Pieces 6 x 1.36 kg," *Nestle Professional.* https://www.nestleprofessional.com/united-states/en/BrandsAndProducts/Brands/NESTLE/Pages/11000354.aspx

483. "Nabisco Oreo Double Stuf Chocolate," *Snackworks.* https://www.snackworks.com/products/product-detail. aspx?product=4400003325

484. "RUFFLES Original Potato Chips," *Frito-Lay.* https://www.fritolay.com/snacks/product-page/ruffles/ruffles-original-potato-chips

485. "TOSTITOS Original Restaurant Style Tortilla Chips," *Frito-Lay.* https://www.fritolay.com/snacks/product-page/tostitos

486. "MUNCHOS Original Potato Crisps," *Frito-Lay.* https://www.fritolay.com/snacks/product-page/munchos

487. "Cheez-It Original Crackers," *Kellogg's.* https://smartlabel.kelloggs.com/Product/Index/00024100122615

488. "SMARTFOOD White Cheddar Cheese Flavored Popcorn," *Frito-Lay.* https://www.fritolay.com/snacks/product-page/smartfood

489. "Goldfish Crackers," Self Nutrition Data. https://nutritiondata.self.com/facts/custom/2307870/2

490. "FUNYUNS Onion Flavored Rings," *Frito-Lay.* https://www.fritolay.com/snacks/product-page/funyuns

491. "BABY RUTH King," Ingredients. *Nestle.* https://products.nestle.ca/en/brands/chocolates/baby-ruth/baby-ruth-king.aspx

492. "SUNCHIPS Original Multigrain Snacks," *Frito-Lay.* https://www.fritolay.com/snacks/product-page/sunchips

493. "Ingredients," Twix Caramel Cookie Bars Single Pack," *Twix.* http://www.twix.com/product/nutrition

494. Strazzullo et al., "Salt Intake, Stroke, and Cardiovascular Disease: Meta- Analysis of Prospective Studies," *British Medical Journal* 339, b4567 (2009). doi: https://dx.doi.org/10.1136/bmj.b4567

495. Stolarz-Skrzypek et al., "Fatal and Nonfatal Outcomes, Incidence of Hypertension, and Blood Pressure Changes in Relation to Urinary Sodium Excretion," *Journal of the American Medical Association* 305, no. 17 (2011): 1777-1785.

496. Bolhuis et al., "Salt Promotes Passive Overconsumption of Dietary Fat in Humans," *Journal of Nutrition* 146, no. 4 (2016): 838-845.

497. "Sodium and Food Sources," Centers for Disease Control and Prevention. https://www.cdc.gov/salt/food. htm

498. "Do You Use Peanut Oil or Soybean Oil in Your Cooking Oil?" FAQs. *McDonald's.* https://www.mcdonalds. com/us/en/your_questions/our_food/do-you-use-peanut-oil-or-soybean-in-your-cooking-oil.html

499. "Ingredient Guide," *Kentucky Fried Chicken.* https://www.kfc.com/nutrition/pdf/kfc_ingredients.pdf

500. "Ingredients Statement," Menu. *Chipotle.* https://www.chipotle.com/en-US/menu/ingredients_statement/ingredients_statement.aspx

501. "Allergen Menu," *Olive Garden.* https://media.olivegarden.com/en_us/pdf/allergen_guide.pdf

502. "Original Popped Corn," *SkinnyPop Popcorn.* https://www.skinnypop.com/our-popcorn/popped-popcorn/original/

503. "Granola Bars, Crunchy Oats n' Dark Chocolate," *Nutritionix.* https://www.nutritionix.com/i/nature-valley/granola-bars-crunchy-oats-n-dark- chocolate/57d8a834964e6128595ca25a

504. "Mixed Berry Nutrition Facts," *Belvita Breakfast.* https://www.belvitabreakfast.com/bites#mixed-berry

505. "Peanut Butter," *KIND Snacks.* https://www.kindsnacks.com/products/breakfast/peanut-butter-breakfast-bar

506. "Nabisco Newtons 100% Whole Grain Fig Cookies, 14 oz," *Walmart.* https://www.walmart.com/ip/Nabisco-Newtons-100-Whole-Grain-Fig-Cookies- 14-oz/13281446

507. "Nabisco Wheat Thins Multi-Grain Baked Snack Crackers, 15 oz," *Walmart.* https://www.walmart.com/ip/Nabisco-Wheat-Thins-Multi-Grain-Baked-Snack-Crackers-15-oz/10292786

508. "Classic Hummus," *Sabra.* https://sabra.com/dips/hummus/classic-hummus.html

509. "LAY'S Over Baked Original Potato Crisps," *Frito-Lay.* https://www.fritolay.com/snacks/product-page/oven-baked

510. "Oats 'n Honey Protein Granola," *Nature Valley.* https://www.naturevalley.com/product/oats-n-honey-protein-granola/

511. "Nutri-Grain Cereal Bars Apple Cinnamon," *Kellogg's.* https://smartlabel.kelloggs.com/Product/Index/00038000356216#ingredients

512. "Whole Grain 100% Whole Wheat," *Pepperidge Farms.* https://www.pepperidgefarm.com/product/whole-grain-100-whole-wheat-bread/

513. "Cashews, Whole, Salted Roasted, Family Pack," *Wegmans.* https://www.wegmans.com/products/grocery-food/chips-and-snacks/cashews/whole-unsalted-roasted-cashews-family-pack.html#

514. Cordain, Loren. "Implications of Plio-Pleistocene Hominin Diets for Modern Humans." In *Evolution of the Human Diet. The Known, the Unknown, and the Unknowable,* edited by P.S. Ungar, 363-83. Oxford, UK: Oxford University Press. 2007.

515. Grosso et al., "Omega-3 Fatty Acids and Depression: Scientific Evidence and Biological Mechanisms," *Oxidative Medicine and Cellular Longevity* (2014): doi: 10.1155/2014/313570

516. Simopoulos, A., "The Importance of the Ratio of Omega-6/Omega-3 Essential Fatty Acids," *Biomedicine & Pharmacotherapy* 56, no. 8 (2002): 365-79.

517. Patterson et al., "Health Implications of High Dietary Omega-6 Polyunsaturated Fatty Acids," *Journal of*

*Nutrition and Metabolism* (2012): doi: 10.1155/2012/539426
518. Ibid.
519. Caterina, R., "N-3 Fatty Acids in Cardiovascular Disease," *New England Journal of Medicine* (2011): 364: 2439-2450 DOI: 10.1056/NEJMra1008153
520. Blasbalg et al., "Changes in Consumption of Omega-3 and Omega-6 Fatty Acids in the United States during the 20th Century," *American Journal of Clinical Nutrition* 93, no. 5 (2011): 950-962.
521. Guyenet, S., and Carlsen, S., "Increase in Adipose Tissue Linoleic Acid of US Adults in the Last Half Century," *Advances in Nutrition* 6, no. 6 (2015): 660-664.
522. Ramsden et al., "N-6 Fatty Acid-Specific and Mixed Polyunsaturate Dietary Interventions Have Different Effects on CHD Risk: A Meta-Analysis of Randomised Controlled Trials," *British Journal of Nutrition* 104, no. 11 (2010): 1586-1600.
523. Mozaffarian et al., "Effects on Coronary Heart Disease of Increasing Polyunsaturated Fat in Place of Saturated Fat: A Systematic Review and Meta-Analysis of Randomized Controlled Trials," *PLOS Medicine* 2010: DOI: 10.1371/journal.pmed.1000252
524. Ramsden et al., "N-6 Fatty Acid-Specific and Mixed Polyunsaturate Dietary Interventions Have Different Effects on CHD Risk: A Meta-Analysis of Randomised Controlled Trials," *British Journal of Nutrition* 104, no. 11 (2010): 1586-1600.
525. Yam et al., "Diet and Disease—The Israeli Paradox: Possible Dangers of a High Omega-6 Polyunsaturated Fatty Acid Diet," *Israel Journal of Medical Science* 32, no. 11 (1996): 1134-1143.
526. "Oil, Vegetable Safflower, Salad or Cooking, Linoleic, (Over 70%)," Self Nutrition Data. https://nutrition-data.self.com/facts/fats-and-oils/573/2
527. "Oil, Vegetable, Corn, Industrial and Retail, All Purpose Salad or Cooking," Self Nutrition Data https://nutritiondata.self.com/facts/fats-and-oils/580/2
528. "Oil, Vegetable, Sunflower, Linoleic, (approx. 65%)," Self Nutrition Data. https://nutritiondata.self.com/facts/fats-and-oils/572/2
529. "Oil, Vegetable, Cottonseed, Salad or Cooking," Self Nutrition Data. https://nutritiondata.self.com/facts/fats-and-oils/571/2
530. "Oil, Soybean, Salad or Cooking," Self Nutrition Data. https://nutritiondata.self.com/facts/fats-and-oils/507/2
531. "Oil, Sesame, Salad or Cooking," Self Nutrition Data. https://nutritiondata.self.com/facts/fats-and-oils/511/2
532. "Oil, Peanut, Salad or Cooking," Self Nutrition Data. https://nutritiondata.self.com/facts/fats-and-oils/506/2
533. "Oil, Vegetable, Canola [Low Erucic Acid Rapeseed Oil]," Self Nutrition Data. https://nutritiondata.self.com/facts/fats-and-oils/621/2
534. "Oil, Olive, Salad or Cooking," Self Nutrition Data. https://nutritiondata.self.com/facts/fats-and-oils/509/2
535. "Oil, Vegetable, Palm," Self Nutrition Data. https://nutritiondata.self.com/facts/fats-and-oils/510/2
536. "Vegetable Oil, Coconut," Self Nutrition Data. https://nutritiondata.self.com/facts/fats-and-oils/508/2
537. "Butter, Without Salt," Self Nutrition Data. https://nutritiondata.self.com/factsdairy-and-egg-products/133/2
538. "Foods Highest in Total Omega-6 Fatty Acids," Self Nutrition Data . https://nutritiondata.self.com/foods-000141000000000000000-w.html
539. Ibid.
540. Ibid.
541. "Glossary of Cooking Oils," *Food Processing: The Information Source for Food and Beverage Manufacturers.* https://www.foodprocessing.com/articles/2009/081/
542. Logan, A., "Omega-3 Fatty Acids and Major Depression: A Primer for the Mental Health Professional," *Lipids in Health and Disease* 3, no. 25 (2004): doi: 10.1186/1476-511X-3-25
543. Haag, A., "Essential Fatty Acids and the Brain," *Canadian Journal of Psychiatry* 48, no. 3 (2008): 195-203.
544. Hubert, A., and Else, P., "Basal Metabolic Rate: History, Composition, Regulation, and Usefulness," *Physiological and Biochemical Zoology: Ecological and Evolutionary Approaches* 77, no. 6 (2004): 869-76.
545. Logan, A., "Omega-3 Fatty Acids and Major Depression: A Primer for the Mental Health Professional," *Lipids in Health and Disease* 3, no. 25 (2004): doi: 10.1186/1476-511X-3-25
546. Su et al., "Omega-3 Fatty Acids in Major Depressive Disorder: A Preliminary Double-Blind, Placebo-Controlled Trial," *European Neuropsychopharmacology* 13, no. 4 (2003): 267-271.
547. Hibbeln et al., "Increasing Homicide Rates and Linoleic Acid Consumption among Five Western Countries, 1961-2000," *Lipids* 39, no. 12 (2004): 1207-13.
548. Stoll et al., "Omega 3 Fatty Acids in Bipolar Disorder: A Preliminary Double-Blind, Placebo-Controlled Trial," *Archives of General Psychiatry* 56, no. 5 (1999): 407-12.
549. Huan et al., "Suicide Attempt and N-3 Fatty Acid Levels in Red Blood Cells: A Case Control Study in China," *Biological Psychiatry* 56, no. 7 (2004): 490-6.
550. St-Onge, M., and Jones, P., "Physiological Effects of Medium-Chain Triglycerides: Potential Agents in the Prevention of Obesity," *The Journal of Nutrition* 132, no. 3 (2002): 329-332.
551. Assunção et al., "Effects of Dietary Coconut Oil on the Biochemical and Anthropometric Profiles of Women Presenting Abdominal Obesity," *Lipids* 44, no. 7 (2009): 593-601.
552. "Bugles Product List," *General Mills.* https://www.generalmills.com/en/Brands/Snacks/bugles/brand-product-list
553. Guyenet, Stephan, "Fat, Added Fat, and Obesity in America," *WholeHealthSource.* https://wholehealthsource.blogspot.com/2015/11/fat-added-fat-and-obesity-in-america.html
554. Ibid.
555. Neuman, William, "Nutrition Plate Unveiled, Replacing Food Pyramid," *The New York Times.* 06-02-2011. https://www.nytimes.com/2011/06/03/business/03plate.html?_r=0
556. "Interview with Walter Willlett, M.D.," Diet Wars. PBS *Frontline*. https://www.pbs.org/wgbh/pages/frontline/shows/diet/interviews/willett.html
557. "Flour," *New World Encyclopedia.* https://www.newworldencyclopedia.org/entry/Flour#Wheat_flour
558. Haard et al., "Major Chemical Components of Cereal Grains," *Fermented Cereals. A Global Perspective,* FAO Agricultural Services Bulletin 138. http://www.fao.org/docrep/x2184e/x2184e00.htm#con
559. "Nutrients in Wheat Flour: Whole, Refined and Enriched," *Whole Grains Council.* https://wholegrainscouncil.org/whole-grains-101/what-is-a-whole-grain
560. "Benzoyl Peroxide," Chemical and Technical Assessment, 61st JECFA. Food and Agriculture Organization.

https://www.fao.org/fileadmin/templates/agns/pdf/jecfa/cta/63/Benzoylperoxide.pdf
561. Wilder, R., "A Brief History of the Enrichment of Flour and Bread," *JAMA* 162, no. 17 (1956): 1539-1541.
562. "Is Food Fortification Necessary? A Historical Perspective," International Food Information Council Foundation. https://www.foodinsight.org/Newsletter/Detail.aspx%3Ftopic%3DIs_Food_Fo
563. Backstrand. J., "The History of Food Fortification in the United States: A Public Health Perspective," *Nutrition Reviews* 60, no. 1 (2002): 15-26.
564. Bishai, D., and Nalubola, R., "The History of Food Fortification in the United States: Its Relevance for Current Fortification Efforts in Developing Countries," *Economic Development and Cultural Change* 51, no. 1 (2002): 37-53.
565. "Wheat Flour, Whole Grain," Self Nutrition Data. https://nutritiondata.self.com/facts/cereal-grains-and-pasta/5744/2
566. "Wheat Flour, White (Industrial), 11.5% Protein, Unbleached, Enriched," Self Nutrition Data. https://nutritiondata.self.com/facts/cereal-grains-and-pasta/9261/2
567. Guallar et al., "Enough Is Enough: Stop Wasting Money on Vitamin and Mineral Supplements," *Annals of Internal Medicine* 159, no. 12 (2013).
568. Ibid.
569. Ibid.
570. Ibid.
571. Hu, F., and Willett, W., "Optimal Diets for Prevention of Coronary Heart Disease," *Journal of the American Medical Association* 288, no. 20 (2002): 2569-2578.
572. Schwingshackl et al., "Food Groups and Risk of All-Cause Mortality: A Systematic Review and Meta-Analysis of Prospective Studies," *The American Journal of Clinical Nutrition* (2017): ajcn153148.
573. Jannasch et al., "Dietary Patterns and Type 2 Diabetes: A Systematic Literature Review and Meta-Analysis of Prospective Studies," *The Journal of Nutrition* (2017): jn242552.
574. "Wheat Flour, White, All-Purpose, Enriched, Bleached," Self Nutrition Data. https://nutritiondata.self.com/facts/cereal- grains-and-pasta/5745/2
575. "Wheat Flour, Whole-Grain," Self Nutrition Data. https://nutritiondata.self.com/facts/cereal-grains-and-pasta/5744/2
576. Holt et al., "A Satiety Index of Common Foods," *European Journal of Clinical Nutrition* 49 (1995): 675-690.
577. Mozaffarian et al., "Changes in Diet and Lifestyle and Long-Term Weight Gain in Women and Men," *New England Journal of Medicine* 364 (2011): 2392-2404.
578. Liu et al., "Relation between Changes in Intakes of Dietary Fiber and Grain Products and Changes in Weight and Development of Obesity Among Middle-Aged Women," *American Journal of Clinical Nutrition* 78, no. 5 (2003): 920-927.
579. Karl et al., "Substituting Whole Grains for Refined Grains in a 6-Wk Randomized Trial Favorably Affects Energy-Balance Metrics in Healthy Men and Postmenopausal Women," *The American Journal of Clinical Nutrition* 105, no. 3 (2017): 589-599.
580. "Grains," United States Department of Agriculture. https://www.choosemyplate.gov/food-groups/grains.html
581. "The State of Food Insecurity in the World 2014," Food and Agriculture Organization of the United Nations. https://www.fao.org/publications/sofi/2014/en/
582. "Hunger and Poverty Fact Sheet," *Feeding America*. https://www.feedingamerica.org/hunger-in-america/impact-of-hunger/hunger-and-poverty/hunger-and-poverty-fact-sheet.html
583. "U.S. and World Population Clock," United States Census Bureau. https://www.census.gov/popclock/
584. Ibid.
585. "Shelf Life of Flour," *EatByDate*. https://www.eatbydate.com/other/baking/how-long-does-flour-last-shelf-life- expiration-date/
586. "What the World Eats," *National Geographic*. https://www.nationalgeographic.com/what-the-world-eats/
587. "Preparation and Use of Food-Based Dietary Guidelines," World Health Organization (1998): Geneva. https://whqlibdoc.who.int/trs/WHO_TRS_880.pdf https://digitalcommons.wayne.edu/cgi/viewcontent.cgi? article=1048&context=humbiol_preprints
588. "Dietary Guidelines for the Brazilian Population," 2nd Edition. Ministry of Health of Brazil. Brazilia—DF 2014. https://www.foodpolitics.com/wp-content/uploads/Brazilian-Dietary-Guidelines-2014.pdf
589. Rohrmann et al., "Meat Consumption and Mortality—Results from the European Prospective Investigation into Cancer and Nutrition," *BMC Medicine* 11, no. 63 (2013): doi: 10.1186/1741-7015-11-63.
590. Schwingshackl et al., "Food Groups and Risk of All-Cause Mortality: A Systematic Review and Meta-Analysis of Prospective Studies," *The American Journal of Clinical Nutrition* (2017): ajcn153148.
591. Larsson, S., and Orsini, N., "Red Meat and Processed Meat Consumption and All-Cause Mortality: A Meta-Analysis," *American Journal of Epidemiology* 179, no. 3 (2014): 282-89.
592. Micha et al., "Red and Processed Meat Consumption and Risk of Incident Coronary Heart Disease, Stroke, and Diabetes Mellitus: A Systematic Review and Meta-Analysis," *Circulation* 121, no. 21 (2010): 2271-2283.
593. Chan et al., "Red and Processed Meat and Colorectal Cancer Incidence: Meta-Analysis of Prospective Studies," *PLOS One* 6, no. 6 (2011): e20456.
594. "Salami, Cooked, Beef and Pork," Self Nutrition Data. https://nutritiondata.self.com/facts/sausages-and-luncheon-meats/1380/2
595. "Bologna, Beef," Self Nutrition Data. https://nutritiondata.self.com/facts/sausages-and-luncheon-meats/1325/2
596. "Pork, Cured, Ham, Boneless, Regular (Approximately 11% Fat), Roasted," Self NutritionData. https://nutritiondata.self.com/facts/pork-products/2216/2
597. "Pork, Cured, Bacon, Raw," Self Nutrition Data. https://nutritiondata.self.com/facts/pork-products/2208/2
598. "Frankfurter, Beef [Frank, Hot Dog, Weiner]," Self Nutrition Data. https://nutritiondata.self.com/facts/sausages-and-luncheon-meats/1338/2
599. Strazzullo et al., "Salt Intake, Stroke, and Cardiovascular Disease: Meta-Analysis of Prospective Studies," *British Medical Journal* 339, b4567 (2009): doi: https://dx.doi.org/10.1136/bmj.b4567.
600. Bolhuis et al., "Salt Promotes Passive Overconsumption of Dietary Fat in Humans," *Journal of Nutrition* 146, no. 4 (2016): 838-845.
601. Paddon-Jones et al., "Protein, Weight Management, and Satiety," *American Journal of Clinical Nutrition* 87, no.5 (2008): 1158S-1561S.
602. "Pork, Cured, Bacon, Raw," Self Nutrition Data. https://nutritiondata.self.com/facts/pork-products/2208/2

603. "Frankfurter, Beef [Frank, Hot Dog, Weiner]," Self Nutrition Data. https://nutritiondata.self.com/facts/sausages-and- luncheon-meats/1338/2
604. "Bologna, Beef," Self Nutrition Data. https://nutritiondata.self.com/facts/sausages-and-luncheon-meats/1325/2
605. "Chicken, Broilers or Fryers, Breast, Meat and Skin, Raw," Self Nutrition Data. https://nutritiondata.self.com/facts/poultry-products/696/2
606. "Sodium Nitrite: The Facts," *American Meat Institute.* https://www.meatinstitute.org/index.php?ht=a/GetDocumentAction/i/44170
607. Hecht, S., and Hoffmann, D., "Tobacco-Specific Nitrosamines, an Important Group of Carcinogens in Tobacco and Tobacco Smoke," *Carcinogenesis* 9, no. 6 (1988): 875-84.
608. Oostindjer et al., "The Role of Red and Processed Meat in Colorectal Cancer Development: A Perspective," *Meat Science* 97, no. 4 (2014): 583-96.
609. Santarelli et al., "Processed Meat and Colorectal Cancer: A Review of Epidemiologic and Experimental Evidence," *Nutrition and Cancer* 60, no. 2 (2008): 131-44.
610. Larsson et al., "Processed Meat Consumption, Dietary Nitrosamines and Stomach Cancer Risk in a Cohort of Swedish Women," *International Journal of Cancer* 119, no. 4 (2006): 915-919.
611. Kessler, David. *The End of Overeating: Taking Control of the Insatiable American Appetite.* New York: Rodale Books, 2010. Pages 112-113.
612. Ibid., 19.
613. Ibid., 70-71.
614. Ibid., 71.
615. "Frank's Red Hot Pepper Sauce, Original," *Wegmans.* https://www.wegmans.com/webapp/wcs/stores/servlet/ProductDisplay?langId=-1&storeId=10052&catalogId=10002&productId=376124
616. "Heinz Tomato Ketchup," *CalorieKing.* https://www.calorieking.com/foods/calories-in-sauces-toma-to-ketchup_f-ZmlkPTU4OTY2.html
617. "A1 Sauce, Original," *Wegmans.* https://www.wegmans.com/webapp/wcs/stores/servlet/ProductDisplay?productId=379241&storeId=10052&langId=-1
618. "Sweet Baby Ray's Barbecue Sauce," *CalorieLab.* https://calorielab.com/brands/sweet-baby-rays-barbecue-sauce/136/2005455
619. "McDonald's USA Ingredients Listing for Popular Menu Items," *McDonald's.* https://nutrition.mcdonalds.com/getnutrition/ingredientslist.pdf
620. "Wegmans Sliced Hot Dog Rolls, FAMILY PACK," *Wegmans.* https://www.wegmans.com/webapp/wcs/stores/servlet/ProductDisplay? productId=720391&storeId=10052&langId=-1
621. "Calories in General Tso's Chicken," *Calorie Count.* https://www.caloriecount.com/calories-general-tsos-chicken- i111989
622. "McDonald's, Chicken McNuggets," Self Nutrition Data. https://nutritiondata.self.com/facts/fast-foods-generic/9336/2
623. "Arby's Specialty: Chicken Fingers 4 Pack," Self Nutrition Data. https://nutritiondata.self.com/facts/foods-from-arbys/7855/2
624. Lindeberg et al., "Age Relations of Cardiovascular Risk Factors in a Traditional Melanesian Society: The Kitava Study," *American Journal of Clinical Nutrition* 66, no. 4 (1997): 845-852.
625. Lindeberg, Staffan. *Food and Western Disease: Health and Nutrition from an Evolutionary Perspective.* Hoboken: Wiley-Blackwell, 2010. Kindle File, Chapter 4.5, Location 3081 of 11554.
626. Ibid., Chapter 4.1, Location 2319 of 11554.
627. Benyshek D., and Watson, J., "Exploring the Thrifty Genotype's Food-Shortage Assumptions: A Cross-Cultural Comparison of Ethnographic Accounts of Food Security Among Foraging and Agricultural Societies," *American Journal of Physical Anthropology* 131, no. 1 (2006): 120-6.
628. Lindeberg, Staffan. *Food and Western Disease: Health and Nutrition from an Evolutionary Perspective.* Hoboken: Wiley-Blackwell, 2010. Kindle File, Chapter 4.6, Location 3474.
629. Pontzer et al., "Hunter-Gatherer Energetics and Human Obesity," *PLOS One* 7 (2012): e40503. doi:10.1371/journal.pone.0040503
630. Ogden et al., "NCHS Health E-Stat: Prevalence of Overweight, Obesity, and Extreme Obesity Among Adults: United States, Trends 1960-1962 through 2007-2008," Centers for Disease Control and Prevention, Publications and Information Products. https://www.cdc.gov/nchs/data/hestat/obesity_adult_07_08/obesity_adult_07_0
631. Frayn, Keith. *Metabolic Regulation: A Human Perspective.* Oxford: Wiley Blackwell, 2010 Kindle File, 7.3, Location 4399 of 9142.
632. Johnston et al., "Comparison of Weight Loss Among Named Diet Programs in Overweight and Obese Adults: A Meta-Analysis," *JAMA* 312, no. 9 (2014): 923-933.
633. Sackner-Bernstein et al., "Dietary Intervention for Overweight and Obese Adults: Comparison of Low-Carbohydrate and Low-Fat Diets. A Meta-Analysis," *PLOS One* 10, no. 10 (2015): e0139817.
634. Mansoor et al., "Effects of Low-Carbohydrate v. Low-Fat Diets on Body Weight and Cardiovascular Risk Factors: A Meta-Analysis of Randomised Controlled Trials," *British Journal of Nutrition* 115, no. 3 (2016): 466-479.
635. Leibel et al., "Energy Intake Required to Maintain Body Weight is Not Affected by Wide Variation in Diet Composition," *American Journal of Clinical Nutrition* 55, no. 2 (1992): 350-5.
636. Biss et al., "Some Unique Biologic Characteristics of the Masai of East Africa," *New England Journal of Medicine* 284, no. 13 (1971): 694-9.
637. "Diet/Nutrition," *National Center for Health Statistics.* CDC. https://www.cdc.gov/nchs/fastats/diet.htm
638. Ngoye et al., "Differences in Hypertension Risk Factors between Rural Maasai in Ngorongoro and Urban Maasai in Arusha Municipal: A Descriptive Study," *Journal of Applied Life Sciences International* 1, no. 1 (2014): 17-31.
639. Mouratoff G.J., and Scott E.M., "Diabetes Mellitus in Eskimos After a Decade," *JAMA* 226, no. 11 (1973): 1345-6.
640. Cordain et al., "Plant-Animal Subsistence Ratios and Macronutrient Energy Estimations in Worldwide Hunter-Gatherer Diets," *American Journal of Clinical Nutrition* 71, no. 3 (2000): 682-692.
641. Willet, Walter, "Is Dietary Fat a Major Determinant of Body Fat?" *American Journal of Clinical Nutrition* 67, no. 3 (1998): 556S-562S.
642. "Ask the Expert: Healthy Fats," *The Nutrition Source,* Harvard T. H. Chan School of Public Health. https://

www.hsph.harvard.edu/nutritionsource/2012/06/21/ask-the-expert-healthy-fats/
643. Stubbs et al., "Covert Manipulation of Dietary Fat and Energy Density: Effect on Substrate Flux and Food Intake in Men Eating Ad Libitum," *The American Journal of Clinical Nutrition* 62, no. 2 (1995): 316-329.
644. Tremblay et al., "Impact of Dietary Fat Content and Fat Oxidation on Energy Intake in Humans," *American Journal of Clinical Nutrition* 49, no. 5 (1989): 799-805.
645. Lissner et al., "Dietary Fat and the Regulation of Energy Intake in Human Subjects," *American Journal of Clinical Nutrition* 46, no. 6 (1987): 886-92.
646. Proserpi et al., "Ad Libitum Intake of a High-Carbohydrate or High-Fat Diet in Young Men: Effects on Nutrient Balances," *American Journal of Clinical Nutrition* 66, no. 3 (1997): 539-545.
647. Blundell et al., "Dietary Fat and the Control of Energy Intake: Evaluating the Effects of Fat on Meal Size and Postmeal Satiety," *American Journal of Clinical Nutrition* 57, no. 5 (1993): 772S-777S.
648. Gerhard et al., "Effects of a Low-Fat Diet Compared with Those of a High-Monounsaturated Fat Diet on Body Weight, Plasma Lipids and Lipoproteins, and Glycemic Control in Type 2 Diabetes," *American Journal of Clinical Nutrition* 80, no. 3 (2004): 668-673.
649. Kendall et al., "Weight Loss on a Low-Fat Diet: Consequence of the Imprecision of the Control of Food Intake in Humans," *American Journal of Clinical Nutrition* 53, no. 5 (1991): 1124-1129.
650. Proserpi et al., "Ad Libitum Intake of a High-Carbohydrate or High-Fat Diet in Young Men: Effects on Nutrient Balances," *American Journal of Clinical Nutrition* 66, no. 3 (1997): 539-545.
651. Blundell et al., "Dietary Fat and the Control of Energy Intake: Evaluating the Effects of Fat on Meal Size and Postmeal Satiety," *American Journal of Clinical Nutrition* 57, no. 5 (1993): 772S-777S.
652. Lissner et al., "Dietary Fat and the Regulation of Energy Intake in Human Subjects," *American Journal of Clinical Nutrition* 46, no. 6 (1987): 886-92.
653. Gerhard et al., "Effects of a Low-Fat Diet Compared with Those of a High-Monounsaturated Fat Diet on Body Weight, Plasma Lipids and Lipoproteins, and Glycemic Control in Type 2 Diabetes," *American Journal of Clinical Nutrition* 80, no. 3 (2004): 668-673.
654. Kendall et al., "Weight Loss on a Low-Fat Diet: Consequence of the Imprecision of the Control of Food Intake in Humans," *American Journal of Clinical Nutrition* 53, no. 5 (1991): 1124-1129.
655. Blundell et al., "Dietary Fat and the Control of Energy Intake: Evaluating the Effects of Fat on Meal Size and Postmeal Satiety," *American Journal of Clinical Nutrition* 57, no. 5 (1993): 772S-777S.
656. Lissner et al., "Dietary Fat and the Regulation of Energy Intake in Human Subjects," *American Journal of Clinical Nutrition* 46, no. 6 (1987): 886-92.
657. Gerhard et al., "Effects of a Low-Fat Diet Compared with Those of a High-Monounsaturated Fat Diet on Body Weight, Plasma Lipids and Lipoproteins, and Glycemic Control in Type 2 Diabetes," *American Journal of Clinical Nutrition* 80, no. 3 (2004): 668-673.
658. Wansink, B., "Can 'Low-Fat' Nutrition Labels Lead to Obesity?" *Journal of Marketing Research* 43, no. 4 (2006): 605- 617.
659. Klein, Richard. *The Human Career: Human Biological and Cultural Origins.* Chicago: University of Chicago Press, 1999.
660. He et al., "Changes in Intake of Fruits and Vegetables in Relation to Risk of Obesity and Weight Gain Among Middle-Aged Women," *International Journal of Obesity* 28 (2004): 1569-1574.
661. Bazzano et al., "Intake of Fruit, Vegetables, and Fruit Juices and Risk of Diabetes in Women," *Diabetes Care* 31, no. 7 (2008): 1311-1317.
662. Holt et al., "A Satiety Index of Common Foods," *European Journal of Clinical Nutrition* 49, no. 9 (1996): 675-690.
663. Aune et al., "Fruit and Vegetable Intake and the Risk of Cardiovascular Disease, Total Cancer, and All-Cause Mortality—A Systematic Review and Dose-Response Meta-Analysis of Prospective Studies," *International Journal of Epidemiology* (2016): doi: https://doi.org/10.1093/ije/dyw319
664. Derr, Mark, "Of Tubers, Fire and Human Evolution," *New York Times.* 01-16-2001. https://www.nytimes.com/2001/01/16/science/of-tubers-fire-and-human-evolution.html
665. Lindeberg et al., "Age Relations of Cardiovascular Risk Factors in a Traditional Melanesian Society: The Kitava Study," *American Journal of Clinical Nutrition* 66, no. 4 (1997): 845-852.
666. Ibid.
667. Lindeberg et al., "Cardiovascular Risk Factors in a Melanesian Population Apparently Free from Stroke and Ischaemic Heart Disease: The Kitava Study," *Journal of Internal Medicine* 236, no. 3 (1994): 331-340.
668. Lindeberg, Staffan. *Food and Western Disease: Health and Nutrition from an Evolutionary Perspective.* Hoboken: Wiley-Blackwell, 2010. Kindle File, Chapter 4.5, Location 3103 of 11554.
669. Marlowe et al. "Honey, Hadza, Hunter-Gatherers, and Human Evolution, "*Journal of Human Evolution* 71 (2014): 119- 128.
670. Marlowe, F.W., and Berbesque, J.C., "Tubers as Fallback Foods and their Impact on Hadza Hunter-Gatherers," *American Journal of Physical Anthropology* 4 (2009): 751-8.
671. Trowell, H.C., and Burkitt, D.P. *Western Diseases: Their Emergence and Prevention.* Cambridge: Harvard University Press, 1981. Page 174.
672. Ibid., page 175.
673. Ibid., pages 180-181.
674. Ibid., page 174.
675. "Learn How Many Calories You Burn Every Day," TDEE CALCULATOR. https://tdeecalculator.net/
676. Gaesser, G., "Carbohydrate Quantity and Quality in Relation to Body Mass Index," *Journal of the American Dietetic Association* 107, no. 10 (2007): 1768-80.
677. Merchant et al., "Carbohydrate Intake and Overweight and Obesity Among Healthy Adults," *Journal of the American Dietetic Association* 109, no. 7 (2009): doi: 10.1016/j.jada.2009.04.002.
678. Bueno et al., "Very-Low-Carbohydrate Ketogenic Diet v. Low-Fat Diet for Long-Term Weight Loss: A Meta-Analysis of Randomised Controlled Trials," *British Journal of Nutrition* 110, no. 7 (2013): 1178-1187.
679. Westman et al., "A Review of Low-Carbohydrate Ketogenic Diets," *Current Atherosclerosis Reports* 5, no. 6 (2003): 476-483.
680. Johnston et al., "Ketogenic Low-Carbohydrate Diets Have No Metabolic Advantage over Non-Ketogenic Low-Carbohydrate Diets," *American Journal of Clinical Nutrition* 83, no. 5 (2006): 1055-1061.
681. Hall et al., "Energy Expenditure and Body Composition Changes after an Isocaloric Ketogenic Diet in Overweight and Obese Men," *American Journal of Clinical Nutrition* 104, no. 2 (2016): 324-333.
682. Sumithran et al., "Ketosis and Appetite-Mediating Nutrients and Hormones After Weight Loss," *European*

*Journal of Clinical Nutrition* 67 (2013): 759-764.
683. Mercader, J., "Mozambican Grass Seed Consumption During the Middle Stone Age," *Science* 326 no. 5960 (2009): 1680-1683.
684. "Separating the Wheat from the Chaff," *Whole Grains Council.* https://wholegrainscouncil.org/newsroom/blog/2014/09/separating-the-wheat-from-the-chaff
685. Mummert et al., "Stature and Robusticity during the Agricultural Transition: Evidence from the Bioarchaeological Record," *Economics & Human Biology* 9, no. 3 (2011): 284-301.
686. Ibid.
687. Diamond, Jared, "The Worst Mistake in the History of the Human Race," *Discover.* 05-01-1999. https://discovermagazine.com/1987/may/02-the-worst-mistake-in-the-history-of-the-human-race
688. Laurence, R., "Health and the Life Course at Heculaneum and Pompeii," *Health in Antiquity.* Routledge, 2004. 105-118.
689. Sams, A., and Hawks, J., "Celiac Disease as a Model for the Evolution of Multifactorial Disease in Humans," *Human Biology* 86, no. 1 (2014): 19-36.
690. Cochran, Gregory and Harpending, Henry, *The 10,000 Year Explosion: How Civilization Accelerated Human Evolution.* New York: Basic Books, 2009. Kindle File, Location 79-80.
691. Thavarajah, P., and Thavarajah, D., "Inaccuracies in Phytic Acid Measurement: Implications for Mineral Biofortification and Bioavailability," *American Journal of Plant Sciences* 5, no. 1 (2014).
692. Lopez et al., "Minerals and Phytic Acid Interactions: Is It a Real Problem for Human Nutrition?" *International Journal of Food Science & Technology* 37 (2002): 727-739.
693. Tulchinksy, T., "Micronutrient Deficiency Conditions: Global Health Issues," *Public Health Reviews* 32, no. 1 (2010): 243.
694. Foroutan, R., "The History and Health Benefits of Fermented Food," *Food & Nutrition.* 02-20-2012. https://www.foodandnutrition.org/Winter-2012/The-History-and-Health-Benefits-of-Fermented-Food/
695. Anjum et al., "Effect of Bioprocesses on Phenolic Compounds, Phytic Acid and HCL Extractability of Minerals in Wheat Cultivars," *Food Science and Technology Research* 18, no. 4 (2012): 555-562.
696. Fan et al., "Evidence of Decreasing Mineral Density in Wheat Grain over the Last 160 Years," *Journal of Trace Elements in Medicine and Biology* 22, no. 4 (2008): 315-324.
697. "Eat More, Weigh Less?," *Healthy Weight.* Centers for Disease Control and Prevention. https://www.cdc.gov/healthyweight/healthy_eating/energy_density.html
698. "Whole Grains and Fiber," American Heart Association. https://www.heart.org/HEARTORG/Getting-Healthy/NutritionCenter/HealthyD Leats-and-Fiber_UCM_303249_Article.jsp
699. Anderson, Jane, "How Many People Have Gluten Sensitivity?" *AboutHealth.* 09-03-2013. https://www.verywellhealth.com/how-many-people-have-gluten-sensitivity-562965
700. Catassi et al., "Non-Celiac Gluten Sensitivity: The New Frontier of Gluten-Related Disorders," *Nutrients* 5, no. 10 (2013): 3839-3853.
701. Hadjivassiliou et al., "Gluten Sensitivity: From Gut to Brain," *Lancet Neurology* 9, no. 3 (2010): 318-330.
702. Watson, Ross, Preedy, Victor, and Zibadi, Sherma. *Wheat and Rice in Disease Prevention and Health: Benefits, Risks, and Mechanisms of Whole Grains in Health Promotion.* Waltham: Academic Press, 2014. Page 83.
703. Holt, S., and Miller, J., "Particle Size, Satiety, and the Glycaemic Response," *European Journal of Clinical Nutrition* 48, no. 7 (1994): 496-502.
704. Heaton et al., "Particle Size of Wheat, Maize, and Oat Test Meals: Effects on Plasma Glucose and Insulin Responses and on the Rate of Starch Digestion In Vitro," *American Journal of Clinical Nutrition* 47 (1988): 675-82.
705. Jayasinghe et al., "Effect of Different Milling Methods on Glycaemic Response of Foods Made with Finger Millet (*Eucenea coracana*) Flour," *Ceylon Medical Journal* 58, no. 4 ( 2013): 148-152.
706. Watson, Ross, Preedy, Victor, and Zibadi, Sherma. *Wheat and Rice in Disease Prevention and Health: Benefits, Risks, and Mechanisms of Whole Grains in Health Promotion.* Waltham: Academic Press, 2014. Page 84.
707. Korem et al., "Bread Affects Clinical Parameters and Induces Gut Microbiome-Associated Personal Glycemic Responses," *Cell Metabolism* 25, no. 6 (2017): p1243-p1253.
708. "Wheat Thins Original Crackers," *Walmart.* https://www.walmart.com/ip/Nabisco-Wheat-Thins-Original-Crackers-10-oz/10292628
709. Pol et al., "Whole Grain and Body Weight Changes in Apparently Healthy Adults: A Systematic Review and Meta-Analysis of Randomized Controlled Trials," *American Journal of Clinical Nutrition* 98, no. 4 (2013): 872-884.
710. Mummert et al., "Stature and Robusticity during the Agricultural Transition: Evidence from the Bioarchaeological Record," *Economics & Human Biology* 9, no. 3 (2011): 284-301.
711. Hu et al., "White Rice Consumption and Risk of Type 2 Diabetes: Meta-Analysis and Systematic Review," *British Medical Journal* 344 (2012): e1454.
712. Holt et al., "A Satiety Index of Common Foods," *European Journal of Clinical Nutrition* 49 (1995): 675-690.
713. Hu et al., "White Rice Consumption and Risk of Type 2 Diabetes: Meta-Analysis and Systematic Review," *British Medical Journal* 344 (2012): e1454.
714. Ibid.
715. "Rice, White, Long-Grain, Regular, Cooked," Self Nutrition Data. https://nutritiondata.self.com/facts/cereal-grains-and-pasta/5712/2
716. "Rice, Brown, Long-Grain, Cooked," Self Nutrition Data. https://nutritiondata.self.com/facts/cereal-grains-and-pasta/5707/2
717. Ye et al., "Greater Whole Grain Intake is Associated with Lower Risk of Type 2 Diabetes, Cardiovascular Disease, and Weight Gain," *Journal of Nutrition* 142, no. 7 (2012): 1304-1313.
718. Schwingshackl et al., "Food Groups and Risk of All-Cause Mortality: A Systematic Review and Meta-Analysis of Prospective Studies," *The American Journal of Clinical Nutrition* (2017): ajcn153148.
719. Smith et al., "Behavioural, Attitudinal and Dietary Responses to the Consumption of Wholegrain Foods," *Proceedings of the Nutrition Society* 62 (2003): 455-67.
720. Harland J., and Garton, L., "Whole Grain Intake as a Marker of Healthy Body Weight and Adiposity," *Public Health Nutrition* 11, no. 6 (2008): 554-563.
721. Ye et al., "Greater Whole Grain Intake is Associated with Lower Risk of Type 2 Diabetes, Cardiovascular Disease, and Weight Gain," *Journal of Nutrition* 142, no. 7 (2012): 1304-1313.
722. Ibid.
723. Pol et al., "Whole Grain and Body Weight Changes in Apparently Healthy Adults: A Systematic Review

and Meta-Analysis of Randomized Controlled Trials," *American Journal of Clinical Nutrition* 98, no. 4 (2013): 872-884.

724. Buettner, Dan. *Blue Zones: 9 Lessons for Living Longer from the People Who've Lived the Longest.* Second Edition Washington: National Geographic, 2012. Kindle File.

725. Lindeberg et al., "Cardiovascular Risk Factors in a Melanesian Population Apparently Free from Stroke and Ischaemic Heart Disease: The Kitava Study," *Journal of Internal Medicine* 236, no. 3 (1994): 331-340.

726. Price, Weston. *Nutrition and Physical Degeneration.* Lemon Grove: Price Pottenger Nutrition, 2012. Print.

727. Self Nutrition Data. https://nutritiondata.self.com

728. Tan et al., "A Review of the Effect of Nuts on Appetite, Food Intake, Metabolism, and Body Weight," *American Journal of Clinical Nutrition* 100 Supplement 1 (2014): 412S-422S.

729. "Nuts, Cashew Nuts, Raw," Self Nutrition Data. https://nutritiondata.self.com/facts/nut-and-seed-products/3095/2

730. "Nuts, Almonds, Dry Roasted, Without Salt Added [Includes USDA Commodity Food A255, A263]," Self Nutrition Data. https://nutritiondata.self.com/facts/nut-and-seed-products/3087/2

731. Jackson, C., and Hu, F., "Long-Term Association of Nut Consumption with Body Weight and Obesity," *American Journal of Clinical Nutrition* 100, Supplement 1 (2014): 408S-411S.

732. Grosso et al., "Nut Consumption on All-Cause, Cardiovascular, and Cancer Mortality Risk: A Systematic Review and Meta-Analysis of Epidemiologic Studies," *American Journal of Clinical Nutrition* 101, no. 4 (2015): 783-793.

733. Flores-Mateo et al., "Nut Intake and Adiposity: Meta-Analysis of Clinical Trials," *American Journal of Clinical Nutrition* 97, no. 6 (2013): 1346-1355.

734. Mozaffarian et al., "Changes in Diet and Lifestyle and Long-Term Weight Gain in Men and Women," *New England Journal of Medicine* 364, no. 25 (2011): 2392-2404.

735. Meyer et al., "Some Physiological Effects of a Mainly Fruit Diet in Man," *South African Medical Journal* 45, no. 8 (1971): 191-195.

736. Pear, Robert, "Senate Saves the Potato on School Lunch Menus," *New York Times.* 10-18-2011. https://www.nytimes.com/2011/10/19/us/politics/potatoes-get-senate-protection-on-school-lunch-menus.html

737. Weaver, C., and Marr, E., "White Vegetables: A Forgotten Source of Nutrients: Purdue Roundtable Summary," *Advances in Nutrition* 4 (2013): 318S-326S.

738. Velioglu et al., "Antioxidant Activity and Total Phenolics in Selected Fruits, Vegetables, and Grain Products," *Journal of Agricultural and Food Chemistry* 46, no. 10 (1998): 4113-4117.

739. "Potato, Russet, Flesh and Skin, Baked," Self Nutrition Data. https://nutritiondata.self.com/facts/vegetables-and-vegetable-products/2550/2

740. Ibid.

741. "Bananas, Raw," Self Nutrition Data. https://nutritiondata.self.com/facts/fruits-and-fruit-juices/1846/2

742. Foster-Powell et al., "International Table of Glycemic Index and Glycemic Load Values: 2002," *American Journal of Clinical Nutrition* 76 (2002): 5-56.

743. Zeevi et al., "Personalized Nutrition by Prediction of Glycemic Responses," *Cell* 163, no. 5 (2015): 1079-1094.

744. Moghaddam et al., "The Effect of Fat and Protein on Glycemic Responses in Nondiabetic Humans Vary with Waist Circumference, Fasting Plasma Insulin, and Dietary Fiber Intake," *The Journal of Nutrition* 136, no. 10 (2006): 2506-2511.

745. "Glycemic Index and Glycemic Load for 100+ Foods," *Harvard Health Publications.* Harvard Medical School. https://www.health.harvard.edu/healthy-eating/glycemic_index_and_glycemic_load_for_100_foods

746. Lindeberg, Staffan. *Food and Western Disease: Health and Nutrition from an Evolutionary Perspective.* Hoboken: Wiley-Blackwell, 2010. Kindle File, Chapter 4.1, Location 1695 of 11554.

747. Foster-Powell et al., "International Table of Glycemic Index and Glycemic Load Values: 2002," *American Journal of Clinical Nutrition* 76 (2002): 5-56.

748. Bhupathiraju et al., "Glycemic Index, Glycemic Load, and Risk of Type 2 Diabetes: Results from 3 Large US Cohorts and an Updated Meta-Analysis," *American Journal of Clinical Nutrition* 100, no. 1 (2014): 218-232.

749. Schwingshackl, L., and Hoffmann, G., "Long-Term Effects of Low Glycemic Index/Load vs. High Glycemic Index/Load Diets on Parameters of Obesity and Obesity-Associated Risks: A Systematic Review and Meta-Analysis," *Nutrition, Metabolism, & Cardiovascular Diseases* 23 (2013): 699-706.

750. "Glycemic Index and Glycemic Load for 100+ Foods," *Harvard Health Publications.* Harvard Medical School. https://www.health.harvard.edu/healthy-eating/glycemic_index_and_glycemic_load_for_100_foods

751. Braunstein et al., "Effect of Low-Glycemic Index/Load Diets on Body Weight: A Systematic Review and Meta-Analysis," *The FASEB Journal* 30, no. 1 (2016): Supplement 906.9.

752. Wolever, T., and Mehling, C., "Long-Term Effect of Varying the Source or Amount of Dietary Carbohydrate on Postprandial Plasma Glucose, Insulin, Triacylglycerol, and Free Fatty Acid Concentrations in Subjects with Impaired Glucose Tolerance," *American Journal of Clinical Nutrition* 77, no. 3 (2003): 612-21.

753. Kristo et al., "Effects of Diets Differing in Glycemic Index and Glycemic Load on Cardiovascular Risk Factors: Review of Randomized Controlled-Feeding Trials," *Nutrients* 5, no. 4 (2013): 1071-1080.

754. Borch et al., "Potatoes and Risk of Obesity, Type 2 Diabetes, and Cardiovascular Disease in Apparently Healthy Adults: A Systematic Review of Clinical Intervention and Observational Studies," *American Journal of Clinical Nutrition* (2016): doi: 10.3945/ajcn.116.132332

755. Holt et al., "A Satiety Index of Common Foods," *European Journal of Clinical Nutrition* 49, no. 9 (1996): 675-690.

756. Bao et al., "Pre-Pregnancy Potato Consumption and Risk of Gestational Diabetes Mellitus: Prospective Cohort Study," *BMJ* 352 (2016): doi: https://doi.org/10.1136/bmj.h6898

757. Borgi et al., "Potato Intake and Incidence of Hypertension from Three Prospective US Cohort Studies," *BMJ* 353 (2016): doi:https://doi.org/10.1136/bmj.i2351

758. Kon, S., and Klein, A., "The Value of Whole Potato in Human Nutrition," *Biochemistry Journal* 22, no. 1 (1928): 258-60.

759. Toselli et al., "Body Size, Composition, and Blood Pressure of High-Altitude Quechua from the Peruvian Central Andes (Huancavelica, 3,680 m)," *American Journal of Human Biology* 13, no. 4 (2001): 539-547.

760. Mazess R., and Baker, P., "Diet of Quechua Indians Living at High Altitude: Nunoa, Peru," *American Journal of Clinical Nutrition* 15, no. 6 (1964): 341-351.

761. "Percent Body Fat Calculator: Skinfold Method," Tools and Calculators, *ACE.* https://www.acefitness.org/acefit/healthy_living_tools_content.aspx?id=2

762. Collier, R., "This Spud's for You: A Two-Month, Tuber-Only Diet," *CMAJ* 182, no. 17 (2010): E781-782.
763. Novick, Jeff, "Getting Well on Twenty Potatoes a Day," *Forks Over Knives*. 01-07-2013. https://www.forksoverknives.com/getting-well-on-twenty-potatoes-a-day/#gs.Dlp7HNs
764. "My Story," *Spud Fit*. https://www.spudfit.com/about-spud-fit
765. De Jong, H., "Impact of the Potato on Society," *American Journal of Potato Research* 93, no. 5 (2016): 415-429.
766. Kelleher et al., "Effect of Social Variation on the Irish Diet," *Proceedings of the Nutritional Society* 61 (2002): 527-536.
767. Kon, S., and Klein, A., "The Value of Whole Potato in Human Nutrition," *Biochemistry Journal* 22, no. 1 (1928): 258-60.
768. "Spud We Like: In Praise of the Humble But World-Changing Tuber," *The Economist*. 02-08-2008. https://www.economist.com/node/10766030
769. Engels, Frederick, "Barbarism and Civilization," In *Origins of the Family, Private Property, and the State*. 1884. https://www.marxists.org/archive/marx/works/1884/origin-family/ch09.htm
770. Smith, Adam. *An Inquiry into the Nature and Causes of the Wealth of Nations*. 1776. https://geolib.com/smith.adam/won1-11.html
771. Tivy, Joy, "Roots and Tubers," *Agricultural Ecology*. London: Routledge, 2014.
772. "Nutritive Value," FAO. http://www.fao.org/docrep/t0207e/T0207E04.htm
773. "Spud We Like: In Praise of the Humble But World-Changing Tuber," *The Economist*. 02-08-2008. https://www.economist.com/node/10766030
774. *Scientific Report of the 2015 Dietary Guidelines Advisory Committee: Advisory Report to the Secretary of Health and Human Services and the Secretary of Agriculture*. Part D: Chapter 1: Food and Nutrient Intakes, and Health: Current Status and Trends, Page 17, Line 646. USDA. https://www.health.gov/dietaryguidelines/2015-scientific-report/PDFs/Scientific-Report-of-the-2015-Dietary-Guidelines-Advisory-Committee.pdf
775. Fernandez, M., "Rethinking Dietary Cholesterol," *Current Opinion in Clinical Nutrition & Metabolic Care* 15, no. 2 (2012): 1117-1121.
776. "Egg, Whole, Raw, Fresh," Self Nutrition Data. https://nutritiondata.self.com/facts/dairy-and-egg-products/111/2
777. Griffin, J., and Lichtenstein, A., "Dietary Cholesterol and Plasma Lipoprotein Profiles: Randomized Controlled Trials," *Current Nutrition Reports* 2, no. 4 (2013): 274-282.
778. Alexander et al., "Meta-Analysis of Egg Consumption and Risk of Coronary Heart Disease and Stroke," *Journal of the American College of Nutrition* 35, no. 8 (2016): 704-716.
779. Rong et al., "Egg Consumption and Risk of Coronary Heart Disease and Stroke: Dose-Dependent Meta-Analysis of Prospective Cohort Studies," *British Medical Journal* 346 (2013): e8539. doi: https://dx.doi.org/10.1136/bmj.e8539
780. Shin et al., "Egg Consumption in Relation to Risk of Cardiovascular Disease and Diabetes: A Systematic Review and Meta-Analysis," *American Journal of Clinical Nutrition* 98 (2013): 146-159.
781. *Dietary Guidelines for Americans: 2015-2020*. Page 32. USDA. https://health.gov/dietaryguidelines/2015/guidelines/
782. Trumbo et al., "Dietary Reference Intakes for Energy, Carbohydrate, Fiber, Fat, Fatty Acids, Cholesterol, Protein, and Amino Acids," *Journal of the Academy of Nutrition and Dietetics* 102, no. 11 (2002): 1621-1630.
783. "Egg, White, Raw, Fresh," Self Nutrition Data. https://nutritiondata.self.com/facts/dairy-and-egg-products/112/2
784. "Egg, Yolk, Raw, Fresh," Self Nutrition Data. https://nutritiondata.self.com/facts/dairy-and-egg-products/113/2
785. *Scientific Report of the 2015 Dietary Guidelines Advisory Committee: Advisory Report to the Secretary of Health and Human Services and the Secretary of Agriculture*. Part D: Chapter 1: Line 2784. USDA. https://www.health.gov/dietaryguidelines/2015-scientific-report/PDFs/Scientific-Report-of-the-2015-Dietary-Guidelines-Advisory-Committee.pdf
786. Ibid., Line 828.
787. Zeisel, S., and da Costo, K., "Choline: An Essential Nutrient for Public Health," *Nutrition Reviews* 67, no. 11 (2009): 615-623.
788. "Foods Highest in Choline," Self Nutrition Data. https://nutritiondata.self.com/foods-000144000000000000000-1w.html
789. "Egg, White, Raw, Fresh," Self Nutrition Data. https://nutritiondata.self.com/facts/dairy-and-egg-products/112/2
790. "Egg, Yolk, Raw, Fresh," Self Nutrition Data. https://nutritiondata.self.com/facts/dairy-and-egg-products/113/2
791. "Egg, Whole, Raw, Fresh," Self Nutrition Data. https://nutritiondata.self.com/facts/dairy-and-egg-products/111/2
792. Vander Wal et al., "Egg Breakfast Enhances Weight Loss," *International Journal of Obesity* 32, no. 10 (2008): 1545-51.
793. "The Lipid Bilayer," In *Molecular Biology of the Cell*. 4th Edition. NCBI. https://www.ncbi.nlm.nih.gov/books/NBK26871/
794. Griffin, J., and Lichtenstein, A., "Dietary Cholesterol and Plasma Lipoprotein Profiles: Randomized Controlled Trials," *Current Nutrition Reports* 2, no. 4 (2013): 274-282.
795. Scirica, B., and Cannon, C., "Cardiology Patient Page: Treatment of Elevated Cholesterol," *Circulation* 111 (2005): e360-e363.
796. "The Complex Regulation of Cholesterol Biosynthesis Takes Place at Several Levels," *Biochemistry*. 5th Edition. Section 26.3. https://www.ncbi.nlm.nih.gov/books/NBK22336/
797. "The Lipid Bilayer," In *Molecular Biology of the Cell*. 4th Edition. NCBI. https://www.ncbi.nlm.nih.gov/books/NBK26871/
798. German, B., and Dillard, C., "Saturated Fats: A Perspective from Lactation and Milk Composition," *Lipids* 45, no. 10 (2010): 915-923.
799. Keys. A., "Coronary Heart Disease in Seven Countries," *Circulation* 41, no. 1 (1970): 186-195.
800. Yang et al., "Added Sugar Intake and Cardiovascular Diseases Mortality Among US Adults," *JAMA Internal Medicine* 174, no. 4 (2014): 516-524.
801. Harcombe et al., "Food for Thought: Have We Been Giving the Wrong Dietary Advice?" *Food and Nutrition Sciences* 4 (2013): 240-44.

802. Ravnskov et al., "The Questionable Benefits of Exchanging Saturated Fat with Polyunsaturated Fat," *Mayo Clinic Proceedings* 89, no. 4 (2014): 451-3.
803. Taubes, Gary. *Good Calories, Bad Calories*. New York: Anchor, 2008. Kindle File, Chapter 1. Location 425 of 13,579.
804. Ibid., Location 756 of 13,579.
805. Muller et al., "The Serum LDL/HDL Cholesterol Ratio is Influenced More Favorably by Exchanging Saturated with Unsaturated Fat Than by Reducing Saturated Fat in the Diet of Women," *The Journal of Nutrition* 133, no. 1 (2003): 78-83.
806. "Saturated Fats," American Heart Association. https://www.heart.org/HEARTORG/GettingHealthy/NutritionCenter/HealthyE Fats_UCM_301110_Article.jsp
807. Packard et al., "The Role of Small, Dense Low Density Lipoprotein (LDL): A New Look," *International Journal of Cardiology* 74, Supplement 1 (2000): S17-S22.
808. Gardner et al., "Association of Small Low-Density Lipoprotein Particles with the Incidence of Coronary Artery Disease in Men and Women," *JAMA* 276, no. 11 (1996): 875-881.
809. Siri-Tarino et al., "Saturated Fat, Carbohydrate, and Cardiovascular Disease," *American Journal of Clinical Nutrition* 91, no. 3 (2010): 502-9.
810. Krauss et al., "Separate Effects of Reduced Carbohydrate Intake and Weight Loss on Atherogenic Dyslipidemia," *American Journal of Clinical Nutrition* 83, no. 5 (2006): 1025-1031.
811. Dreon et al., "Change in Dietary Saturated Fat Intake Is Correlated with Change in Mass of Large Low-Density-Lipoprotein Particles in Men," *American Journal of Clinical Nutrition* 67, no. 5 (1998): 828-36.
812. St-Pierre et al., "Low-Density Lipoprotein Subfractions and the Long-Term Risk of Ischemic Heart Disease in Men: 13-Year Follow-Up Data from the Quebec Cardiovascular Study," *Arteriosclerosis, Thrombosis, and Vascular Biology* 25 (2005): 553-9.
813. Mensink R., and Katan, M., "Effect of Dietary Fatty Acids on Serum Lipids and Lipoproteins: A Meta-Analysis of 27 Trials," *Arteriosclerosis, Thrombosis, and Vascular Biology* 12 (1992): 911-19.
814. Mensink et al., "Effects of Dietary Fatty Acids and Carbohydrates on the Ratio of Serum Total to HDL Cholesterol and on Serum Lipids and Apolipoproteins: A Meta-Analysis of 60 Controlled Trials," *American Journal of Clinical Nutrition* 77, no. 5 (2003): 1146-1155.
815. Hoenselaar et al., "Saturated Fat and Cardiovascular Disease: The Discrepancy Between the Scientific Literature and Dietary Advice," *Nutrition* 28, no. 2 (2012): 118-23.
816. Mensink et al., "Effects of Dietary Fatty Acids and Carbohydrates on the Ratio of Serum Total to HDL Cholesterol and on Serum Lipids and Apolipoproteins: A Meta-Analysis of 60 Controlled Trials," *American Journal of Clinical Nutrition* 77, no. 5 (2003): 1146-1155.
817. Morris et al., "Diet and Plasma Cholesterol in 99 Bank Men," *British Medical Journal* 2, no. 1 (1963): 571-76.
818. Ibid.
819. Nichols et al., "Daily Nutritional Intake and Serum Lipid Levels. The Tecumseh Study." *American Journal of Clinical Nutrition* 29, no. 12 (1976): 1384-1392.
820. Mente et al., "A Systematic Review of the Evidence Supporting a Causative Link Between Dietary Factors and Coronary Artery Disease," *JAMA Internal Medicine* 169, no. 7 (2009): 659-669.
821. Siri-Tarino et al., "Meta-Analysis of Prospective Cohort Studies Evaluating the Association of Saturated Fat with Cardiovascular Disease," *American Journal of Clinical Nutrition* 91, no. 3 (2010): 535-546.
822. Hooper et al., "Reduced or Modified Dietary Fat for Preventing Cardiovascular Disease," *Cochrane Database Systematic Reviews* 7 (2011): CD002137. doi: 10.1002/14651858.CD002137.pub2
823. Hamley, S., "The Effect of Replacing Saturated Fat with Mostly n-6 Polyunsaturated Fat on Coronary Heart Disease: A Meta-Analysis of Randomised Controlled Trials," *Nutrition Journal* 16, no. 1 (2017): 30. https://doi.org/10.1186/s12937-017-0254-5
824. Hoenselaar et al., "Saturated Fat and Cardiovascular Disease: The Discrepancy Betweenthe Scientific Literature and Dietary Advice," *Nutrition* 28, no. 2 (2012): 118-123.
825. Malhorta, A., "Saturated Fat Is Not the Major Issue: Let's Bust the Myth of Its Role in Heart Disease," *British Medical Journal* 347 (2013): f6340. doi: https://dx.doi.org/10.1136/bmj.f6340
826. Chowdhury et al., "Association of Dietary, Circulating, and Supplement Fatty Acids with Coronary Risk: A Systematic Review and Meta-Analysis," *Annals of Internal Medicine* 160 (2014): 398-406.
827. Ferrieres, J., "The French Paradox: Lessons for Other Countries," *Heart* 90 no. 1 (2004): 107-111.
828. Palaniappan et al., "Fruit and Vegetable Consumption is Lower and Saturated Fat Intake is Higher Among Canadians Reporting Smoking," *The Journal of Nutrition* 131, no. 7 (2001): 1952-1958.
829. Ibid.
830. Salmeron et al., "Dietary Fat Intake and Risk of Type 2 Diabetes in Women," *American Journal of Clinical Nutrition* 73, no. 6 (2001): 1019-1026.
831. Hu et al., "Dietary Fat Intake and the Risk of Coronary Heart Disease in Women," *The New England Journal of Medicine* 337 (1997): 1491-1499.
832. Yamagishi et al., "Dietary Intake of Saturated Fatty Acids and Mortality from Cardiovascular Disease in Japan: The Japan Collaborative Cohort Study for Evaluation of Cancer Risk (JACC) Study," *American Journal of Clinical Nutrition* (2010): ajcn.2009.29146v1.
833. "USA vs Japan: Top 10 Causes of Death," *World Life Expectancy*. https://www.worldlifeexpectancy.com/usa-vs-japan-top-10-causes-of-death
834. "Trends in Intake of Energy and Macronutrients—United States, 1971- 2000," Centers for Disease Control and Prevention. *Morbidity and Mortality Weekly Report* 53, no. 4 (2004): 80-82.
835. Ibid.
836. Klein, Richard. *The Human Career: Human Biological and Cultural Origins*. Third Edition. Chicago: University of Chicago Press, 2009. Digital Editions. Page 97.
837. Ibid, 82.
838. Milton, K., "A Hypothesis to Explain the Role of Meat-Eating in Human Evolution," *Evolutionary Anthropology* 8, no. 1 (1999): 11-21.
839. Stanford, C., "The Predatory Behavior and Ecology of Wild Chimpanzees," University of Southern California. https://www-bcf.usc.edu/~stanford/chimphunt.html
840. Milton, K., "A Hypothesis to Explain the Role of Meat-Eating in Human Evolution," *Evolutionary Anthropology* 8, no. 1 (1999): 11-21.
841. "Comparison of Digestive Systems," *Saylor Academy*. https://www.saylor.org/site/wp-content/uploads/2012/07/BIO309-OC-3.8.1-Comparison-of-Digestive-Systems-FINAL.pdf

842. Milton, K., "A Hypothesis to Explain the Role of Meat-Eating in Human Evolution," *Evolutionary Anthropology* 8, no. 1 (1999): 11-21.
843. "Homo neanderthalensis," *What Does It Mean to Be Human?* Smithsonian Institution. https://humanorigins. si.edu/evidence/human-fossils/species/homo-neanderthalensis
844. Klein, Richard. *The Human Career: Human Biological and Cultural Origins.* Third Edition. Chicago: University of Chicago Press, 2009. Digital Editions. Page 433.
845. Than, K., "Neanderthals, Humans Interbred—First Solid DNA Evdence," *National Geographic.* https://news. nationalgeographic.com/news/2010/05/100506-science-neanderthals-humans-mated-interbred-dna-gene/
846. Green et al., "Draft Sequence of the Neandertal Genome," *Science* 328, no. 5979 (2010): 710-22.
847. Klein, Richard. *The Human Career: Human Biological and Cultural Origins.* Third Edition. Chicago: University of Chicago Press, 2009. Digital Editions. Page 551.
848. Ibid, 422.
849. Pobiner, B., "Evidence for Meat-Eating by Early Humans," *Nature Education* 2013. Knowledge Project. https://www.nature.com/scitable/knowledge/library/evidence-for-meat-eating-by-early-humans-103874273
850. Klein, Richard. *The Human Career: Human Biological and Cultural Origins.* Third Edition. Chicago: University of Chicago Press, 2009. Digital Editions. Page 269.
851. Ibid., 725.
852. Ibid.
853. Carmody, R., and Wrangham, R., "The Energetic Significance of Cooking," *Journal of Human Evolution* 57, no. 4 (2009): 379-91.
854. Klein, Richard. *The Human Career: Human Biological and Cultural Origins.* Third Edition. Chicago: University of Chicago Press, 2009. Digital Editions. Pages 261-262.
855. Ibid., 713.
856. Ibid., 711-713.
857. Cordain et al., "Plant-Animal Subsistence Ratios and Macronutrient Energy Estimations in Worldwide Hunter-Gatherer Diets," *American Journal of Clinical Nutrition* 71, no. 3 (2000): 682-692.
858. Kaplan et al., "A Theory of Human Life History Evolution: Diet, Intelligence, and Longevity," *Evolutionary Anthropology* 9 (2000): 156-85.
859. Charles, D., "The Making of Meat-Eating America," National Public Radio. *The Salt.* 06-26-2012. https:// www.npr.org/sections/thesalt/2012/06/26/155720538/the-making-of-meat-eating-america
860. Eaton et al., "Stone-Agers in the Fast Lane: Chronic Degenerative Diseases in Evolutionary Perspective," *American Journal of Medicine* 84, no. 4 (1988): 739-49.
861. Lindeberg, Staffan. *Food and Western Disease: Health and Nutrition from an Evolutionary Perspective.* Hoboken: Wiley-Blackwell, 2010. Kindle File, Chapter 4.5, Location 3062.
862. Ibid, Chapter 4.11, Location 4583.
863. Gurven, M., and Kaplan, H., "Longevity among Hunter-Gatherers: A Cross-Cultural Examination," *Population and Development Review* 33, no. 2 (2007): 321-65.
864. Ibid.
865. Lindeberg, Staffan. *Food and Western Disease: Health and Nutrition from an Evolutionary Perspective.* Hoboken: Wiley-Blackwell, 2010. Kindle File, Chapter 4.1, Location 1717.
866. Huang et al., "Cardiovascular Disease Mortality and Cancer Incidence in Vegetarians: A Meta-Analysis and Systematic Review," *Annals of Nutrition and Metabolism* 60, no. 4 (2012): 233-40.
867. Ibid.
868. Key et al., "Mortality in Vegetarians and Nonvegetarians: Detailed Findings from a Collaborative Analysis of 5 Prospective Cohort Studies," *American Journal of Clinical Nutrition* 70, no. 3 (1999): 516s-524s.
869. Orlich et al., "Patterns of Food Consumption Among Vegetarians and Non-Vegetarians," *British Journal of Nutrition* 112, no. 10 (2014): 1644-53.
870. Key et al., "Dietary Habits and Mortality in 11,000 Vegetarians and Health Conscious People: Results of a 17 Year Follow Up," *British Medical Journal* 313 (1996): 775-779.
871. Buettner, Dan. *Blue Zones: 9 Lessons for Living Longer from the People Who've Lived the Longest.* Second Edition. Washington: National Geographic, 2012. Kindle File.
872. Key et al., "Mortality in Vegetarians and Nonvegetarians: Detailed Findings from a Collaborative Analysis of 5 Prospective Cohort Studies," *American Journal of Clinical Nutrition* 70, no. 3 (1999): 516s-524s.
873. Burkert et al., "Nutrition and Health—The Association Between Eating Behavior and Various Health Parameters: A Matched Sample Study," *PLOS One* 9, no. 2 (2014): DOI:10.1371/journal.pone.0088278.
874. Watanabe et al., "Biologically Active B12 Compounds in Foods for Preventing Deficiency among Vegetarians and Elderly Subjects," *Journal of Agricultural and Food Chemistry* 61, no. 28 (2013): 6769-75.
875. "Vitamin B12," *Micronutrient Information Center.* Linus Pauling Institute. https://lpi.oregonstate.edu/mic/vitamins/vitamin-B12
876. "Vitamin B12: Fact Sheet for Consumers," *Office of Dietary Supplements.* National Institutes of Health. https://ods.od.nih.gov/factsheets/VitaminB12-Consumer/#h2
877. Louwman et al., "Signs of Impaired Cognitive Function in Adolescents with Marginal Cobalamin Status," *American Journal of Clinical Nutrition* 72, no. 3 (2000): 762-769.
878. Pawlak et al., "How Prevalent is Vitamin B12 Deficiency Among Vegetarians?" *Nutrition Reviews* 71, no. 2 (2013): 110-117.
879. Herrmann et al., "Vitamin B-12 Status, Particularly Holotranscobalamin II and Methylmalonic Acid Concentrations, and Hyperhomocysteinemia in Vegetarians," *American Journal of Clinical Nutrition* 78, no. 1 (2003): 131-6.
880. Foster et al., "Effect of Vegetarian Diets on Zinc Status: A Systematic Review and Meta-Analysis of Studies in Humans," *Journal of the Science of Food and Agriculture* 93, no. 10 (2013): 2362-2371.
881. Davey et al., "EPIC-Oxford: Lifestyle Characteristics and Nutrient Intakes in a Cohort of 33,383 Meat-Eaters and 31,546 Non Meat-Eaters in the UK," *Public Health Nutrition* 6, no. 3 (2003): 259-268.
882. Ibid.
883. Rosell et al., "Long-Chain n-3 Polyunsaturated Fatty Acids in Plasma in British Meat-Eating, Vegetarian, and Vegan Men," *American Journal of Clinical Nutrition* 82, no. 2 (2005): 327-334.
884. "U.S. Could Feed 800 Million People with Grain that Livestock Eat, Cornell Ecologist Advises Animal Scientists," *Cornell Chronicle.* 08-07-97. https://www.news.cornell.edu/stories/1997/08/us-could-feed-800-million-people-grain-livestock-eat
885. Sugimura et al., "Heterocyclic Amines: Mutagens/Carcinogens Produced During Cooking of Meat and

Fish," *Cancer Science* 95, no. 4 (2004): 290-99.
886. Li et al., "Dietary Mutagen Exposure and Risk of Pancreatic Cancer," *Cancer Epidemiology, Biomarkers & Prevention* 16, no. 4 (2007): 655-61.
887. Puangsombat et al., "Occurrence of Heterocyclic Amines in Cooked Meat Products," *Meat Science* 90, no. 3 (2012): 739-46.
888. "Polycyclic Aromatic Hydrocarbons in Food: Scientific Opinion of the Panel of Contaminants in the Food Chain," *The EFSA Journal* 724 (2008): 1-114. 5.1.2.
889. "ToxFAQs for Polycyclic Aromatic Hydrocarbons (PAHs)," Agency for Toxic Substances and Disease Registry. https://www.atsdr.cdc.gov/toxfaqs/tf.asp?id=121&tid=25
890. "Polycyclic Aromatic Hydrocarbons," *Tox Town*. U.S. National Library of Medicine. https://www.toxtown.nlm.nih.gov/text_version/chemicals.php?id=80
891. Knize, M., and Felton, J., "Formation and Human Risk of Carcinogenic Heterocyclic Amines Formed from Natural Precursors in Meat," *Nutrition Reviews* 63, no. 5 (2005): 158-165.
892. Smith et al., "Effect of Marinades on the Formation of Heterocyclic Amines in Grilled Beef Steaks," *Journal of Food Science* 73, no. 6 (2008): T100-T105.
893. Salmon et al., "Effects of Marinating on Heterocyclic Amine Carcinogen Formation in Grilled Chicken," *Food and Chemical Toxicology* 35, no. 5 (1997): 433-41.
894. Sinha et al., "Meat Intake and Mortality: A Prospective Study of over Half a Million People," *Archives of Internal Medicine* 169, no. 6 (2009): 562-71.
895. Ibid.
896. Cross et al., "A Prospective Study of Red and Processed Meat Intake in Relation to Cancer Risk," *PLOS One* (2007): doi: 10.1371/journal.pmed.0040325
897. Flood et al., "Meat, Fat, and Their Subtypes as Risk Factors for Colorectal Cancer in a Prospective Cohort of Women," *American Journal of Epidemiology* 158, no.1 (2003): 59-68.
898. "McDonald's USA Ingredients Listing for Popular Menu Items," *McDonald's*. https://nutrition.mcdonalds.com/getnutrition/ingredientslist.pdf
899. "Classic Hot Dog Buns," *Franz Buns*. https://franzbakery.com/product/franz-classic-hot-dog-buns/
900. "Simply Heinz Ketchup (34 OZ)," *Heinz*. https://www.heinzketchup.com/Products/Simply%20Heinz%20Ketchup%2034
901. Sinha et al., "Meat Intake and Mortality: A Prospective Study of over Half a Million People," *Archives of Internal Medicine* 169, no. 6 (2009): 562-71.
902. Cross et al., "A Prospective Study of Red and Processed Meat Intake in Relation to Cancer Risk," *PLOS One* (2007): doi: 10.1371/journal.pmed.0040325
903. Flood et al., "Meat, Fat, and Their Subtypes as Risk Factors for Colorectal Cancer in a Prospective Cohort of Women," *American Journal of Epidemiology* 158, no.1 (2003): 59-68.
904. Giovannucci et al., "Intake of Fat, Meat, and Fiber in Relation to Risk of Colon Cancer in Men," *Cancer Research* 54 (1994): 2390-7.
905. Schwingshackl et al., "Food Groups and Risk of All-Cause Mortality: A Systematic Review and Meta-Analysis of Prospective Studies," *The American Journal of Clinical Nutrition* (2017): ajcn153148.
906. Larsson, S., and Orsini, N., "Red Meat and Processed Meat Consumption and All-Cause Mortality: A Meta-Analysis," *American Journal of Epidemiology* 179, no. 3 (2014): 282-89.
907. Rohrmann et al., "Meat Consumption and Mortality—Results from the European Prospective Investigation into Cancer and Nutrition," *BMC Medicine* 11, no. 63 (2013): doi:10.1186/1741-7015-11-63.
908. Halton et al., "Potato and French Fry Consumption and Risk of Type 2 Diabetes in Women," *American Journal of Clinical Nutrition* 83, no. 2 (2006): 284-290.
909. Micha et al., "Red and Processed Meat Consumption and Risk of Incident Coronary Heart Disease, Stroke, and Diabetes Mellitus: A Systematic Review and Meta-Analysis," *Circulation* 121, no. 21 (2010): 2271-2283.
910. Rohrmann et al., "Meat Consumption and Mortality—Results from the European Prospective Investigation into Cancer and Nutrition," *BMC Medicine* 11, no. 63 (2013): doi:10.1186/1741-7015-11-63.
911. Ibid.
912. "Red Meat and Colon Cancer," *Family Health Guide*. Harvard Health Publications. https://www.health.harvard.edu/family_health_guide/red-meat-and-colon-cancer
913. Alexander et al., "Meta-Analysis of Prospective Studies of Red Meat Consumption and Colorectal Cancer," *European Journal of Cancer Prevention* 20, no. 4 (2011): 293-307.
914. Norat et al., "Meat, Fish, and Colorectal Cancer Risk: The European Prospective Investigation into Cancer and Nutrition," *Journal of the National Cancer Institute* 97, no. 12 (2005): 906-16.
915. Ibid.
916. Leslie et al., "Weight Management: A Comparison of Existing Dietary Approaches in a Work-Site Setting," *International Journal of Obesity* 26 (2002): 1469-1475.
917. Paddon-Jones et al., "Protein, Weight Management, and Satiety," *American Journal of Clinical Nutrition* 87, no.5 (2008): 1158S-1561S.
918. Westerterp-Plantenga et al., "Dietary Protein-Its Role in Satiety, Energetics, Weight Loss and Health," *British Journal of Nutrition* 108 (2012): S105-S112.
919. Paddon-Jones et al., "Protein, Weight Management, and Satiety," *American Journal of Clinical Nutrition* 87, no.5 (2008): 1158S-1561S.
920. Speth, J., and Spielmann, K., "Energy Source, Protein Metabolism, and Hunter-Gatherer Subsistence Strategies," *Journal of Anthropological Archeology* 2 (1983): 1-31.
921. Noli, D., and Avery, G., "Protein Poisoning and Coastal Subsistence," *Journal of Archaeological Science* 15 (1988): 395-401.
922. Bilsborough S., and Mann, N., "A Review of Issues of Dietary Protein Intake in Humans," *International Journal of Sport Nutrition and Exercise Metabolism* 16, no. 2 (2006): 129-52.
923. "Game Meat, Rabbit, Wild, Raw," Self Nutrition Data. https://nutritiondata.self.com/facts/lamb-veal-and-game-products/4649/2
924. Speth, J., and Spielmann, K., "Energy Source, Protein Metabolism, and Hunter-Gatherer Subsistence Strategies," *Journal of Anthropological Archeology* 2 (1983): 1-31.
925. Ibid.
926. Darwin, Charles. *The Voyage of the Beagle*, Volume 29. New York: P.F. Collier & Son Company, 1909. Page 123.
927. Key et al., "Dietary Habits and Mortality in 11,000 Vegetarians and Health Conscious People: Results of a

17 Year Follow Up," *British Medical Journal* 313 (1996): 775-779.

928. Rohrmann et al., "Meat Consumption and Mortality—Results from the European Prospective Investigation into Cancer and Nutrition," *BMC Medicine* 11, no. 63 (2013): doi:10.1186/1741-7015-11-63.

929. Cordain et al., "Plant-Animal Subsistence Ratios and Macronutrient Energy Estimations in Worldwide Hunter-Gatherer Diets," *American Journal of Clinical Nutrition* 71, no. 3 (2000): 682-692.

930. "Beef, Variety Meats and By-Products, Brain, Raw," Self Nutrition Data. https://nutritiondata.self.com/facts/beef-products/3461/2

931. "Beef, Variety Meats and By-Products, Pancreas, Raw," Self Nutrition Data. https://nutritiondata.self.com/facts/beef- products/3474/2

932. "Pork, Fresh, Variety Meats and By-Products, Stomach, Raw," Self Nutrition Data. https://nutritiondata.self.com/facts/pork-products/2204/2

933. "Beef, Variety Meats and By-Products, Tongue, Raw," Self Nutrition Data. https://nutritiondata.self.com/facts/beef- products/3481/2

934. "Caribou, Bone Marrow, Raw," Self Nutrition Data. https://nutritiondata.self.com/facts/ethnic-foods/8088/2

935. Price, Weston. *Nutrition and Physical Degeneration.* Lemon Grove: Price Pottenger Nutrition, 2012. Chapter 15, page 232.

936. "By-Product Feeds for Alabama Beef Cattle," Alabama A&M and Auburn Universities, Extension. https://store.aces.edu/ItemDetail.aspx?ProductID=13835

937. Duckett et al., "Effects of Winter Stocker Growth Rate and Finishing System on: III. Tissue Proximate, Fatty Acid, Vitamin, and Cholesterol Content," *Journal of Animal Science* 87, no. 9 (2009): 2961-2970.

938. Leheska et al., "Effects of Conventional and Grass-Feeding Systems on the Nutrient Composition of Beef," *Journal of Animal Science* 86, no. 12 (2008): 3575-3585.

939. Valvo et al., "Effect of Ewe Feeding System (Grass v. Concentrate) on Intramuscular Fatty Acids of Lambs Raised Exclusively on Maternal Milk," *Animal Science* 81, no. 3 (2005): 431-36.

940. Karsten et al., "Vitamins A, E and Fatty Acid Composition of the Eggs of Caged Hens and Pastured Hens," *Renewable Agriculture and Food Systems* 25, no. 1 (2010): 45-54.

941. "Beef, Grass-Fed, Ground, Raw," Self Nutrition Data. https://nutritiondata.self.com/facts/beef-products/10526/2

942. "Fish, Salmon, Atlantic, Farmed, Raw," Self Nutrition Data. https://nutritiondata.self.com/facts/finfish-and-shellfish- products/4258/2

943. Hauswirth et al., "High ω-3 Fatty Acid Content in Alpine Cheese," *Circulation* 109 (2004): 103-107.

944. Leheska et al., "Effects of Conventional and Grass-Feeding Systems on the Nutrient Composition of Beef," *Journal of Animal Science* 86, no. 12 (2008): 3575-3585.

945. Kratz et al., "The Relationship Between High-Fat Dairy Consumption and Obesity, Cardiovascular, and Metabolic Disease," *European Journal of Nutrition* 52 (2013): 1-24.

946. Namazi et al., "The Effects of Supplementation with Conjugated Linoleic Acid on Anthropometric Indices in Overweight and Obese Patients: A Systematic Review and Meta-Analysis," *Critical Reviews in Food Science and Nutrition* (2018): 1-39.

947. Kratz et al., "The Relationship Between High-Fat Dairy Consumption and Obesity, Cardiovascular, and Metabolic Disease," *European Journal of Nutrition* 52 (2013): 1-24.

948. Ibid.

949. Ibid.

950. Gillma et al., "Margarine Intake and Subsequent Coronary Heart Disease in Men," *Epidemiology* 8, no. 2 (1997): 144-9.

951. Holt et al., "A Satiety Index of Common Foods," *European Journal of Clinical Nutrition* 49, no. 9 (1996): 675-690.

952. "Black Cherry," *Chobani*. https://www.chobani.com/products/greek/fruit- on-the-bottom/black-cherry/

953. Buettner, Dan. *Blue Zones: 9 Lessons for Living Longer from the People Who've Lived the Longest.* Second Edition Washington: National Geographic, 2012. Kindle File, Chapter 2.

954. Kratz et al., "The Relationship Between High-Fat Dairy Consumption and Obesity, Cardiovascular, and Metabolic Disease," *European Journal of Nutrition* 52 (2013): 1-24.

955. Yang et al., "Added Sugar Intake and Cardiovascular Diseases Mortality Among US Adults," *JAMA Internal Medicine* 174, no. 4 (2014): 516-524.

956. Basu et al., "The Relationship of Sugar to Population-Level Diabetes Prevalence: An Econometric Analysis of Repeated Cross-Sectional Data," *PLOS One* (2013): doi: 10.1371/journal.pone.0057873.

957. "Basic Report: 01211, Milk, Whole, 3.25% Milkfat, Without Added Vitamin A and Vitamin D," *National Nutrient Database for Standard Reference Release 27*, USDA. https://ndb.nal.usda.gov/ndb/foods/show/180?fgcd=Dairy+and+Egg+Products&manu=&facet=&format=&count=&max=3

958. "Basic Report: 01151, Milk, Nonfat, Fluid, Without Added Vitamin A and Vitamin D (Fat Free or Skim)," *National Nutrient Database for Standard Reference Release 27*, USDA. https://ndb.nal.usda.gov/ndb/foods/show/134? fgcd=&manu=&facet=&format=&count=&max=35&offset=&sort=&qlooku

959. Guyton, Arthur and Hall, John. *Textbook of Medical Physiology.* Eleventh Edition. Philadelphia: Elsevier Saunders, 2006. Pages 464, 873, 991.

960. Brown et al., "Carotenoid Bioavailability is Higher from Salads with Full-Fat Than with Fat-Reduced Salad Dressings as Measured with Electrochemical Detection," *American Journal of Clinical Nutrition* 80, no. 2 (2004): 396-403.

961. Melia et al., "The Effect of Orlistat, an Inhibitor of Dietary Fat Absorption, on the Absorption of Vitamins A and E in Healthy Volunteers," *The Journal of Clinical Pharmacology* 36, no. 7 (1996): 647-53.

962. "Foods Highest in Calcium (Based on Levels Per 100-Gram Serving)," Self Nutrition Data. https://nutritiondata.self.com/foods- 000118000000000000000-4w.html?

963. "Yogurt, Plain, Whole Milk, 8 Grams Protein Per 8 Ounce," Self Nutrition Data. https://nutritiondata.self.com/facts/dairy-and-egg-products/104/2

964. "Cheese, Mozzarella, Whole Milk," Self Nutrition Data. https://nutritiondata.self.com/facts/dairy-and-egg-products/25/2

965. "Cheese, Cheddar," Self Nutrition Data. https://nutritiondata.self.com/facts/dairy-and-egg-products/8/2

966. "Cheese, Parmesan, Grated," Self Nutrition Data. https://nutritiondata.self.com/facts/dairy-and-egg-products/31/2

967. "Milk, Whole, 3.25% Milkfat," Self Nutrition Data. https://nutritiondata.self.com/facts/dairy-and-egg-products/69/2

968. "Yogurt, Plain, Whole Milk, 8 Grams Protein Per 8 Ounce," Self Nutrition Data. https://nutritiondata.self.com/facts/dairy-and-egg-products/104/2

969. Paddon-Jones et al., "Protein, Weight Management, and Satiety," *American Journal of Clinical Nutrition* 87, no.5 (2008): 1158S-1561S.

970. Self Nutrition Data. https://nutritiondata.self.com

971. Skov et al., "Randomized Trial on Protein vs Carbohydrate in Ad Libitum Fat Reduced Diet for Treatment of Obesity," *International Journal of Obesity* 23 (1999): 528-36.

972. Wycherley et al., "Effects of Energy-Restricted High-Protein, Low-Fat Compared with Standard-Protein, Low-Fat Diets: A Meta-Analysis of Randomized Controlled Trials," *American Journal of Clinical Nutrition* 96, no. 6 (2012): 1281-98.

973. Leidy et al., "The Role of Protein in Weight Loss and Maintenance," *American Journal of Clinical Nutrition* 101, no. 6 (2015): 1320S-1329S.

974. Ibid.

975. Ibid.

976. Ibid.

977. Bray et al., "Effect of Protein Overfeeding on Energy Expenditure Measured in a Metabolic Chamber," *American Journal of Clinical Nutrition* 101, no. 3 (2015): 496-505.

978. Wycherley et al., "Effects of Energy-Restricted High-Protein, Low-Fat Compared with Standard-Protein, Low-Fat Diets: A Meta-Analysis of Randomized Controlled Trials," *American Journal of Clinical Nutrition* 96, no. 6 (2012): 1281-98.

979. Leidy et al., "The Effects of Consuming Frequent, Higher Protein Meals on Appetite and Satiety During Weight Loss in Overweight/Obese Men," *Obesity* 19, no. 4 (2011): 818-24.

980. Due et al., "Effect of Normal-Fat Diets, Either Medium or High in Protein, on Body Weight in Overweight Subjects: A Randomized 1-Year Trial," *International Journal of Obesity and Related Metabolic Disorders* 28, no. 10 (2004): 1283-90.

981. Westerterp-Plantenga et al., "High Protein Intake Sustains Weight Maintenance after Body Weight Loss in Humans," *International Journal of Obesity and Related Metabolic Disorders* 28, no. 1 (2004): 57-64.

982. Ibid.

983. Soenen et al., "Relative High-Protein or 'Low-Carb' Energy-Restricted Diets for Body Weight Loss and Body Weight Maintenance?" *Physiology & Behavior* 107, no. 3 (2012): 374-80.

984. Holt et al., "A Satiety Index of Common Foods," *European Journal of Clinical Nutrition* 49, no. 9 (1996): 675-690.

985. Martin et al., "Dietary Protein Intake and Renal Function," *Nutrition & Metabolism* 2, no. 2 (2005): doi:10.1186/1743-7075-2-25.

986. Blum et al., "Protein Intake and Kidney Function in Humans: Its Effect on 'Normal Aging'," *Archives of Internal Medicine* 149, no. 1 (1989): 211-212.

987. Poortmans, J., and Dellalieux, O., "Do Regular High Protein Diets Have Potential Health Risks on Kidney Function in Athletes?" *International Journal of Sports Nutrition* 10, no. 1 (2000): 28-38.

988. Ayyad C., and Andersen, T., "Long-Term Efficacy of Dietary Treatment of Obesity: A Systematic Review of Studies Published Between 1931 and 1999," *Obesity Reviews* 1, no. 2 (2000): 113-119.

989. Diaz et al., "Metabolic Response to Experimental Overfeeding in Lean and Overweight Healthy Volunteers," *American Journal of Clinical Nutrition* 56, no. 4 (1992): 641-655.

990. Pasquet, P., and Apfelbaum, M., "Recovery of Initial Body Weight and Composition after Long-Term Massive Overfeeding in Men," *American Journal of Clinical Nutrition* 60, no. 6 (1994): 861-863.

991. Frayn, Keith. *Metabolic Regulation: A Human Perspective.* Oxford: Wiley Blackwell, 2010. Kindle File, 12.4.2, Location 7824-40.

992. Marlowe, F., and Berbesque, J., "Tubers as Fallback Foods and Their Impact on Hadza Hunter-Gatherers," *American Journal of Physical Anthropology* 4 (2009): 751-8.

993. Lindeberg, Staffan. *Food and Western Disease: Health and Nutrition from an Evolutionary Perspective.* Hoboken: Wiley-Blackwell, 2010. Kindle File, Chapter 4.5, Location 3065.

994. Ngoye et al., "Differences in Hypertension Risk Factors between Rural Maasai in Ngorongoro and Urban Maasai in Arusha Municipal: A Descriptive Study," *Journal of Applied Life Sciences International* 1, no. 1 (2014): 17-31.

995. Levin, B., and Dunn-Meynell, A., "Defense of Body Weight Depends on Dietary Composition and Palatability in Rats with Diet-Induced Obesity," *American Journal of Physiology: Regulatory, Integrative and Comparative Physiology* 282, no. 1 (2002): R46-R54.

996. Levin, B., and Keesey, R., "Defense of Differing Body Weight Set Points in Diet-Induced Obese and Resistant Rats," *American Journal of Physiology* 274 (1998): R412-R419.

997. Larson et al., "Spontaneous Overfeeding with a 'Cafeteria Diet' in Men: Effects on 24-Hour Energy Expenditure and Substrate Oxidation," *International Journal of Obesity and Related Metabolic Disorders* 19, no. 5 (1995): 331-7.

998. Larson et al., "Ad Libitum Food Intake on a 'Cafeteria Diet' in Native American Women: Relations with Body Composition and 24-H Energy Expenditure," *American Journal of Clinical Nutrition* 62, no. 5 (1995): 911-917.

999. Risling et al., "Food Intake Measured by an Automated Food-Selection System: Relationship to Energy Expenditure," *American Journal of Clinical Nutrition* 55, no. 2 (1992): 343-9.

1000. Cabanac, M., and Rabe, E., "Influence of a Monotonous Food on Body Weight Regulation in Humans," *Physiology & Behavior* 17, no. 4 (1976): 675-678.

1001. Hashim, S., and Van Itallie, T., "Studies in Normal and Obese Subjects with a Monitored Food Dispensing Device," *Annals of the New York Academy of Sciences* 131, no. 1 (1965): 654-661.

1002. Ibid.

1003. "NWCR Facts," National Weight Control Registry. https://www.nwcr.ws/Research/default.htm

1004. Wing, R., and Phelan, S., "Long-Term Weight Loss Maintenance," *American Journal of Clinical Nutrition* 82, no. 1 (2005): 222S-225S.

1005. Ibid.

1006. Stroebele, N., and De Castro, J., "Effect of Ambience on Food Intake and Choice," *Nutrition* 20, no. 9 (2004): 821-838.

1007. Wansink, B., "Environmental Factors That Increase the Food Intake and Consumption Volume of Unknowing Consumers," *Annual Review of Nutrition* 24 (2004): 455-479.

1008. Painter, J., and Wansink, B., "How Visibility and Convenience Influence Candy Consumption," *Appetite* 38, no. 3 (2002): 237-238.
1009. Westenhoefer et al., "Cognitive and Weight-Related Correlates of Flexible and Rigid Restrained Eating Behavior," *Eating Behaviors* 14, no. 1 (2013): 69-72.
1010. Smith et al., "Flexible vs. Rigid Dieting Strategies: Relationship with Adverse Behavioral Outcomes," *Appetite* 32, no. 3 (1999): 295-305.
1011. Ibid.
1012. Westenhoefer et al., "Validation of the Flexible and Rigid Control Dimensions of Dietary Restraint," *International Journal of Eating Disorders* 26, no. 1 (1999): 53-64.
1013. Rubinstein, Sarah, "The Michael Phelps Diet: Don't Try It at Home," Health Blog, *The Wall Street Journal.* 08-13-2008.
1014. Janssen et al., "Food Intake and Body Composition in Novice Athletes During a Training Period to Run a Marathon," *International Journal of Sports Medicine* 10 (1989): S17-S21.
1015. Ibid.
1016. Dahl, Mellisa, "I Am Training for a Marathon. So Why Am I Getting Fat?" *New York Times Magazine.* 10-12-2015. https://nymag.com/scienceofus/2015/10/on-the-mysteries-of-marathon-weight-gain.html
1017. Swift et al., "The Role of Exercise and Physical Activity in Weight Loss and Maintenance," *Progress in Cardiovascular Diseases* 56, no. 4 (2014): 441-447.
1018. Thorogood et al., "Isolated Aerobic Exercise and Weight Loss: A Systematic Review and Meta-Analysis of Randomized Controlled Trials," *The American Journal of Medicine* 124, no. 8 (2011): 747-755.
1019. Ibid.
1020. Bateman et al., "Comparison of Aerobic versus Resistance Exercise Training Effects on Metabolic Syndrome (from the Studies of a Targeted Risk Reduction Intervention through Defined Exercise – STRRIDE-AT/RT)," *The American Journal of Cardiology* 108, no. 6 (2011): 838-844.
1021. Sigal et al., "Effects of Aerobic Training, Resistance Training, or Both on Glycemic Control in Type 2 Diabetes: A Randomized Trial," *Annals of Internal Medicine* 147, no. 6 (2007): 357-369.
1022. Church et al., "Effects of Aerobic and Resistance Training on Hemoglobin A1c Levels in Patients with Type 2 Diabetes," *JAMA* 304, no. 20 (2010): 2253-2262.
1023. "Eric Ravussin," *Research and Faculty*, Pennington Biomedical Research Center. https://www.pbrc.edu/research-and- faculty/faculty/?faculty=1264
1024. Reynolds, Gretchen, "Weighing the Evidence on Exercise," *New York Times Magazine.* 04-16-2010. https://www.nytimes.com/2010/04/18/magazine/18exercise-t.html?pagewanted=all
1025. Franz et al., "Weight-Loss Outcomes: A Systematic Review and Meta-Analysis of Weight-Loss Clinical Trials with a Minimum 1-Year Follow-Up," *Journal of the Academy of Nutrition and Dietetics* 107, no. 10 (2007): 1755-1767.
1026. Miller et al., "A Meta-Analysis of the Past 25 Years of Weight Loss Research Using Diet, Exercise, or Diet Plus Exercise Intervention," *International Journal of Obesity* 21 (1997): 941-947.
1027. Franz et al., "Weight-Loss Outcomes: A Systematic Review and Meta-Analysis of Weight-Loss Clinical Trials with a Minimum 1-Year Follow-up," *Journal of the Academy of Nutrition and Dietetics* 107, no. 10 (2007): 1755-1767.
1028. Miller et al., "A Meta-Analysis of the Past 25 Years of Weight Loss Research Using Diet, Exercise, or Diet Plus Exercise Intervention," *International Journal of Obesity* 21 (1997): 941-947.
1029. Miller et al., "The Effects of Exercise Training in Addition to Energy Restriction on Functional Capacities and Body Composition in Obese Adults during Weight Loss: A Systematic Review," *PLOS One* (2013): doi: 10.1371/journal.pone.0081692.
1030. Johns et al., "Diet or Exercise Interventions vs Combined Behavioral Weight Management Programs: A Systematic Review and Meta-Analysis of Direct Comparisons," *Journal of the Academy of Nutrition and Dietetics* 114, no. 10 (2014): 1557-1568.
1031. "BMR Calculator," *BMR Calculator.* https://www.bmrcalculator.org
1032. Ibid.
1033. Frayn, Keith. *Metabolic Regulation: A Human Perspective.* Oxford: Wiley Blackwell, 2010. Kindle File, 12.3.2, Location 7743.
1034. Hubert, A., and Else, P., "Basal Metabolic Rate: History, Composition, Regulation, and Usefulness," *Physiological and Biochemical Zoology: Ecological and Evolutionary Approaches* 77, no. 6 (2004): 869-76.
1035. Durnin, J., "Basal Metabolic Rate in Man," Joint FAO/WHO/UNU Expert Consultation on Energy and Protein Requirements, 1981. https://www.fao.org/3/contents/3079f916-ceb8-591d-90da-02738d5b0739/M2845E00.HTM
1036. Frayn, Keith. *Metabolic Regulation: A Human Perspective.* Oxford: Wiley Blackwell, 2010. Kindle File, 5.6.2, Location 3266.
1037. Durnin, J., "Basal Metabolic Rate in Man," Joint FAO/WHO/UNU Expert Consultation on Energy and Protein Requirements, 1981. https://www.fao.org/3/contents/3079f916-ceb8-591d-90da-02738d5b0739/M2845E00.HTM
1038. Speakman, J. and Selman, C., "Physical Activity and Resting Metabolic Rate," *Proceedings of the Nutrition Society* 62 (2003): 621-634.
1039. "BMR Calculator," *BMR Calculator.* https://www.bmrcalculator.org
1040. "Calorie Calculator," *MapMyRun.* https://www.mapmyrun.com/improve/calorie_calculator/
1041. King et al., "Individual Variability Following 12 Weeks of Supervised Exercise: Identification and Characterization of Compensation for Exercise-Induced Weight Loss," *International Journal of Obesity* 32 (2008): 177-84.
1042. Finlayson et al., "Acute Compensatory Eating Following Exercise Is Associated with Implicit Hedonic Wanting For Food," *Physiology & Behavior* 97, no. 1 (2009): 62-67.
1043. Thomas et al., "Why Do Individuals Not Lose More Weight from an Exercise Intervention at a Defined Dose? An Energy Balance Analysis," *Obesity Reviews* 13, no. 10 (2012): 835-47.
1044. Finlayson et al., "Acute Compensatory Eating Following Exercise Is Associated with Implicit Hedonic Wanting For Food," *Physiology & Behavior* 97, no. 1 (2009): 62-67.
1045. "Calorie Calculator," *MapMyRun.* https://www.mapmyrun.com/improve/calorie_calculator/
1046. "Nutrition Information," *Subway.* https://www.subway.com/nutrition/nutritionlist.aspx?id=soup
1047. King et al., "Individual Variability Following 12 Weeks of Supervised Exercise: Identification and Characterization of Compensation for Exercise-Induced Weight Loss," *International Journal of Obesity* 32 (2008):

177-84.

1048. Thomas et al., "Why Do Individuals Not Lose More Weight from an Exercise Intervention at a Defined Dose? An Energy Balance Analysis," *Obesity Reviews* 13, no. 10 (2012): 835-47.

1049. Frayn, Keith. *Metabolic Regulation: A Human Perspective.* Oxford: Wiley Blackwell, 2010. Kindle File, 12.4.2, Location 7824-40.

1050. The National Weight Control Registry. https://www.nwcr.ws/default.htm

1051. Wing, R. and Hill, J., "Successful Weight Loss Maintenance," *Annual Review of Nutrition* 21 (2001): 323-41.

1052. "NWCR Facts," National Weight Control Registry. https://www.nwcr.ws/Research/default.htm

1053. Dulloo, A., and Montani, J., "Pathways from Dieting to Weight Regain, to Obesity and the Metabolic Syndrome: An Overview," *Obesity Reviews* 16, S1 (2015): 1-6.

1054. Ayyad C., and Andersen, T., "Long-Term Efficacy of Dietary Treatment of Obesity: A Systematic Review of Studies Published Between 1931 and 1999," *Obesity Reviews* 1, no. 2 (2000): 113-119.

1055. Dombrowski et al., "Long Term Maintenance of Weight Loss with Non-Surgical Interventions in Obese Adults: Systematic Review and Meta-Anaylses of Randomised Controlled Trials," *BMJ* 348 (2014): doi: https://dx.doi.org/10.1136/bmj.g2646

1056. Anderson et al., "Long-Term Weight Loss Maintenance: Meta-Analysis of US Studies," *American Journal of Clinical Nutrition* 74 (2001): 579-584.

1057. Franz et al., "Weight-Loss Outcomes: A Systematic Review and Meta-Analysis of Weight-Loss Clinical Trials with a Minimum 1-Year Follow-Up," *Journal of the American Dietetic Association* 107 (2007): 1755-1767.

1058. Ewbank et al., "Physical Activity as a Predictor of Weight Maintenance in Previously Obese Subjects," *Obesity Research* 3, no. 3 (1995): 257-263.

1059. Pronk. N., and Wing, R., "Physical Activity and Long-Term Maintenance of Weight Loss," *Obesity Research* 2, no. 6 (1994): 587-599.

1060. Hensrud et al., "A Prospective Study of Weight Maintenance in Obese Subjects Reduced to Normal Body Weight without Weight-Loss Training," *American Journal of Clinical Nutrition* 60, no. 5 (1994): 688-694.

1061. Sciamanna et al., "Practices Associated with Weight Loss versus Weight Loss Maintenance," *American Journal of Preventive Medicine* 41, no. 2 (2011): 159-166.

1062. Donnelly et al., "The Role of Exercise for Weight Loss and Maintenance," *Best Practice and Research: Clinical Gastroenterology* 18, no. 6 (2004): 1009-29.

1063. "Physical Activity for a Healthy Weight," Centers for Disease Control and Prevention. https://www.cdc.gov/healthyweight/physical_activity/

1064. "NWCR Facts," National Weight Control Registry. https://www.nwcr.ws/Research/default.htm

1065. Catenacci et al., "Physical Activity Patterns Using Accelerometry in the National Weight Control Registry," *Obesity* 19 (2011): 1163-1170.

1066. "NWCR Facts," National Weight Control Registry. https://www.nwcr.ws/Research/default.htm

1067. Wing, R., and Phelan, S., "Long-Term Weight Loss Maintenance," *American Journal of Clinical Nutrition* 82, no. 1 (2005): 222S-225S.

1068. Fogelholm, M., and Kukkonen-Harjula, K., "Does Physical Activity Prevent Weight Gain—A Systematic Review," *Obesity Reviews* 1, no. 2 (2000): 95-111.

1069. I-Min Lee et al., "Physical Activity and Weight Gain Prevention," *JAMA* 303, no. 12 (2010): 1173-79.

1070. Saris et al., "How Much Physical Activity Is Enough to Prevent Unhealthy Weight Gain? The Outcome of the IASO 1st Stock Conference and Consensus Statement," *Obesity Reviews* 4, no. 2 (2003): 101-114.

1071. Catenacci et al., "Physical Activity Patterns in the National Weight Control Registry," *Obesity* 16 (2008): 153-161.

1072. Sumithran et al., "Long-Term Persistence of Hormonal Adaptations to Weight Loss," *New England Journal of Medicine* 365 (2011): 1597-1604.

1073. Catenacci et al., "Physical Activity Patterns in the National Weight Control Registry," *Obesity* 16 (2008): 153-161.

1074. Catenacci et al., "Dietary Habits and Weight Maintenance Success in High versus Low Exercisers in the National Weight Control Registry," *Journal of Physical Activity and Health* 11, no. 8 (2014): 1540-1548.

1075. Cordain et al., "Plant-Animal Subsistence Ratios and Macronutrient Energy Estimations in Worldwide Hunter-Gatherer Diets," *American Journal of Clinical Nutrition* 71, no. 3 (2000): 682-692.

1076. Cordain et al., "Evolutionary Aspects of Exercise," *World Review of Nutrition and Dietetics* 81 (1997): 49-60.

1077. Stearns et al., "Measuring Selection in Contemporary Human Populations," *Nature Reviews Genetics* 11 (2010): 611- 622.

1078. Milot et al., "Evidence for Evolution in Response to Natural Selection in a Contemporary Human Population," *Proceedings of the National Academy of Sciences of the United States of America* 108, no. 41 (2011): 17040-17045.

1079. Lindeberg, Staffan. *Food and Western Disease: Health and Nutrition from an Evolutionary Perspective.* Hoboken: Wiley-Blackwell, 2010. Kindle File, Chapter 4.6, Location 3474.

1080. Malina, R., and Little, B., "Physical Activity: The Present in the Context of the Past," *American Journal of Human Biology* 20 (2008): 373-391.

1081. Schneider et al., "Effects of a 10,000 Steps per Day Goal in Overweight Adults," *American Journal of Health Promotion* 21, no. 2 (2006): 85-89.

1082. Masataka et al., "Walking 10,000 Steps/Day or More Reduces Blood Pressure and Sympathetic Nerve Activity in Mild Essential Hypertension," *Hypertension Research* 23, no. 6 (2000): 573-580.

1083. Basset et al., "Physical Activity in an Old Order Amish Community," *Medicine and Science In Sports and Exercise* 36, no. 1 (2004): 79-85.

1084. Pontzer et al., "Hunter-Gatherer Energetics and Human Obesity," *PLOS One* 7 (2012): e40503. doi:10.1371/journal.pone.0040503

1085. "Historical Timeline—Farmers and the Land," Growing a Nation: The Story of American Agriculture. https://www.agclassroom.org/gan/timeline/farmers_land.htm

1086. "The 20th Century Transformation of U.S. Agriculture and Farm Policy," *Economic Information Bulletin 3.* USDA. https://www.ers.usda.gov/media/259572/eib3_1_.pdf

1087. Archer et al., "45-Year Trends in Women's Use of Time and Household Management Energy Expenditure," *PLOS One* (2013): doi: 10.1371/journal.pone.0056620

1088. Ibid.

1089. "Exercise: The Miracle Cure and the Role of the Doctor in Promoting It," *Academy of Medical Royal Colleges*. February 2015. https://www.aomrc.org.uk/wp-content/uploads/2016/05/Exercise_the_Miracle_Cure_0215.pdf

1090. Booth et al., "Waging War on Modern Chronic Diseases: Primary Prevention Through Exercise Biology," *Journal of Applied Physiology* 88, no. 2 (2000): 774-787.

1091. Nieman, D., "Clinical Implications of Exercise Immunology," *Journal of Sport and Health Science* 1, no. 1 (2012): 12-17.

1092. Nieman et al., "Upper Respiratory Tract Infection Is Reduced in Physically Fit and Active Adults," *British Journal of Sports Medicine* 45 (2011): 987-992.

1093. Mattusch et al., "Reduction of the Plasma Concentration of C-Reactive Protein Following Nine Months of Endurance Training," *International Journal of Sports Medicine* 21, no. 1 (2000): 21-24.

1094. Kodama et al., "Effect of Aerobic Exercise Training on Serum Levels of High-Density Lipoprotein Cholesterol: A Meta-Analysis," *JAMA Internal Medicine* 167, no. 10 (2007): 999-1008.

1095. Halbert et al., "Exercise Training and Blood Lipids in Hyperlipidemic and Normolipidemic Adults: A Meta-Analysis of Randomized, Controlled Trials," *European Journal of Clinical Nutrition* 53, no. 7 (1999): 514-522.

1096. Lamprecht et al., "Effects of a Single Bout of Walking Exercise on Blood Coagulation Parameters in Obese Women," *Journal of Applied Physiology* 115, no. 1 (2013): 57-63.

1097. Kupchak et al., "Beneficial Effects of Habitual Resistance Exercise Training on Coagulation and Fibrinolytic Responses," *Thrombosis Research* 131, no. 6 (2013): e227-e234.

1098. Whelton et al., "Effect of Aerobic Exercise on Blood Pressure: A Meta-Analysis of Randomized, Controlled Trials," *Annals of Internal Medicine* 136, no. 7 (2002): 493-503.

1099. Cornelissen, V., and Smart, N., "Exercise Training for Blood Pressure: A Systematic Review and Meta-Analysis," *Hypertension* (2013): doi: 10.1161/JAHA.112.004473.

1100. Lee et al., "Physical Activity and Stroke Risk: A Meta-Analysis," *Stroke* 34 (2003): 2475-2781.

1101. Berlin, J., and Colditz, G., "A Meta-Analysis of Physical Activity in the Prevention of Coronary Heart Disease," *American Journal of Epidemiology* 132, no. 4 (1990): 612-628.

1102. Sattelmair et al., "Dose Response between Physical Activity and Risk of Coronary Heart Disease: A Meta-Analysis," *Circulation* 124 (2011): 789-795.

1103. Lee, I., "Physical Activity and Cancer Prevention—Data from Epidemiologic Studies," *Medicine and Science in Sports and Exercise* 35, no. 11 (2003): 1823-1827.

1104. Steindorf et al., "Physical Activity and Primary Cancer Prevention," Chapter 6: *Physical Activity and Primary Cancer Prevention. Exercise, Energy Balance, and Cancer*. New York: Springer Science+Business Media, 2013.

1105. Hu et al., "Epidemiological Studies of Exercise in Diabetes Prevention," *Applied Physiology, Nutrition, and Metabolism* 32, no. 3 (2007): 583-595.

1106. Boule et al., "Effects of Exercise on Glycemic Control and Body Mass in Type 2 Diabetes Mellitus: A Meta-Analysis of Controlled Clinical Trials," *JAMA* 286, no. 10 (2001): 1218-1227.

1107. White, L., and Dressendorfer, R., "Exercise and Multiple Sclerosis," *Sports Medicine* 34, no. 15 (2004): 1077-1100.

1108. Cheng et al., "Physical Activity and Erectile Dysfunction: Meta-Analysis of Population-Based Studies," *International Journal of Impotence Research* 19 (2007): 245-252.

1109. Hayden et al., "Meta-Analysis: Exercise Therapy for Nonspecific Low Back Pain," *Annals of Internal Medicine* 142, no. 9 (2005): 765-775.

1110. Freiberger et al., "Physical Activity, Exercise, and Sarcopenia—Future Challenges," *Wiener Medizinische Wochenschrift* 161, no. 17 (2011): 416-425.

1111. Kasch et al., "The Effect of Physical Activity and Inactivity on Aerobic Power in Older Men (A Longitudinal Study)," *Physician and Sports Medicine* 18, no. 4 (1990): 73-83.

1112. Gregg et al., "Physical Activity, Falls, and Fractures Among Older Adults: A Review of the Epidemiologic Evidence," *Journal of the American Geriatrics Society* 48, no. 8 (2000): 883-893.

1113. Brosseau et al., "Efficacy of Aerobic Exercises for Osteoarthritis (Part II): A Meta-Analysis," *Physical Therapy Reviews* 9, no. 3 (2004): 125-145.

1114. Baillet et al., "Efficacy of Cardiorespiratory Aerobic Exercise in Rheumatoid Arthritis: Meta-Analysis of Randomized Controlled Trials," *Arthritis Care & Research* 62, no. 7 (2010): 984-992.

1115. Howe et al., "Exercise for Preventing and Treating Osteoporosis in Postmenopausal Women," *Cochrane Database of Systematic Reviews* (2011): doi: 10.1002/14651858.CD000333.pub2.

1116. Roig et al., "The Effects of Cardiovascular Exercise on Human Memory: A Review with Meta-Analysis," *Neuroscience and Biobehavioral Reviews* 37 (2013): 1645-1666.

1117. Chang et al., "The Effects of Acute Exercise on Cognitive Performance: A Meta-Analysis," *Brain Research* 1453 (2012): 87-101.

1118. Radak et al., "Exercise Plays a Preventive Role against Alzheimer's Disease," *Journal of Alzheimer's Disease* 20 (2010): 777-783.

1119. Chen et al., "Physical Activity and the Risk of Parkinson Disease," *Neurology* 64, no. 4 (2005): 664-669.

1120. Silveira et al., "Physical Exercise and Clinically Depressed Patients: A Systematic Review and Meta-Analysis," *Neuropsychobiology* 67 (2013): 61-68.

1121. Craft et al., "The Benefits of Exercise for the Clinically Depressed," *Primary Care Companion to the Journal of Clinical Psychiatry* 6, no. 3 (2004): 104-111.

1122. Yang et al., "Exercise Training Improves Sleep Quality in Middle-Aged and Older Adults with Sleep Problems: A Systematic Review," *Journal of Physiotherapy* 58, no. 3 (2012): 157-163.

1123. Campbell, A., and Hausenblas, H., "Effects of Exercise Interventions on Body Image: A Meta-Analysis," *Journal of Health Psychology* 14, no. 6 (2009): 780-793.

1124. Wegner et al., "Effects of Exercise on Anxiety and Depression Disorders: Review of Meta-Analyses and Neurobiological Mechanisms," *CNS & Neurological Disorders—Drug Targets* 13 (2014): 1002-1014.

1125. Penedo, F., and Dahn, J., "Exercise and Well-Being: A Review of Mental and Physical Health Benefits Associated with Physical Activity," *Current Opinion in Psychiatry* 18, no. 2 (2005): 189-193.

1126. Stephens, T., "Physical Activity and Mental Health in the United States and Canada: Evidence from Four Population Surveys," *Preventive Medicine* 17, no. 1 (1988): 35-47.

1127. Ahn, S., and Fedewa, A., "A Meta-Analysis of the Relationship Between Children's Physical Activity and Mental Health," *Journal of Pediatric Psychology* (2011): doi: 10.1093/jpepsy/jsq107.

1128. Hopkins et al., "Differential Effects of Acute and Regular Physical Exercise on Cognition and Affect," *Neuroscience* 215 (2013): 59-68.
1129. Delextrat et al., "An 8-Week Exercise Intervention Based on Zumba® Improves Aerobic Fitness and Psychological Well Being in Healthy Women," *Journal of Physical Activity & Health* 13, no. 2 (2016): 131-139.
1130. Khazaee-pool et al., "Effects of Physical Exercise Programme on Happiness Among Older People," *Journal of Psychiatric and Mental Health Nursing* 22, no. 1 (2015): 47-57.
1131. Woodcock et al., "Non-Vigorous Physical Activity and All-Cause Mortality: Systematic Review and Meta-Analysis of Cohort Studies," *International Journal of Epidemiology* 40, no. 1 (2011): 121-138.
1132. Ross et al., "Exercise-Induced Reduction in Obesity and Insulin Resistance in Women: A Randomized Controlled Trial," *Obesity Research* 12, no. 5 (2004): 789-798.
1133. Ibid.
1134. Catenacci et al., "The Role of Physical Activity in Producing and Maintaining Weight Loss," *Nature Clinical Practice Endocrinology & Metabolism* 3 (2007): 518-529.
1135. Rottensteiner et al., "Physical Activity, Fitness, Glucose Homeostasis, and Brain Morphology in Twins," *Medicine & Science in Sports & Exercise* 47, no. 3 (2015): 509-518.
*1136. ACSM's Advanced Exercise Physiology.* Edited by Peter Farrell, Michael Joyner, and Vincent Caiozzo. Second Edition. Lippincott Williams & Wilkins, 2012. Page 693.
1137. Ibid., 520.
1138. Ibid., 690.
1139. Ibid., 695.
1140. Chau et al., "Daily Sitting Time and All-Cause Mortality: A Meta-Analysis," *PLOS One* (2013): doi: 10.1371/journal.pone.0080000.
1141. Biswas et al., "Sedentary Time and Its Association with Risk for Disease Incidence, Mortality, and Hospitalization in Adults: A Systematic Review and Meta-Analysis," *Annals of Internal Medicine* 162, no. 2 (2015): 123-132.
1142. Katzmarzyk, P., "Standing and Mortality in a Prospective Cohort of Canadian Results," *Medicine & Science in Sports & Exercise* 46, no. 5 (2014): 940-946.
1143. Kaplan, H., and Hill, K., "Hunting Ability and Reproductive Success Among Male Ache Foragers: Preliminary Results," *Current Anthropology* 26, no. 1 (1985): 131-133.
1144. Altman, J., "Hunter-Gatherer Subsistence Production in Arnhem Land: The Original Affluence Hypothesis Re-Examined," *The Australian Journal of Anthropology* 14, no. 3 (1984): 179-190.
1145. Winterhalder, B., "Work, Resources and Population in Foraging Societies," *Man* 28, no. 2 (1993): 321-340.
1146. Gurven et al., "Physical Activity and Modernization Among Bolivian Amerindians," *PLOS One* (2013): doi: 10.1371/journal.pone.0055679.
1147. Basset et al., "Physical Activity in an Old Order Amish Community," *Medicine and Science In Sports and Exercise* 36, no. 1 (2004): 79-85.
1148. Malina, R., and Little., B., "Physical Activity: The Present in the Context of the Past," *American Journal of Human Biology* 20 (2008): 373-391.
1149. Frith et al., "Orthostatic Intolerance Is Common in Chronic Disease—A Clinical Cohort Study," *International Journal of Cardiology* 174, no. 3 (2014): 861-863.
1150. Reiff et al., "Difference in Caloric Expenditure in Sitting Versus Standing Desks," *Journal of Physical Activity and Health* 9 (2012): 1009-1011.
1151. Tuchsen et al., "Standing at Work and Varicose Veins," *Scandinavian Journal of Work, Environment, & Health* 26, no. 5 (2000): 414-420.
1152. Krause et al., "Standing at Work and Progression of Carotid Atherosclerosis," *Scandinavian Journal of Work, Environment, & Health* 26, no. 3 (2000): 227-236.
1153. Buckley et al., "The Sedentary Office: An Expert Statement on the Growing Case for Change Towards Better Health and Productivity," *British Journal of Sports Medicine* 49 (2015): 1357-1362.
1154. Bailey, D., and Locke, C., "Breaking up Prolonged Sitting with Light-Intensity Walking Improves Postprandial Glycemia, but Breaking up Sitting with Standing Does Not," *Journal of Science and Medicine in Sport* 18, no. 3 (2015): 294-298.
1155. Mummery et al., "Occupational Sitting Time and Overweight and Obesity in Australian Workers," *American Journal of Preventive Medicine* 29, no. 2 (2005): 91-97.
1156. Martinez-Gonzalez et al., "Physical Inactivity, Sedentary Lifestyle and Obesity in the European Union," *International Journal of Obesity and Related Metabolic Disorders* 23, no. 11 (1999): 1192-1201.
1157. Chau et al., "Cross-Sectional Associations Between Occupational and Leisure-Time Sitting, Physical Activity and Obesity in Working Adults," *Preventive Medicine* 54, no. 3-4 (2012): 195-200.
1158. Herman et al., "Keeping the Weight Off: Physical Activity, Sitting Time, and Weight Loss Maintenance in Bariatric Surgery Patients 2 to 16 Years Postsurgery," *Obesity Surgery* 24, no. 7 (2014): 1064-1072.
1159. Henson et al., "Associations of Sedentary Time with Fat Distribution in a High-Risk Population," *Medicine & Science in Sports & Exercise* 47, no. 8 (2015): 1727-1734.
1160. Shuval et al., "Standing, Obesity, and Metabolic Syndrome: Findings from the Cooper Center Longitudinal Study," *Mayo Clinic Proceedings* 90, no. 11 (2015): 1524-1532.
1161. Owen et al., "Too Much Sitting: Health Risks for Sedentary Behavior and Opportunities for Change," *President's Council on Fitness, Sports, & Nutrition. Research Digest* 13, no. 3 (2012): https://www.presidentschallenge.org/informed/digest/docs/201212digest.pdf
1162. Buckley et al., "The Sedentary Office: An Expert Statement on the Growing Case for Change Towards Better Health and Productivity," *British Journal of Sports Medicine* 49 (2015): 1357-1362.
1163. Dunstan et al., "Breaking up Prolonged Sitting Reduces Postprandial Glucose and Insulin Responses," *Diabetes Care* 35, no. 5 (2012): 976-983.
1164. Latouche et al., "Effects of Breaking up Prolonged Sitting on Skeletal Muscle Gene Expression," *Journal of Applied Physiology* 114, no. 4 (2013): 453-460.
1165. Healy et al., "Breaks in Sedentary Time: Beneficial Associations with Metabolic Risk," *Diabetes Care* 31, no. 4 (2008): 661-666.
1166. "2008 Physical Activity Guidelines for Americans," US Department of Health and Human Services. https://health.gov/paguidelines/pdf/paguide.pdf
1167. Ibid.
1168. Zheng et al., "Quantifying the Dose-Response of Walking in Reducing Coronary Heart Disease Risk: Meta-Analysis," *European Journal of Epidemiology* 24, no. 4 (2009): 181-192.

1169. Murphy et al., "The Effect of Walking on Fitness, Fatness and Resting Blood Pressure: A Meta-Analysis of Randomised, Controlled Trials," *Preventive Medicine* 44 (2007): 377-385.

1170. Wing, R., and Phelan, S., "Long-Term Weight Loss Maintenance," *American Journal of Clinical Nutrition* 82, no. 1 (2005): 222S-225S.

1171. Marlowe, F., "Hunter-Gatherers and Human Evolution," *Evolutionary Anthropology* 14 (2005): 54-67.

1172. Pontzer et al., "Hunter-Gatherer Energetics and Human Obesity," *PLOS One* 7 (2012): e40503. doi:10.1371/journal.pone.0040503.

1173. O'Keefe et al., "Organic Fitness: Physical Activity Consistent with Our Hunter-Gatherer Heritage," *The Physician and Sportsmedicine* 38, no. 4 (2010): 11-18.

1174. Malina, R., and Little., B., "Physical Activity: The Present in the Context of the Past," *American Journal of Human Biology* 20 (2008): 373-391.

1175. Holick, M., "Vitamin D and Sunlight: Strategies for Cancer Prevention and Other Health Benefits," *Clinical Journal of the American Society of Nephrology* 3, no. 5 (2008): 1548-1554.

1176. Ibid.

1177. Coon et al., "Does Participating in Physical Activity in Outdoor Natural Environments Have a Greater Effect on Physical and Mental Wellbeing Than Physical Activity Indoors? A Systematic Review," *Environmental Science and Technology* 45, no. 5 (2011): 1761-1772.

1178. Powers, S. and Howley, E. *Exercise Physiology : Theory and Application to Fitness and Performance*. Eighth Edition. McGraw-Hill, 2012. Page 431.

1179. Saris et al., "How Much Physical Activity Is Enough to Prevent Unhealthy Weight Gain? The Outcome of the IASO 1st Stock Conference and Consensus Statement," *Obesity Reviews* 4, no. 2 (2003): 101-114.

1180. Powers, S. and Howley, E. *Exercise Physiology : Theory and Application to Fitness and Performance*. Eighth Edition. McGraw-Hill, 2012. Page 357.

1181. Ibid., 431.

1182. "Strength and Resistance Exercise," *Getting Healthy*, The American Heart Association. Updated: March 24, 2015. https://www.heart.org/HEARTORG/GettingHealthy/PhysicalActivity/FitnessBand-Resistance-Training-Exercise_UCM_462357_Article.jsp#.VoS7ELRmj8E

1183. "What We Recommend," American Diabetes Association. Last Edited: May 19, 2015. https://www.diabetes.org/food-and-fitness/fitness/types-of-activity/what-we-recommend.html

1184. "Resistance Training for Health and Fitness," *ACSM Information On...*, American College of Sports Medicine. https://www.prescriptiontogetactive.com/app/uploads/resistance-training-ACSM.pdf

1185. Malina, R., and Little., B., "Physical Activity: The Present in the Context of the Past," *American Journal of Human Biology* 20 (2008): 373-391.

1186. Eaton, S., and Eaton III, S., "Hunter-Gatherers and Human Health," (1999): In: Lee, R. and Daly, R., *The Cambridge Encyclopedia of Hunters and Gatherers*. Cambridge: Cambridge University Press, pp. 449-456.

1187. Ibid.

1188. Brightman, R., "The Sexual Division of Foraging Labor: Biology, Taboo, and Gender Politics," *Comparative Studies in Society and History* 38, no. 4 (1996): 687-729.

1189. Malina, R., and Little., B., "Physical Activity: The Present in the Context of the Past," *American Journal of Human Biology* 20 (2008): 373-391.

1190. Ibid.

1191. Snowling, N., and Hopkins, W., "Effects of Different Modes of Exercise Training on Glucose Control and Risk Factors for Complications in Type 2 Diabetic Patients: A Meta-Analysis," *Diabetes Care* 29, no. 11 (2006): 2518-2527.

1192. Marzolini et al., "Effect of Combined Aerobic and Resistance Training versus Aerobic Training Alone in Individuals with Coronary Artery Disease: A Meta-Analysis," *European Journal of Preventive Cardiology* (2011): 1741826710393197. https://cpr.sagepub.com/content/early/2011/02/19/1741826710393197. abstract

1193. Ho et al., "The Effect of 12 Weeks of Aerobic, Resistance or Combination Exercise Training on Cardiovascular Risk Factors in the Overweight and Obese in a Randomized Trial," *BMC Public Health* 12 (2012): 704: doi: 10.1186/1471-2458-12-704.

1194. Mekary et al., "Weight Training, Aerobic Physical Activities, and Long-Term Waist Circumference Change in Men," *Obesity* 23, no. 2 (2015): 461-467.

1195. Powers, S. and Howley, E. *Exercise Physiology: Theory and Application to Fitness and Performance*. Eighth Edition. McGraw-Hill, 2012. Page 38.

1196. Morton et al., "Resistance Training vs. Static Stretching: Effects on Flexibility and Strength," *Journal of Strength and Conditioning Research* 25, no. 12 (2011): 3391-3398.

1197. Cheema et al., "Safety and Efficacy of Progressive Resistance Training in Breast Cancer: A Systematic Review and Meta-Analysis," *Breast Cancer Research and Treatment* 148, no. 2 (2014): 249-268.

1198. Liu-Ambrose et al., "Resistance Training and Executive Functions: A 12-Month Randomized Controlled Trial," *JAMA Internal Medicine* 170, no. 2 (2010): 170-178.

1199. Netz et al., "Physical Activity and Psychological Well-Being in Advanced Age: A Meta-Analysis of Intervention Studies," *Psychology and Aging* 20, no. 2 (2005): 272-284.

1200. Prabhakaran et al., "Effects of 14 Weeks of Resistance Training on Lipid Profile and Body Fat Percentage in Premenopausal Women," *British Journal of Sports Medicine* 33 (1999): 190-195.

1201. Schmitz et al., "Strength Training for Obesity Prevention in Midlife Women," *International Journal of Obesity and Related Metabolic Disorders* 27, no. 3 (2003): 326-333.

1202. Kelley et al., "Resistance Training and Bone Mineral Density in Women: A Meta-Analysis of Controlled Trials," *American Journal of Physical Medicine & Rehabilitation* 80, no. 1 (2001): 65-77.

1203. Ryan et al., "Regional Bone Mineral Density After Resistive Training in Young and Older Men and Women," *Scandinavian Journal of Medicine & Science in Sports* 14, no. 1 (2004): 16-23.

1204. Dawson et al., "Potential Benefits of Improved Protein Intake in Older People," *Nutrition and Dietetics* 65 (2008): 151-156.

1205. Fiatarone et al., "High-Intensity Strength Training in Nonagenarians: Effects on Skeletal Muscle," *JAMA* 263, no. 22 (1990): 3029-3034.

1206. Ibid.

1207. Powers, S. and Howley, E. *Exercise Physiology: Theory and Application to Fitness and Performance*. Eighth Edition. McGraw-Hill, 2012. Page 183.

1208. Volaklis et al., "Muscular Strength as a Strong Predictor of Mortality: A Narrative Review," *European*

*Journal of Internal Medicine* 26, no. 5 (2015): 303-310.

1209. Straight et al., "Effects of Resistance Training on Lower-Extremity Power in Middle Aged and Older Adults: A Systematic Review and Meta-Analysis of Randomized Controlled Trials," *Sports Medicine* (2015): https://www.ncbi.nlm.nih.gov/pubmed/26545362

1210. Lo et al., "Training and Detraining Effects of the Resistance vs. Endurance Program on Body Composition, Body Size, and Physical Performance in Young Men," *Journal of Strength & Conditioning Research* 25, no. 8 (2011): 2246-2254.

1211. Braith, R., and Stewart, K., "Resistance Exercise Training: Its Role in the Prevention of Cardiovascular Disease," *Circulation* 113 (2006): 2642-2650.

1212. *ACSM's Advanced Exercise Physiology*. Edited by Peter Farrell, Michael Joyner, and Vincent Caiozzo. Second Edition. Lippincott Williams & Wilkins, 2012. Page 673.

1213. DeFronzo, R., and Tripathy, D., "Skeletal Muscle Insulin Resistance Is the Primary Defect in Type 2 Diabetes," *Diabetes Care* 32 (2009): S157-S163.

1214. Sayer et al., "Type 2 Diabetes, Muscle Strength, and Impaired Physical Function: The Tip of the Iceberg?" *Diabetes Care* 28, no. 10 (2005): 2541-2542.

1215. Ginsberg, H., "Insulin Resistance and Cardiovascular Disease," *Journal of Clinical Investigation* 106, no. 4 (2000): 453-458.

1216. Wolfe, R., "The Underappreciated Role of Muscle in Health and Disease," *American Journal of Clinical Nutrition* 84, no. 3 (2006): 475-482.

1217. Ibid.

1218. Ibid.

1219. Tisdale, M., "Cachexia in Cancer Patients," *Nature Reviews Cancer* 2 (2002): 862-871.

1220. Anker, S., and Coats, A., "Cardiac Cachexia: A Syndrome with Impaired Survival and Immune and Neuroendocrine Activation," *Chest* 115, no. 3 (1999): 836-847.

1221. Snowling, N., and Hopkins, W., "Effects of Different Modes of Exercise Training on Glucose Control and Risk Factors for Complications in Type 2 Diabetic Patients: A Meta-Analysis," *Diabetes Care* 29, no. 11 (2006): 2518-2527.

1222. Marzolini et al., "Effect of Combined Aerobic and Resistance Training Versus Aerobic Training Alone in Individuals with Coronary Artery Disease: A Meta-Analysis," *European Journal of Preventive Cardiology* (2011): 1741826710393197. https://cpr.sagepub.com/content/early/2011/02/19/1741826710393197.abstract

1223. Ho et al., "The Effect of 12 Weeks of Aerobic, Resistance or Combination Exercise Training on Cardiovascular Risk Factors in the Overweight and Obese in a Randomized Trial," *BMC Public Health* 12 (2012): 704: doi: 10.1186/1471-2458-12-704.

1224. Mekary et al., "Weight Training, Aerobic Physical Activities, and Long-Term Waist Circumference Change in Men," *Obesity* 23, no. 2 (2015): 461-467.

1225. Prabhakaran et al., "Effects of 14 Weeks of Resistance Training on Lipid Profile and Body Fat Percentage in Premenopausal Women," *British Journal of Sports Medicine* 33 (1999): 190-195.

1226. Schmitz et al., "Strength Training for Obesity Prevention in Midlife Women," *International Journal of Obesity and Related Metabolic Disorders* 27, no.3 (2003): 326-333.

1227. Hunter et al., "Resistance Training and Intra-Abdominal Adipose Tissue in Older Men and Women," *Medicine & Science in Sports & Exercise* 34, no. 6 (2002): 1023-1028.

1228. Nicklas et al., "Effects of Resistance Training with and without Caloric Restriction on Physical Function and Mobility in Overweight and Obese Older Adults: A Randomized Controlled Trial," *American Journal of Clinical Nutrition* 101, no. 5 (2015): 991-999.

1229. Botero et al., "Effects of Long-Term Periodized Resistance Training on Body Composition, Leptin, Resistin and Muscle Strength in Elderly Post-Menopausal Women," *The Journal of Sports Medicine and Physical Fitness* 53, no. 3 (2013): 289-294.

1230. Wang et al., "Evaluation of Specific Metabolic Rates of Major Organs and Tissues: Comparison Between Men and Women," *American Journal of Human Biology* 23, no. 3 (2011): 333-338.

1231. Wolfe, R., "The Underappreciated Role of Muscle in Health and Disease," *American Journal of Clinical Nutrition* 84, no. 3 (2006): 475-482.

1232. Williamson, D., and Kirwan, J., "A Single Bout of Concentric Resistance Exercise Increases Basal Metabolic Rate 48 Hours After Exercise in Healthy 59–77-Year-Old Men," *Journal of Gerontology Series A: Biological Sciences and Medical Sciences* 52, no. 6 (1997): M352-M355.

1233. *ACSM's Advanced Exercise Physiology*. Edited by Peter Farrell, Michael Joyner, and Vincent Caiozzo. Second Edition. Lippincott Williams & Wilkins, 2012. Page 433.

1234. Schuenke et al., "Effect of an Acute Period of Resistance Exercise on Excess Post-Exercise Oxygen Consumption: Implications for Body Mass Management," *European Journal of Applied Physiology* 86 (2002): 411-417.

1235. Borsheim, E., and Bahr, R., "Effect of Exercise Intensity, Duration and Mode on Post-Exercise Oxygen Consumption," *Sports Medicine* 33, no. 14 (2003): 1037-1060.

1236. Heymsfield et al., "Weight Loss Composition Is One-Fourth Fat-Free Mass: A Critical Review and Critique of This Widely Cited Rule," *Obesity Reviews* 15, no. 4 (2014): 310-321.

1237. Dixon et al., "Fat-Free Mass Loss Generated with Weight Loss in Overweight and Obese Adults: What May We Expect?" *Diabetes, Obesity and Metabolism* 17, no. 1 (2015): 91-93.

1238. Schwartz et al., "Greater than Predicted Decrease in Resting Energy Expenditure and Weight Loss: Results from a Systematic Review," *Obesity* 20, no. 11 (2012): 2307-2310.

1239. Campbell et al., "Resistance Training Preserves Fat-Free Mass Without Impacting Changes in Protein Metabolism After Weight Loss in Older Women," *Obesity* 17, no. 7 (2009): 1332-1339.

1240. Ryan et al., "Resistive Training Increases Fat-Free Mass and Maintains RMR despite Weight Loss in Postmenopausal Women," *Journal of Applied Physiology* 79, no. 3 (1995): 818-823.

1241. Bryner et al., "Effects of Resistance vs. Aerobic Training Combined with an 800 Calorie Liquid Diet on Lean Body Mass and Resting Metabolic Rate," *Journal of the American College of Nutrition* 18, no. 2 (1999): 115-121.

1242. Pavlou et al., "Effects of Dieting and Exercise on Lean Body Mass, Oxygen Uptake, and Strength," *Medicine and Science in Sports and Exercise* 17, no. 4 (1985): 466-471.

1243. Frey-Hewitt et al., "The Effect of Weight Loss by Dieting or Exercise on Resting Metabolic Rate in Overweight Men," *International Journal of Obesity* 14, no. 4 (1990): 327-334.

1244. Bryner et al., "Effects of Resistance vs. Aerobic Training Combined with an 800 Calorie Liquid Diet on Lean Body Mass and Resting Metabolic Rate," *Journal of the American College of Nutrition* 18, no. 2 (1999): 115-121.

1245. Hunter et al., "Resistance Training Conserves Fat-Free Mass and Resting Energy Expenditure Following Weight Loss," *Obesity* 16, no. 5 (2008): 1045-1051.

1246. Geliebter et al., "Effects of Strength or Aerobic Training on Body Composition, Resting Metabolic Rate, and Peak Oxygen Consumption in Obese Dieting Subjects," *American Journal of Clinical Nutrition* 66, no. 3 (1997): 557-563.

1247. Hulens et al., "Exercise Capacity in Lean versus Obese Women," *Scandinavian Journal of Medicine & Science in Sports* 11, no. 5 (2001): 305-309.

1248. Forbes, G., and Welle, S., "Lean Body Mass in Obesity," *International Journal of Obesity* 7, no. 2 (1982): 99-107.

1249. Hibbert et al., "Determinants of Free-Living Energy Expenditure in Normal Weight and Obese Women Measured by Doubly Labeled Water," *Obesity Research* 2, no. 1 (1994): 44-53.

1250. Lafortuna et al., "Gender Variations of Body Composition, Muscle Strength and Power Output in Morbid Obesity," *International Journal of Obesity* 29 (2005): 833-841.

1251. Schoenfield, Brad, "Squatting Kinematics and Kinetics and Their Application to Exercise Performance," *Journal of Strength and Conditioning Research* 24, no. 12 (2010): 3497-3506.

1252. Maddalozzo et al., "The Effects of Hormone Replacement Therapy and Resistance Training on Spine Bone Mineral Density in Early Postmenopausal Women," *Bone* 40, no. 5 (2007): 1244-1251.

1253. Keogh et al., "Retrospective Injury Epidemiology of One Hundred One Competitive Oceania Power Lifters: The Effects of Age, Body Mass, Competitive Standard, and Gender," *Journal of Strength and Conditioning Research* 20, no. 3 (2006): 672-681.

1254. Ibid.

1255. Siewe et al., "Injuries and Overuse Syndromes in Powerlifting," *International Journal of Sports Medicine* 32, no. 9 (2011): 703-711.

1256. Hespanhol Jr. et al., "Previous Injuries and Some Training Characteristics Predict Running-Related Injuries in Recreational Runners: A Prospective Cohort Study," *Journal of Physiotherapy* 59, no. 4 (2013): 263-269.

1257. "Safety of the Squat Exercise," *ACSM Current Comment*, American College of Sports Medicine. https://www.acsm.org/docs/current-comments/safetysquat.pdf

1258. Fleck, S., and Falkel, J., "Value of Resistance Training for the Reduction of Sports Injuries," *Sports Medicine* 3, no. 1 (1986): 61-68.

1259. "Safety of the Squat Exercise," *ACSM Current Comment*, American College of Sports Medicine. https://www.acsm.org/docs/current-comments/safetysquat.pdf

1260. "Progression Models in Resistance Training for Healthy Adults," *Medicine & Science in Sports & Exercise* 41, no. 3 (2009): 687-708.

1261. *ACSM's Advanced Exercise Physiology.* Edited by Peter Farrell, Michael Joyner, and Vincent Caiozzo. Second Edition. Lippincott Williams & Wilkins, 2012. Page 487.

1262. Sinha-Hikim et al., "Testosterone Induced Increase in Muscle Size in Healthy Young Men Is Associated with Muscle Fiber Hypertrophy," *American Journal of Physiology-Endocrinology and Metabolism* 283, no. 1 (2002): E154-E164.

1263. Vingren et al., "Testosterone Physiology in Resistance Exercise and Training," *Sports Medicine* 40, no. 12 (2010): 1037-1053.

1264. O'Keefe et al., "Exercise Like a Hunter-Gatherer: A Prescription for Organic Physical Fitness," *Progress in Cardiovascular Diseases* 53 (2011): 471-479.

1265. Liebenberg, L., "Persistence Hunting by Modern Hunter-Gatherers," *Current Anthropology* 47, no. 6 (2006): 1017-1025.

1266. Pickering, T., and Bunn, H., "The Endurance Running Hypothesis and Hunting and Scavenging in Savanna-Woodlands," *Journal of Human Evolution* 53 (2007): 434-438.

1267. Steudel-Numbers, K., and Wall-Scheffler, C., "Optimal Running Speed and the Evolution of Hominin Hunting Strategies," *Journal of Human Evolution* 56, no. 4 (2009): 355-360.

1268. Lieberman et al., "The Evolution of Endurance Running and the Tyranny of Ethnography: A Reply to Pickering and Bunn," *Journal of Human Evolution* 53 (2007): 434-437.

1269. Churchill, Steven, "Weapon Technology, Prey Size Selection, and Hunting Methods in Modern Hunter-Gatherers: Implications for Hunting in the Palaeolithic and Mesolithic," *Archeological Papers of the American Anthropological Association* 4, no. 1 (1993): 11-24.

1270. Brightman, Robert, "The Sexual Division of Foraging Labor: Biology, Taboo, and Gender Politics," *Comparative Studies in Society and History* 38, no. 4 (1996): 687-729.

1271. Malina, R., and Little., B., "Physical Activity: The Present in the Context of the Past," *American Journal of Human Biology* 20 (2008): 373-391.

1272. Ireland, M., "Anterior Cruciate Ligament Injury in Female Athletes: Epidemiology," *Journal of Athletic Training* 34, no. 2 (1999): 150-154.

1273. Malina, R., and Little., B., "Physical Activity: The Present in the Context of the Past," *American Journal of Human Biology* 20 (2008): 373-391.

1274. Ruff, C., "Mechanical Determinants of Bone Form: Insights from Skeletal Remains," *Journal of Musculoskeletal and Neuronal Interactions* 5, no. 3 (2005): 202-212.

1275. Pitsiladis et al., "The Dominance of Kenyans in Distance Running," *Equine and Comparative Exercise Physiology* 1, no. 4 (2004): 285-291.

1276. "What Is Moderate and Vigorous Cardio?" *Choices*, National Health Service. https://www.nhs.uk/chq/Pages/2419.aspx?CategoryID=52

1277. Powers, S. and Howley, E. *Exercise Physiology: Theory and Application to Fitness and Performance.* Eighth Edition. McGraw-Hill, 2012. Pages 355-356.

1278. "American Heart Association Recommendations for Physical Activity in Adults," *Healthy Living*, American Heart Association. https://www.heart.org/HEARTORG/HealthyLiving/PhysicalActivity/FitnessBasics/American-Heart-Association-Recommendations-for-Physical-Activity-in-Adults_UCM_307976_Article.jsp#.VqEHJLRmj8E

1279. Garber et al., "Quantity and Quality of Exercise for Developing and Maintaining Cardiorespiratory, Musculoskeletal, and Neuromotor Fitness in Apparently Healthy Adults: Guidance for Prescribing Exercise," *Medicine & Science in Sports & Exercise* 43, no. 7 (2011): 1334-1359.

1280. Gormley et al., "Effect of Intensity of Aerobic Training on VO2 Max," *Medicine & Science in Sports & Exercise* 40, no. 7 (2008): 1336-1343.
1281. Kodama et al., "Cardiorespiratory Fitness as a Quantitative Predictor of All-Cause Mortality and Cardiovascular Events in Healthy Men and Women: A Meta-Analysis," *JAMA* 301, no. 19 (2009): 2024-2035.
1282. Swain, D., and Franklin, B., "Comparison of Cardioprotective Benefits of Vigorous Versus Moderate Intensity Aerobic Exercise," *The American Journal of Cardiology* 97, no. 1 (2006): 141-147.
1283. Ibid.
1284. Boule et al., "Meta-Analysis of the Effect of Structured Exercise Training on Cardiorespiratory Fitness in Type 2 Diabetes Mellitus," *Diabetologia* 46, no. 8 (2003): 1071-1081.
1285. Hu et al., "Walking Compared with Vigorous Physical Activity and Risk of Type 2 Diabetes in Women: A Prospective Study," *JAMA* 282, no. 15 (1999): 1433-1439.
1286. Slattery, M., "Physical Activity and Colorectal Cancer," *Sports Medicine* 34, no. 4 (2004): 239-252.
1287. Proper et al., "Dose-Response Relation Between Physical Activity and Sick Leave," *British Journal of Sports Medicine* 40, no. 2 (2006): 173-178.
1288. Lee, I., and Paffenbarger, R., "Associations of Light, Moderate, and Vigorous Intensity Physical Activity with Longevity: The Harvard Alumni Health Study," *American Journal of Epidemiology* 151, no. 3 (2000): 293-299.
1289. Samitz et al., "Domains of Physical Activity and All-Cause Mortality: Systematic Review and Dose-Response Meta-Analysis of Cohort Studies," *International Journal of Epidemiology* 40, no. 5 (2011): 1382-1400.
1290. Lahti et al., "Leisure-Time Physical Activity and All-Cause Mortality," *PLOS One* (2014): doi: 10.1371/journal.pone.0101548
1291. De Feo, P., "Is High-Intensity Exercise Better than Moderate-Intensity Exercise for Weight Loss?" *Nutrition, Metabolism & Cardiovascular Diseases* 23 (2013): 1037-1042.
1292. Swift et al., "The Role of Exercise and Physical Activity in Weight Loss and Maintenance," *Progress in Cardiovascular Diseases* 56, no. 4 (2014): 441-447.
1293. Jakicic et al., "Effect of Exercise Duration and Intensity on Weight Loss in Overweight, Sedentary Women: A Randomized Trial," *JAMA* 290, no. 10 (2003): 1323-1330.
1294. O'Donovan et al., "Changes in Cardiorespiratory Fitness and Coronary Heart Disease Risk Factors Following 24 Wk of Moderate- or High-Intensity Exercise of Equal Energy Cost," *Journal of Applied Physiology* 98, no. 5 (2005): 1619-1625.
1295. Kraus et al., "Effects of the Amount and Intensity of Exercise on Plasma Lipoproteins," The New England Journal of Medicine 347 (2002): 1483-1492.
1296. Bryner et al., "The Effects of Exercise Intensity on Body Composition, Weight Loss, and Dietary Composition in Women," *Journal of the American College of Nutrition* 16, no. 1 (1997): 68-73.
1297. Powers, S. and Howley, E. *Exercise Physiology: Theory and Application to Fitness and Performance.* Eighth Edition. McGraw-Hill, 2012. Page 363.
1298. Lee, B., and Oh, D., "Effect of Regular Swimming Exercise on the Physical Composition, Strength, and Blood Lipid of Middle-Aged Women," *Journal of Exercise Rehabilitation* 11, no. 5 (2015): 266-271.
1299. Powers, S. and Howley, E. *Exercise Physiology: Theory and Application to Fitness and Performance.* Eighth Edition. McGraw-Hill, 2012. Page 558.
1300. Hofmann et al., "The Reduction of Metabolic Cost While Using Handrail Support during Inclined Treadmill Walking Is Dependent on the Handrail-Use Instruction," *International Journal of Exercise Science* 7, no. 4 (2014): 339-345.
1301. Perri et al., "Adherence to Exercise Prescriptions: Effects of Prescribing Moderate versus Higher Levels of Intensity and Frequency," *Health Psychology* 21, no. 5 (2002): 452-458.
1302. Tabata et al., "Effects of Moderate-Intensity Endurance and High-Intensity Intermittent Training on Anaerobic Capacity and VO2 Max," *Medicine & Science in Sports & Exercise* 28, no. 10 (1996): 1327-1330.
1303. Boutcher, S., "High-Intensity Intermittent Exercise and Fat Loss," *Journal of Obesity* (2011): doi:10.1155/2011/868305.
1304. Engh et al., "Effects of High-Intensity Aerobic Exercise on Psychotic Symptoms and Neurocognition in Outpatients with Schizophrenia: Study Protocol for a Randomized Controlled Trial," *Trials* 16, no. 1 (2015): 557.
1305. "High-Intensity Interval Training," *ACSM Information On…, American College of Sports Medicine.* https://www.acsm.org/docs/brochures/high-intensity-interval-training.pdf
1306. Boutcher, S., "High-Intensity Intermittent Exercise and Fat Loss," *Journal of Obesity* (2011): doi: 10.1155/2011/868305.
1307. Little et al., "Low-Volume High-Intensity Interval Training Reduces Hyperglycemia and Increases Mitochondrial Capacity in Patients with Type 2 Diabetes," *Journal of Applied Physiology* 111, no. 6 (2011): 1554-1560.
1308. Tjønna et al., "Aerobic Interval Training versus Continuous Moderate Exercise as a Treatment for the Metabolic Syndrome: A Pilot Study," *Circulation* 118, no. 4 (2008): 346-354.
1309. Danladi et al., "The Effect of a High-Intensity Interval Training Program on High-Density Lipoprotein Cholesterol in Young Men," *Journal of Strength and Conditioning Research* 23, no. 2 (2009): 587-592.
1310. Weston et al., "High-Intensity Interval Training in Patients with Lifestyle-Induced Cardiometabolic Disease: A Systematic Review and Meta-Analysis," *British Journal of Sports Medicine* 48 (2014): 1227-1234.
1311. Boutcher, S., "High-Intensity Intermittent Exercise and Fat Loss," *Journal of Obesity* (2011): doi: 10.1155/2011/868305.
1312. Ibid.
1313. Tremblay et al., "Impact of Exercise Intensity on Body Fatness and Skeletal Muscle Metabolism," *Metabolism* 43, no. 7 (1994): 814-818.
1314. Trapp et al., "The Effects of High-Intensity Intermittent Exercise Training on Fat Loss and Fasting Insulin Levels of Young Women," *Obesity* 32 (2008): 684-691.
1315. Keating et al., "Continuous Exercise but Not High-Intensity Interval Training Improves Fat Distribution in Overweight Adults," *Journal of Obesity* (2014): 834865.
1316. Kemmler et al., "High Versus Moderate Intense Running Exercise- Effects on Cardiometabolic Risk Factors in Untrained Males," *Deutsche medizinische Wochenschrift* 140, no. 1 (2015): e7-e13.
1317. Ciolac et al., "Effects of High-Intensity Aerobic Interval Training vs. Moderate Exercise on Hemodynamic, Metabolic, and Neuro-Hormonal Abnormalities of Young Normotensive Women at High Familial Risk for Hypertension," *Hypertension Research* 33 (2010): 836-843.

1318. Tjønna et al., "Aerobic Interval Training versus Continuous Moderate Exercise as a Treatment for the Metabolic Syndrome: A Pilot Study," *Circulation* 118 (2008): 346-354.
1319. Terada et al., "Feasibility and Preliminary Efficacy of High Intensity Interval Training in Type 2 Diabetes," *Diabetes Research and Clinical Practice* 99 (2013): 120-129.
1320. Almenning et al., "Effects of High Intensity Interval Training and Strength Training on Metabolic, Cardiovascular and Hormonal Outcomes in Women with Polycystic Ovary Syndrome: A Pilot Study," *PLOS One* 10, no. 9 (2015): doi: 10.1371/journal.pone.0138793.
1321. Jelleyman et al., "The Effects of High-Intensity Interval Training on Glucose Regulation and Insulin Resistance: A Meta-Analysis," *Obesity Reviews* 16, no. 11 (2015): 942-961.
1322. Liou et al., "High Intensity Interval Versus Moderate Intensity Continuous Training in Patients with Coronary Artery Disease: A Meta-Analysis of Physiological and Clinical Parameters," *Heart, Lung and Circulation* 25, no. 2 (2016): 166-174.
1323. Tremblay et al., "Impact of Exercise Intensity on Body Fatness and Skeletal Muscle Metabolism," *Metabolism* 43, no. 7 (1994): 814-818.
1324. Ibid.
1325. Ibid.
1326. Sloth et al., "Effects of Sprint Interval Training on VO2max and Aerobic Exercise Performance: A Systematic Review and Meta-Analysis," *Scandinavian Journal of Medicine & Science in Sports* 23 (2013): e341-e352.
1327. Gist et al., "Sprint Interval Training Effects on Aerobic Capacity: A Systematic Review and Meta-Analysis," *Sports Medicine* 44, no. 2 (2014): 269-279.
1328. Sandvei et al., "Sprint Interval Running Increases Insulin Sensitivity in Young Healthy Subjects," *Archives of Physiology and Biochemistry* 118, no. 3 (2012): 139-147.
1329. Rakobowchuk et al., "Sprint Interval and Traditional Endurance Training Induce Similar Improvements in Peripheral and Arterial Stiffness and Flow-Mediated Dilation in Healthy Humans," *American Journal of Physiology—Regulatory, Integrative and Comparative Physiology* 295, no. 1 (2008): R236-R242.
1330. Hazell et al., "Two Minutes of Sprint-Interval Exercise Elicits 24-hr Oxygen Consumption Similar to That of 30 min of Continuous Endurance Exercise," *International Journal of Sport Nutrition and Exercise Metabolism* 22 (2012): 276-283.
1331. Hazell et al., "Running Sprint Interval Training Induces Fat Loss in Women," *Applied Physiology, Nutrition, and Metabolism* 39, no. 8 (2014): 944-950.
1332. Zelt et al., "Reducing the Volume of Sprint Interval Training Does Not Diminish Maximal and Submaximal Performance Gains in Healthy Men," *European Journal of Applied Physiology* 114, no. 11 (2014): 2427-2436.
1333. "Facts About Physical Activity," Centers for Disease Control and Prevention. https://www.cdc.gov/physicalactivity/data/facts.html
1334. "Physical Inactivity," *Statistical Fact Sheet*, 2013 Update. American Heart Association. https://www.heart.org/idc/groups/heart-public/@wcm/@sop/@smd/documents/downloadable/ucm_319589.pdf
1335. Stern et al., "Short Sleep Duration Is Associated with Decreased Serum Leptin, Increased Energy Intake and Decreased Diet Quality in Postmenopausal Women," *Obesity* 22, no. 5 (2014): E55-E61.
1336. Robertson et al., "Effects of Three Weeks of Mild Sleep Restriction Implemented in the Home Environment on Multiple Metabolic and Endocrine Markers in Healthy Young Men," *Metabolism* 62, no. 2 (2013): 204-211.
1337. Higgins et al., "Ghrelin, the Peripheral Hunger Hormone," *The Annals of Medicine* 39, no. 2 (2007): 116-136.
1338. Broussard et al., "Elevated Ghrelin Predicts Food Intake During Experimental Sleep Restriction," *Obesity* 24, no. 1 (2016): 132-138.
1339. Brondel et al., "Acute Partial Sleep Deprivation Increases Food Intake in Healthy Young Men," *American Journal of Clinical Nutrition* 91, no. 6 (2010): 1550-1559.
1340. Spaeth et al., "Effects of Experimental Sleep Restriction on Weight Gain, Caloric Intake, and Meal Timing in Healthy Adults," *Sleep* 36, no. 7 (2013): 981-990.
1341. Greer et al., "The Impact of Sleep Deprivation on Food Desire in the Human Brain," *Nature Communications* 4 (2013): 2259.
1342. Hanlon et al., "Sleep Restriction Enhances the Daily Rhythm of Circulating Levels of Endocannabinoid 2-Arachidonoylglycerol," *Sleep* 39, no. 3 (2016): 653-664.
1343. Ibid.
1344. Christian, M., and Ellis, A., "Examining the Effect of Sleep Deprivation on Workplace Deviance: A Self-Regulatory Perspective," *Academy of Management Journal* 54, no. 5 (2011): 913-934.
1345. Wu et al., "The Effect of Sleep Deprivation on Cerebral Glucose Metabolic Rate in Normal Humans Assessed with Positron Emission Tomography," *Sleep* 14, no. 2 (1991): 155-162.
1346. Venkatraman et al., "Sleep Deprivation Elevates Expectation of Gains and Attenuates Response to Losses Following Risky Decisions," *Sleep* 30, no. 5 (2007): 603-609.
1347. Meldrum et al., "Sleep Deprivation, Low Self-Control, and Delinquency: A Test of the Strength Model of Self-Control," *Journal of Youth and Adolescence* 44, no. 2 (2015): 465-477.
1348. Cappuccio et al., "Meta-Analysis of Short Sleep Duration and Obesity in Children and Adults," *Sleep* 31, no. 5 (2008): 619-626.
1349. Wu et al., "Sleep Duration and Obesity Among Adults: A Meta-Analysis of Prospective Studies," *Sleep Medicine* 15, no. 12 (2014): 1456-1462.
1350. Watson et al., "A Twin Study of Sleep Duration and Body Mass Index," *Journal of Clinical Sleep Medicine* 6, no. 1 (2010): 11-17.
1351. Chaput et al., "Risk Factors for Adult Overweight and Obesity in the Quebec Family Study: Have We Been Barking Up the Wrong Tree?" *Obesity* 17, no. 10 (2009): 1964-1970.
1352. Buxton et al., "Association with Sleep Adequacy with More Healthful Food Choices and Positive Workplace Experiences Amongst Motor Freight Workers," *American Journal of Public Health* 99, Supplement 3 (2009): S636-S643.
1353. "Summary of Findings," *Sleep in America Poll*, 2005. National Sleep Foundation. https://sleepfoundation.org/sites/default/files/2005_summary_of_findings.pdf
1354. "Summary of Findings," *Sleep in America Poll*, 2009. National Sleep Foundation. https://sleepfoundation.org/sites/default/files/2009%20SLEEP%20IN%20AM
1355. "Obesity Rates and Trends Overview," Better Policies for a Healthier America. https://stateofobesity.org/obesity-rates-trends-overview/

1356. Hirschkowitz et al., "National Sleep Foundation's Sleep Time Duration Recommendations: Methodology and Results Summary," *Sleep Health* 1, no. 1 (2015): 40-43.
1357. Arendt, J., "Melatonin, Circadian Rhythms, and Sleep," *New England Journal of Medicine* 343 (2000): 1114-1116.
1358. Dijk, D., and Archer, S., "Light, Sleep, and Circadian Rhythms: Together Again," *PLOS Biology* 7, no. 6 (2009): e1000145.
1359. Burkhart, K., and Phelps, J., "Amber Lenses to Block Blue Light and Improve Sleep: A Randomized Trial," *Chronobiology International* 26, no.8 (2009): 1602-1612.
1360. Yang et al., "Exercise Training Improves Sleep Quality in Middle-Aged and Older Adults with Sleep Problems: A Systematic Review," *Journal of Physiotherapy* 58, no. 3 (2012): 157-163.
1361. Smith. S., and Trinder, J., "Morning Sunlight Can Advance the Circadian Rhythms of Young Adults," *Sleep and Biological Rhythms* 3, no. 1 (2005): 39-41.
1362. Holick, M., "Vitamin D and Sunlight: Strategies for Cancer Prevention and Other Health Benefits," *Clinical Journal of the American Society of Nephrology* 3, no. 5 (2008): 1548-1554.
1363. Statland, B., and Demas, T., "Serum Caffeine Half-Lives: Healthy Subjects vs. Patients Having Alcoholic Hepatic Disease," *American Journal of Clinical Pathology* 73, no. 3 (1980): 390-393.
1364. Kotagal, S., and Pianosi, P., "Sleep Disorders in Children and Adolescents," *BMJ* 332 (2006): 828-832.
1365. Ibid.
1366. Konsta et al., "Stress Management Techniques in Primary Insomnia: A Randomized Controlled Trial," *Sleep Medicine* 14, Supplement 1 (2013): e173.
1367. De Niet et al., "Music-Assisted Relaxation to Improve Sleep: A Meta-Analysis," *Journal of Advanced Nursing* 65, no. 7 (2009): 1356-1364.
1368. Konsta et al., "Stress Management Techniques in Primary Insomnia: A Randomized Controlled Trial," *Sleep Medicine* 14, Supplement 1 (2013): e173.
1369. Butler et al., "The Empirical Status of Cognitive Behavioral Therapy: A Review of Meta-Analyses," *Clinical Psychology Review* 26, no. 1 (2006): 17-31.
1370. Trauer et al., "Cognitive Behavioral Therapy for Chronic Insomnia: A Systematic Review and Meta-Analysis," *Annals of Internal Medicine* 163, no. 3 (2015): 191-204.
1371. Sumithran et al., "Long-Term Persistence of Hormonal Adaptations to Weight Loss," *New England Journal of Medicine* 365 (2011): 1597-1604.
1372. Ochner et al., "Biological Mechanisms That Promote Weight Regain Following Weight Loss in Obese Humans," *Physiology & Behavior* 120 (2013): 106-113.
1373. Jampolis, Melina, "Expert Q&A," *Health*, CNN. 09-30-2011. https://www.cnn.com/2011/HEALTH/expert.q.a/09/30/body.fat.testing.jampolis/index.html
1374. Mahon et al., "Measurement of Body Composition Changes with Weight Loss in Postmenopausal Women: Comparison of Methods," *The Journal of Nutrition and Healthy Aging* 11, no. 3 (2007): 203-213.
1375. Pateyjohns et al., "Comparison of Three Bioelectrical Impedance Methods with DXA in Overweight and Obese Men," *Obesity* 14, no. 11 (2006): 2064-2070.
1376. Lichtenbelt et al., "Body Composition Changes in Bodybuilders: A Method Comparison," *Medicine & Science in Sports & Exercise* 36, no. 3 (2004): 490-497.
1377. Ibid.
1378. Peterson et al., "Development and Validation of Skinfold-Thickness Prediction Equations with a 4-Compartment Model," *American Journal of Clinical Nutrition* 77, no. 5 (2003): 1186-1191.
1379. Ohlson et al., "The Influence of Body Fat Distribution on the Incidence of Diabetes Mellitus. 13.5 Years of Follow-Up of the Participants in the Study of Men Born in 1913," *Diabetes* 34, no. 10 (1985): 1055-58.
1380. De Koning et al., "Waist Circumference and Waist-To-Hip Ratio as Predictors of Cardiovascular Events: Meta-Regression Analysis of Prospective Cohort Studies," *European Heart Journal* 28, no. 7 (2007): 850-856.
1381. Pischon et al., "General and Abdominal Obesity and Risk of Death in Europe," *New England Journal of Medicine* 359, no. 20 (2008): 2105-2120.
1382. De Koning et al., "Waist Circumference and Waist-To-Hip Ratio as Predictors of Cardiovascular Events: Meta-Regression Analysis of Prospective Cohort Studies," *European Heart Journal* 28, no. 7 (2007): 850-856.
1383. Ruderman et al., "The Metabolically Obese, Normal-Weight Individual Revisted," *Diabetes* 47, no. 5 (1998): 669-713.
1384. Zhang et al., "Abdominal Obesity and the Risk of All-Cause, Cardiovascular, and Cancer Mortality: Sixteen Years of Follow-Up in US Women," *Circulation* 117, no. 13 (2008): 1658-1667.
1385. Zhang et al., "Abdominal Adiposity and Mortality in Chinese Women," *Archives of Internal Medicine* 167, no. 9 (2007): 886-892.
1386. "Body Mass Index (BMI) in Adults," American Heart Association. https://www.heart.org/en/healthy-living/healthy-eating/losing-weight/bmi-in-adults
1387. "Assessing Your Weight and Health Risk," National Heart, Lung, and Blood Institute. https://www.nhlbi.nih.gov/health/educational/lose_wt/risk.htm
1388. "Waist Circumference and Waist-Hip Ratio: Report of a WHO Expert Consulation," World Health Organization, 2008. https://apps.who.int/iris/bitstream/handle/10665/44583/9789241501491_eng.pdf;jsequence=1
1389. Tchernof, A., and Despres, J.P., "Pathophysiology of Human Visceral Obesity: An Update," *Physiology Reviews* 93, no. 1 (2013): 359-404.
1390. "NWCR Facts," National Weight Control Registry. https://www.nwcr.ws/Research/default.htm
1391. Wing, R., and Phelan, S., "Long-Term Weight Loss Maintenance," *American Journal of Clinical Nutrition* 82, no. 1 (2005): 222S-225S.
1392. Zheng et al., "Self-Weighing in Weight Management: A Systematic Literature Review," *Obesity* 23, no. 2 (2015): 256-265.
1393. Linde et al., "Self-Weighing in Weight Gain Prevention and Weight Loss Trials," *Annals of Behavioral Medicine* 30, no. 3 (2005): 210-216.
1394. Linde et al., "Relation of Body Mass Index to Depression and Weighing Frequency in Overweight Women," *Preventive Medicine* 45, no. 1 (2007): 75-79.
1395. VanWormer et al., "The Impact of Regular Self-Weighing on Weight Management: A Systematic Literature Review," *International Journal of Behavioral Nutrition and Physical Activity* 5 (2008): 54.

1396. Frayn, Keith. *Metabolic Regulation: A Human Perspective*. Oxford: Wiley Blackwell, 2010. Kindle File. 12.3.2, Location 7782 of 9142.
1397. Keys, A., Brozek, J., Henschel, A., Mickelsen, O., and Taylor, H. *The Biology of Human Starvation*. Oxford, England: University of Minnesota Press, 1950.
1398. Miller et al., "A Meta-Analysis of the Past 25 Years of Weight Loss Research Using Diet, Exercise, or Diet Plus Exercise Intervention," *International Journal of Obesity* 21 (1997): 941-947.
1399. Freedman et al., "Popular Diets: A Scientific Review," *Obesity Research* 9, Supplement 1 (2001): 24S-33S.
1400. Franz et al., "Weight-Loss Outcomes: A Systematic Review and Meta-Analysis of Weight-Loss Clinical Trials with a Minimum 1-Year Follow-Up," *Journal of the Academy of Nutrition and Dietetics* 107, no. 10 (2007): 1755-1767.
1401. Leibel et al., "Energy Intake Required to Maintain Body Weight Is Not Affected by Wide Variation in Diet Composition," *American Journal of Clinical Nutrition* 55, no. 2 (1992): 350-355.
1402. Bogardus et al., "Comparison of Carbohydrate-Containing and Carbohydrate-Restricted Hypocaloric Diets in the Treatment of Obesity," *Journal of Clinical Investigation* 68, no. 2 (1981): 399-404.
1403. Stein et al., "Effect of Reduced Dietary Intake on Energy Expenditure, Protein Turnover, and Glucose Cycling in Man," *Metabolism* 40, no. 5 (1991): 478-483.
1404. Wycherley et al., "Effects of Energy-Restricted High-Protein, Low-Fat Compared with Standard-Protein, Low-Fat Diets: A Meta-Analysis of Randomized Controlled Trials," *American Journal of Clinical Nutrition* 96, no. 6 (2012): 1281-98.
1405. Davy et al., "Water Consumption Reduces Energy Intake at a Breakfast Meal in Older Adults," *Journal of the American Dietetic Association* 108, no. 7 (2008): 1236-1239.
1406. Boschmann et al., "Water-Induced Thermogenesis," *Journal of Clinical Endocrinology and Metabolism* 88, no. 12 (2003): 6015-6019.
1407. Frayn, Keith. *Metabolic Regulation: A Human Perspective*. Oxford: Wiley Blackwell. 2010. Print. 9.2.2, page 237.
1408. Stewart, W., and Fleming, L., "Features of a Successful Therapeutic Fast of 382 Day's Duration," *Postgraduate Medical Journal* 49 (1973): 203-209.
1409. Kerndt et al., "Fasting: The History, Pathophysiology, and Complications," *The Western Journal of Medicine* 137, no. 5 (1982): 379-399.
1410. Gilliland, I., "Total Fasting in the Treatment of Obesity," *Postgraduate Medical Journal* 507, no. 44 (1968): 58-61.
1411. Al-Arouj et al., "Recommendations for Management of Diabetes During Ramadan: Update 2010," *Diabetes Care* 33, no. 8 (2010): 1895-1902.
1412. Cahill, G., "President's Address. Starvation," *Transactions of the American Clinical and Climatological Association* 94 (1983): 1-21.
1413. Ibid.
1414. Chaston et al., "Changes in Fat-Free Mass During Significant Weight Loss: A Systematic Review," *International Journal of Obesity* 31 (2007): 743-750.
1415. Berg, J., Tymoczko, J., and Stryer, L. *Biochemistry*. 5th edition. New York: WH Freeman. 2002. 30.3.1.
1416. Heilbronn et al., "Alternate-Day Fasting in Nonobese Subjects: Effects on Body Weight, Body Composition, and Energy Metabolism," *American Journal of Clinical Nutrition* 81, no. 1 (2005): 69-73.
1417. Webber, J., and McDonald, I., "The Cardiovascular, Metabolic and Hormonal Changes Accompanying Acute Starvation in Men and Women," *British Journal of Nutrition* 71 (1994): 437-447.
1418. Zauner et al., "Resting Energy Expenditure in Short-Term Starvation Is Increased as a Result of an Increase in Serum Norephinephrine," *American Journal of Clinical Nutrition* 71, no. 6 (2000):1511-1515.
1419. Mansell et al., "Enhanced Thermogenic Response to Epinephrine after 48-H Starvation in Humans," *American Journal of Physiology–Regulatory, Integrative and Comparative Physiology* 258, no. 1 (1990): R87-R93.
1420. Benedict et al. *A Study of Prolonged Fasting*. No. 203, Carnegie Institute of Washington. 1915. Google Books: Digital Edition.
1421. Major et al., "Clinical Significance of Adaptive Thermogenesis," *International Journal of Obesity* 31 (2007): 204-212.
1422. Rosenbaum et al., "Long-Term Persistence of Adaptive Thermogenesis in Subjects Who Have Maintained a Reduced Body Weight," *American Journal of Clinical Nutrition* 88, no. 4 (2008): 906-912.
1423. Mehta et al., "Impact of Weight Cycling on Risk of Morbidity and Mortality," *Obesity Reviews* 15, no. 11 (2014): 870-881.
1424. Vink et al., "The Effect of Rate of Weight Loss on Long-Term Weight Regain in Adults with Overweight and Obesity," *Obesity* 24, no. 2 (2016): 321-327.
1425. Moffitt et al., "A Gradient of Childhood Self-Control Predicts Health, Wealth, and Public Safety," *Proceedings of the National Academy of Sciences* 108, no. 7 (2011): 2693-2698.
1426. Shenhav et al., "The Expected Value of Control: An Integrative Theory of Anterior Cingulate Cortex Function," *Neuron* 79, no. 2 (2013): 217-240.
1427. Gailliot M., and Baumeister R., "The Physiology of Willpower: Linking Blood Glucose to Self-Control," *Personality and Social Psychology Review* 11, no. 4 (2007): 303-327.
1428. Durnin, J., "Basal Metabolic Rate in Man," Joint FAO/WHO/UNU Expert Consultation on Energy and Protein Requirements, 1981. https://www.fao.org/3/contents/3079f916-ceb8-591d-90da-02738d5b0739/M2845E00.HTM
1429. Gailliot, M., and Baumeister R., "The Physiology of Willpower: Linking Blood Glucose to Self-Control," *Personality and Social Psychology Review* 11, no. 4 (2007): 303-327.
1430. Ibid.
1431. Ibid.
1432. Ibid.
1433. Ibid.
1434. Baumeister et al., "Ego Depletion: Is the Active Self a Limited Resource?" *Journal of Personality and Social Psychology* 74, no. 5 (1998): 1252-65.
1435. Vohs et al., "Making Choices Impairs Subsequent Self-Control: A Limited-Resource Account of Decision Making, Self-Regulation, and Active Initiative," *Motivation Science* 1S (2014): 19-42.
1436. Danziger et al., "Extraneous Factors in Judicial Decisions," *Proceedings of the National Academy of Sciences* 108, no. 17 (2011): 6689-92.
1437. Gailliot et al., "Self-Control Relies on Glucose as a Limited Energy Source: Willpower Is More Than a

Metaphor," *Journal of Personality and Social Psychology* 92, no. 2 (2007): 325-336.

1438. Hagger et al, "Ego Depletion and the Strength Model of Self-Control: A Meta-Analysis," *Psychological Bulletin* 136, no. 4 (2010): 495-525.

1439. Loewenstein G., and Adler D., "A Bias in the Prediction of Tastes," *The Economic Journal* 105, no. 431 (1995): 929-937.

1440. Read D., and Van Leeuwen, B., "Time and Desire: The Effects of Anticipated and Experienced Hunger and Delay to Consumption on the Choice between Healthy and Unhealthy Snack Food." *Organizational Behavior and Human Decision Processes* 76 (1998): 189–205.

1441. Ariely D., and Loewenstein G, "The Heat of the Moment: The Effect of Sexual Arousal on Sexual Decision Making," *Journal of Behavioral Decision Making* 19, no. 2 (2006): 87-98.

1442. Tanner, R., and Carlson, K., "Unrealistically Optimistic Consumers: A Selective Hypothesis Testing Account for Optimism in Predictions of Future Behavior," *Journal of Consumer Research* 35, no. 5 (2009): 810-822.

1443. Oaten, M., and Chang, K., "Longitudinal Gains in Self-Regulation from Regular Physical Exercise," *British Journal of Health Psychology* 11 (2006): 717-733.

1444. Christian, M., and Ellis, A., "Examining the Effect of Sleep Deprivation on Workplace Deviance: A Self-Regulatory Perspective," *Academy of Management Journal* 54, no. 5 (2011): 913-934.

1445. Wu et al., "The Effect of Sleep Deprivation on Cerebral Glucose Metabolic Rate in Normal Humans Assessed with Positron Emission Tomography," *Sleep* 14, no. 2 (1991): 155-162.

1446. Venkatraman et al., "Sleep Deprivation Elevates Expectation of Gains and Attenuates Response to Losses Following Risky Decisions," *Sleep* 30, no. 5 (2007): 603-609.

1447. Meldrum et al., "Sleep Deprivation, Low Self-Control, and Delinquency: A Test of the Strength Model of Self-Control," *Journal of Youth and Adolescence* 44, no. 2 (2015): 465-477.

1448. Friese et al., "Mindfulness Meditation Counteracts Self-Control Depletion," *Consciousness and Cognition* 21, no. 2 (2012): 1016-1022.

1449. Tice et al., "Restoring the Self: Positive Affect Helps Improve Self-Regulation Following Ego Depletion," *Journal of Experimental and Social Psychology* 43 (2007): 379-384.

1450. Fujita et al., "Construal Levels and Self-Control," *Journal of Personality and Social Psychology* 90, no. 3 (2006): 351-67.

1451. Vohs et al., "Motivation, Personal Beliefs, and Limited Resources All Contribute to Self-Control," *Journal of Experimental Social Psychology* 48, no. 4 (2012): 943-947.

1452. Hagger et al, "Ego Depletion and the Strength Model of Self-Control: A Meta-Analysis," *Psychological Bulletin* 136, no. 4 (2010): 495-525.

1453. Job et al., "Ego Depletion—Is It All in Your Head? Implicit Theories About Willpower Affect Self-Regulation," *Psychological Science* 21, no. 11 (2010): 1686-93.

1454. Bernecker et al., "Implicit Theories About Willpower Predict Subjective Well-Being," *Journal of Personality* 85, no. 2 (2017): 136-150.

1455. Vohs et al., "Motivation, Personal Beliefs, and Limited Resources All Contribute to Self-Control," *Journal of Experimental Social Psychology* 48 (2012): 943-947.

1456. Korbontis et al., "Refeeding David Blaine—Studies After a 44-Day Fast," *New England Journal of Medicine* 353, no. 21 (2005): 2306-7.

1457. Sharples, Tiffany, "How David Blaine Held His Breath," *Time*. 05-01-2008. https://content.time.com/time/health/article/0,8599,1736834,00.html

1458. Baumeister, Roy, and Tierney, John. *Willpower: Rediscovering the Greatest Human Strength*. New York: Penguin, 2011. Print. Page 140.

1459. Nordgren et al., "The Restraint Bias: How the Illusion of Self-Restraint Promotes Impulsive Behavior," *Psychological Science* 20, no. 12 (2009): 1523-8.

1460. Wood et al, "Habits in Everyday Life: Thought, Emotion, and Action," *Journal of Personality and Social Psychology* 83, no. 6 (2002): 1281-1297.

1461. Wansink B., and Sobel J., "Mindless Eating: The 200 Daily Food Decisions We Overlook," *Environment and Behavior* 39, no. 1 (2007): 106-23.

1462. De Ridder et al., "Taking Stock of Self-Control: A Meta-Analysis of How Trait Self-Control Relates to a Wide Range of Behaviors," *Personality and Social Psychology Review* 16, no. 1 (2012): 76-99.

1463. Muraven et al., "Conserving Self-Control Strength," *Journal of Personality and Social Psychology* 91, no. 3 (2006): 524-537.

1464. Tranel et al., "Asymmetric Functional Roles of Right and Left Ventromedial Prefrontal Cortices in Social Conduct, Decision-Making, and Emotional Processing," *Cortex* 38, no. 4 (2002): 589-612.

1465. Bechara et al., "Emotion, Decision Making and the Orbitofrontal Cortex," *Cerebral Cortex* 10, no. 3 (2000): 295-307.

1466. Seger C., and Spiering B., "A Critical Review of Habit Learning and the Basal Ganglia," *Frontiers in Systems Neuroscience* 66, no. 5 (2011). doi: 10.3389/fnsys.2011.00066.

1467. Yin H., and Knowlton B., "The Role of the Basal Ganglia in Habit Formation," *Nature Reviews Neuroscience* 7, no. 6 (2006): 464-476.

1468. "Original," Product Facts. *Coca-Cola*. https://www.coca-colaproductfacts.com/en/products/coca-cola/original/12-oz/?&gclid=EAIaIQobChMIyNf6hOvS2wIV1bbACh3UmAqXEAAYASAAEgIK

1469. "Basic Report: 09206, Orange Juice, Raw (Includes Foods for USDA's Food Distribution)," USDA. https://ndb.nal.usda.gov/ndb/foods/show/09206?n1=%7BQy%3D1%7D&fgcd=&man=&lfacet=&count=&max-=25&sort=default&qlookup=Orange+juice%7C+raw+%28Includes+foods+for+USDA%27s+Food+Distribution+Program%29&offset=&format=Full&new=&measureby=&Qv=1&ds=SR&qt=&qp=&qa-=&qn=&q=&ing=

1470. Duhigg, Charles. *The Power of Habit: Why We Do What We Do in Life and Business*. New York: Random House, 2012. Print.

1471. Lally et al., "How Habits Are Formed: Modelling Habit Formation in the Real World," *European Journal of Social Psychology* 40, no. 6 (2010): 998-1009.

1472. Ibid.

1473. Wenzlaff R., and Wegner D., "Thought Suppression," *Annual Review of Psychology* 51, no. 1 (2000): 59–91.

1474. Ibid.

1475. Ibid.

1476. Dean, Jeremy. *Making Habits, Breaking Habits: Why We Do Things, Why We Don't, and How to Make Any*

*Change Stick*. Cambridge: De Capo Press, 2013. Print.
1477. Chapman et al, "Comparing Implementation Intention Interventions in Relation to Young Adults' Intake of Fruit and Vegetables," *Psychology & Health* 24, no. 3 (2009): 317-32.
1478. Gollwitzer P, "Implementation Intentions: Strong Effects of Simple Plans," *American Psychologist* 54, no. 7 (1999): 493-503.
1479. Luszczynska et al., "Planning to Lose Weight: Randomized Controlled Trial of an Implementation Intention Prompt to Enhance Weight Reduction among Overweight and Obese Women," *Health Psychology* 26, no. 4 (2007): 507-512.
1480. Gollwitzer P., "Implementation Intentions: Strong Effects of Simple Plans," *American Psychologist* 54, no. 7 (1999): 493-503.
1481. "Obesity and Overweight," Centers for Disease Control and Prevention. https://www.cdc.gov/nchs/fastats/obesity-overweight.htm
1482. Flegal et al., "Association of All-Cause Mortality with Overweight and Obesity Using Standard Body Mass Index Categories: A Systematic Review and Meta-Analysis," *JAMA* 309, no. 1 (2013): 71-82.
1483. Corrada et al., "Association of Body Mass Index and Weight Change with All-Cause Mortality in the Elderly," *American Journal of Epidemiology* 163, no. 10 (2006): 938-949.
1484. Volaklis et al., "Muscular Strength as a Strong Predictor of Mortality: A Narrative Review," *European Journal of Internal Medicine* 26, no. 5 (2015): 303-310.
1485. Berrington de Gonzalez et al., "Body-Mass Index and Mortality Among 1.46 Million White Adults," *New England Journal of Medicine* 363 (2010): 2211-2219.
1486. Willet et al., *Eat, Drink, and Be Healthy: The Harvard Medical School Guide to Healthy Eating*. New York: Simon & Schuster, 2001, p. 35.
1487. Bogers et al., "Association of Overweight with Increased Risk of Coronary Heart Disease Partly Independent of Blood Pressure and Cholesterol Levels: A Meta-Analysis of Cohort Studies Including More Than 300,000 Persons," *JAMA Internal Medicine* 167, no. 16 (2007): 1720-1728.
1488. Ibid.
1489. Abdullah et al., "The Magnitude of Association between Overweight and Obesity and the Risk of Diabetes: A Meta-Analysis of Prospective Cohort Studies," *Diabetes Research and Clinical Practice* 89, no. 3 (2010): 309-319.
1490. Luppino et al., "Overweight, Obesity, and Depression: A Systematic Review and Meta-Analysis of Longitudinal Studies," *JAMA Psychiatry* 67, no. 3 (2010): 220-229.
1491. Wang et al., "Association between Obesity and Kidney Disease: A Systematic Review and Meta-Analysis," *Kidney International* 73, no. 1 (2008): 19-33.
1492. Beuther, D., and Sutherland, R., "Overweight, Obesity, and Incident Asthma: A Meta-Analysis of Prospective Epidemiologic Studies," *American Journal of Respiratory and Critical Care Medicine* 175, no. 7 (2007): 661-666.
1493. Nguyen et al., "Men's Body Mass Index and Infertility," *Human Reproduction* 22, no. 9 (2007): 2488-2493.
1494. Guh et al., "The Incidence of Comorbidities Related to Obesity and Overweight: A Systematic Review and Meta- Analysis," *BMC Public Health* 9 (2009): 88: doi: 10.1186/1471-2458-9-88.
1495. Ibid.
1496. Ibid.
1497. Larsson, S., and Wolk, A., "Obesity and the Risk of Gallbladder Cancer: A Meta-Analysis," *British Journal of Cancer* 96 (2007): 1457-1461.
1498. Beydoun et al., "Obesity and Central Obesity as Risk Factors for Incident Dementia and Its Subtypes: A Systematic Review and Meta-Analysis," *Obesity Reviews* 9, no. 3 (2008): 204-218.
1499. Schwartz et al., "Obesity and Obstructive Sleep Apnea: Pathogenic Mechanisms and Therapeutic Approaches," *Proceedings of the American Thoracic Society* 5, no. 2 (2008): 185-192.
1500. Derby et al., "Modifiable Risk Factors and Erectile Dysfunction: Can Lifestyle Changes Modify Risk?" *Urology* 56, no. 2 (2000): 302-306.
1501. Balen et al., "Obesity and Reproductive Health: Impact on Obesity on Female Reproductive Health: British Fertility Society, Policy and Practice Guidelines," *Human Fertility* 10, no. 4 (2007): 195-206.
1502. Mendall et al., "Is Obesity a Risk Factor for Crohn's Disease?" *Digestive Diseases and Sciences* 56, no. 3 (2011): 837- 844.
1503. Scheen, A., and Luyckx, F., "Obesity and Liver Disease," *Best Practice & Research Clinical Endocrinology and Metabolism* 16, no. 4 (2002): 703-716.
1504. Scheinfeld, Noah, "Obesity and Dermatology," *Clinics in Dermatology* 22, no. 4 (2004): 303-309.
1505. Kramer et al., "Are Metabolically Healthy Overweight and Obesity Benign Conditions? A Systematic Review and Meta-Analysis," *Annals of Internal Medicine* 159 (2013): 758-769.
1506. Hansen et al., "Metabolically Healthy Obesity and Ischemic Heart Disease: A 10-Year Follow-Up of the Inter99 Study," *The Journal of Clinical Endocrinology and Metabolism* 102, no. 6 (2017): 1934-1942.
1507. Hashimoto et al., "Metabolically Healthy Obesity without Fatty Liver and Risk of Incident Type 2 Diabetes: A Meta-Analysis of Prospective Cohort Studies," *Obesity Research & Clinical Practice* 12, no. 1 (2018): 4-15.
1508. Abdullah et al., "The Magnitude of Association Between Overweight and Obesity and the Risk of Diabetes: A Meta-Analysis of Prospective Cohort Studies," *Diabetes Research and Clinical Practice* 89, no. 3 (2010): 309-319.
1509. Farag, Y., and Gaballa, M., "Diabesity: An Overview of a Rising Epidemic," *Nephrology Dialysis Transplantation* 26, no. 1 (2011): 28-35.
1510. Astrup, A., and Finer, N., "Redefining Type 2 Diabetes: 'Diabesity' or 'Obesity Dependent Diabetes Mellitus?'" *Obesity Reviews* 1, no. 2 (2000): 57-59.
1511. Pemberton, Max, "As a Doctor, I'd Rather Have HIV Than Diabetes," *The Spectator*. 04-19-2014. https://www.spectator.co.uk/2014/04/why-id-rather-have-hiv-than-diabetes/
1512. Harris, Mary, "Is Love Seen as Different for the Obese?" *Journal of Applied Social Psychology* 20, no. 15 (1990): 1209-1224.
1513. Lieberman et al., "Disgust Sensitivity, Obesity Stigma, and Gender: Contamination Psychology Predicts Weight Bias for Women, Not Men," *Obesity* 20, no. 9 (2012): 1803-1814.
1514. Sitton, S., and Blanchard, S., "Men's Preferences in Romantic Partners: Obesity vs Addiciton," *Psychological Reports* 77, no. 3 part 2 (1995): 1185-1186.
1515. Chen, E., and Brown, M., "Obesity Stigma in Sexual Relationships," *Obesity Research* 13, no. 8 (2005):

1393-1397.

1516. Puhl., R., and Heuer, C., "The Stigma of Obesity: A Review and Update," *Obesity* 17, no. 5 (2009): 941-964.

1517. Puhl, R., and Brownell, K., "Bias, Discrimination, and Obesity," *Obesity Research* 9, no. 12 (2001): 788-805.

1518. Kersbergen, I., and Robinson, E., "Blatant Dehumanization of People with Obesity," *Obesity* (2019): https://doi.org/10.1002/oby.22460.

1519. Puhl., R., and Heuer, C., "The Stigma of Obesity: A Review and Update," *Obesity* 17, no. 5 (2009): 941-964.

1520. Dor et al., "A Heavy Burden: The Individual Costs of Being Overweight and Obese in the United States," The George Washington University School of Public Health and Services, 2010.

1521. Carr, D., and Friedman, M., "Is Obesity Stigmatizing? Body Weight, Perceived Discrimination, and Psychological Well-Being in the United States," *Journal of Health and Social Behavior* 46, no. 3 (2005): 244-259.

1522. Luppino et al., "Overweight, Obesity, and Depression: A Systematic Review and Meta-Analysis of Longitudinal Studies," *JAMA Psychiatry* 67, no. 3 (2010): 220-229.

Made in the USA
Columbia, SC
14 May 2020